PART II. COSMETICS AND PERSONAL CARE PRODUCTS

CHAPTER 8. EYE AND FACE MAKEUP   201

<small>T
H
E</small> Safe Shopper's

B I B L E

THE Safe

Shopper's

BIBLE

A Consumer's Guide to Nontoxic Household Products, Cosmetics, and Food

David Steinman &
Samuel S. Epstein, M.D.

MACMILLAN • USA

This book is dedicated to Terri Steinman and Catherine Epstein.

MACMILLAN
A Simon & Schuster Macmillan Company
1633 Broadway
New York, NY 10019

Library of Congress Cataloging-in-Publication Data
Steinman, David.
   The safe shopper's bible: a consumer's guide to nontoxic household products,
cosmetics, and food/David Steinman & Samuel S. Epstein.
      p.   cm.
   Includes bibliographical references and index.
   ISBN 0-02-082085-2 (permanent paper)
   1. Marketing (Home economics)   2. Household supplies—Toxicology.
3. Consumer goods—Toxicology.   I. Epstein, Samuel S.   II. Title.
TX356.S74   1995   95-2841
640 ' .73—dc20   CIP

Manufactured in the United States of America
10 9 8 7 6 5 4 3 2 1

Illustrations by Terri Steinman

C●ntents

16. FOOD SAFETY ISSUES   373

APPENDIXES

Authors' Note

There will always be honest differences of opinion in science—especially in the evaluation and interpretation of information about short-term and long-term health effects arising from chemical exposures such as allergies; eye, skin, or respiratory irritation; cancer; nervous system damage; and birth defects. This book represents our views as to product safety based on facts obtained from a variety of sources.

In evaluating product brands of household products and cosmetics as well as foods and determining which are safest, the authors have endeavored to be thorough and conscientious in their review of the information provided by the federal government, international agencies, and industry. A primary source for information on consumer products is Material Safety Data Sheets, which are mandated by a government agency but are created by the manufacturers themselves. We have not independently tested products, so any errors or omissions in the information on which we rely could affect the validity of our findings. Also, manufacturers modify their product ingredients from time to time, and there may be variations within products. Anyone who knows of data that may alter the evaluation of the products and foods reviewed in this book is encouraged to make this information available to the authors by writing them in care of Macmillan Publishing Company, 1633 Broadway, New York, NY 10019. The authors will consider all such information so that any revisions, if necessary, can be made in future editions.

Furthermore, we would like readers to let us know what they think about the *The Safe Shopper's Bible*. What did you like? Where could it be improved? If there are other household products, cosmetics, personal care products, food or beverages, or categories of consumer products (e.g., over-the-counter medicines) you would like evaluated in future editions, send the name of the product or food and its manufacturer to the authors at the above address.

Acknowledgments

We gratefully acknowledge help of the following for reviewing all or portions of the manuscript: Phillip Dickey of the Washington Toxics Coalition for advice on product evaluations; Dr. William Lijinsky for assistance with carcinogenicity evaluations; Laura Yeomans of Citizen Action for helpful advice in improving the readability of the manuscript; Ira Arlook, Ed Hopkins, and Sandra Buchanan of Citizen Action for public policy recommendations on labeling and disclosure of hazardous chemicals in consumer products and foods.

We also thank the following for their advice and interviews: Dr. John Bailey, acting director of the Food and Drug Administration (FDA) Office of Cosmetics and Colors, whose personal correspondence and interviews provided invaluable regulatory insight; Dr. Stan Milstein, special assistant to the director of the FDA Office of Cosmetics and Colors, for cosmetics and personal care products; Dr. Umberto Saffiotti, chief of the National Cancer Institute (NCI) Laboratory for Experimental Pathology, for discussions on silica in cosmetics; Drs. Aaron Blar and Shelia Hoar Zahm, Ph.D., of the NCI for comments on cancer hazards of permanent and semi-permanent hair dyes; Dr. Ernest Sternglass, professor emeritus of radiological physics at the University of Pittsburgh School of Medicine, for his information on the hazards of nuclear emission products in food and water; Marie Ardita, of Earth Science, Inc., for discussion on natural fragrances; Dr. Richard A. Ford of the Research Institute for Fragrance Materials for information on hazardous ingredients in fragrances; and Congressman Ron Wyden, who supplied documentation on the cosmetics industry.

We also acknowledge the following whose own writings provided background to this book: Aubrey Hampton and Tom Conry on cosmetics; Annie Berthold-Bond, a pioneer in nontoxic cleaning; Debra Lynn Dadd on safe and effective consumer products; Ralph Nader on citizen rights to know and on consumer product safety; Ed Begley, Jr., whose 1994 *Los Angeles Times* essay crystallized the idea that the most powerful weapon of consumers, beyond their vote, is their shopping dollars.

We also thank the following for publishing various early versions of sections of this book:

Tom Rawls, former editor of *Harrowsmith-Country Life* and *Natural Health*; Mark Bittman, former editor of *Natural Health*; Bill Thomson, senior editor at *Natural Health*; Sharon Bloyd Pleshkin and Karin Horgan at *Vegetarian Times*; James Sogg, Alex Demyanenko, and Danny Feingold at the *L.A. Village View*; James Vowell of the *Los Angeles Reader*; Jay Levin of *L.A. Weekly*; David Camp of *Veggie Life*.

We also pay tribute to the following members of Congress for their longtime support of the authors' efforts in the area of the right to know of toxic hazards in consumer products and of their efforts to reduce such hazards and of need for reform in federal cancer policy:

Congressmen Henry Waxman (D-CA), David Ongy (D-WI), John Conyers (D-MI), and Bernie Sanders, member at large (VT); Senator Ted Kennedy (D-MA); and former Senators Gaylord Nelson (D-WI) and Howard Metzenbaum (D-OH).

Finally we thank Natalie Chapman of Macmillan Books for her highly skilled editing and enthusiasm.

Foreword

The American household consumes, uses, applies, or attaches products that make up a large portion of the American economy. As more and more family functions spill out into the marketplace (e.g., pest control) and as more wants are created by persistent advertising and marketing, the exposure of people to a multiplicity of products, many of them serving similar purposes, grows markedly. If the choice that stresses health, safety, and one's money's worth is to be a product of consumer knowledge, then brand names need to be recommended or given comparative caution designations. Unfortunately, neither the marketplace nor the mandated government agencies are providing such point-of-sale information. The authors of *The Safe Shopper's Bible* make this quite clear in the early pages of the book, where they provide a broader frame of reference for what is fortunately much practical advice.

Because most shoppers patronize supermarkets, this book wades right into the brand-name arena with easy-to-use visual charts and written summaries for each food, cosmetic, and product category. Of particular interest is the number of times in which safer, old-fashioned alternatives, such as baking soda or white vinegar, can substitute for more complex, synthetic chemicals. If these alternatives are not found in most stores but available through mail-order catalogs, the places and addresses are given. Often the safest foods and products are competitively priced with the most hazardous. Indeed, some of the superior materials are often cheaper than the highly advertised and thereby highly priced brands.

In evaluating risks, the authors lean to the side of caution—especially since history shows that what some researchers don't know may harm you, and there is no downside to such caution when there are so many other better ways to perform the same tasks. There is little "alternative life style" exhortation in this book, but readers cannot help but be stimulated into asking on more than a few occasions, "Who needs some of these products or foods or cosmetics anyhow?"

The wise advice about prevention rather than cure finds much material to mine. From safer drinking water to pots and pans to household cleaners to sources of indoor air pollution to safer baby food, the inventory of prevention for your household is deep and diverse. If this book saves you money, prevents illness and aggravation, and thereby saves you time, it is well worth a quick read and a prominent place on your reference shelf to draw upon its contents as your needs dictate. But should these pages further stimulate you to reflect on the waste, the mindless claims and duplications, and the deep dependency-inducing strategy of the contemporary marketplace, your civic role comes forward alongside your shopper's function. In that case, the authors have wittingly or unwittingly provided you with a doubleheader between one pair of book covers.

—Ralph Nader
Washington, D.C.
February 1995

Introduction

THE CASE FOR CONCERN

What is in that product? Is it safe?

Can my hair color cause breast cancer? How can I find a conditioner that does not sting my eyes?

How can I tell which bathroom cleaner brand is gentlest and safest?

Will the chemicals, hormones, and pesticides contaminating some foods and beverages give me cancer? Is this apple juice safe for my baby?

These are some of the questions consumers ask most often when shopping for foods, beverages, cosmetics, personal care products, and household products.

We all use them. We all need them. They are the myriad cleaners, deodorizers, polishers, fabric protectants, glues, paints, pesticides, cosmetics, and personal care products that we use daily.

Yet, shoppers share an escalating concern for making sound shopping decisions that will bring them the safest household products, cosmetics, and foods and beverages.

Of course, we all know about some of the most commonly cited health maladies, which include:

- Allergic reactions
- Breathing difficulty
- Dizziness, lethargy, confusion
- Dry, roughened hands
- Eye irritation

But in recent years the public is beginning to recognize that food and consumer products contain undisclosed ingredients and contaminants that pose hidden, long-term health hazards.

Risks of twenty different environmental problems were compared for their relative threat to human health in a 1989 Environmental Protection Agency report. Indoor air pollution and pesticide residues on foods posed two of the greatest health risks.

A National Academy of Sciences workshop concluded that some 15 percent of the American population suffers from chemical sensitivity. Researchers have traced this increased sensitivity to the proliferation of synthetic chemicals in consumer products and furnishings.

Residues of more than four hundred toxic chemicals—some found in household products and foods—have been identified in human blood and fat tissue. Some of those chemicals cause cancer and nervous system damage. Others cause birth defects and other damaging reproductive effects.

At least some 4 percent of leukemia and non-Hodgkin's lymphoma cases in the U.S. general population may be associated with exposure to hair color products. Other experts put the proportion of non-Hodgkin's lymphoma cases among women in particular, attributable to their use of hair dyes, at 20 percent.

The risk for leukemia increases by four to seven times for children, ages ten and under, whose parents use home or garden pesticides.

The risk of childhood brain cancer is associated with the use of pesticide "bombs" in the home, pesticides to control termites, flea collars on pets, insecticides in the garden or orchard, and herbicides to control weeds, including exposure to two common pesticides available in garden shops, carbaryl and diazinon.

The Safe Shopper's Bible isn't just for "environmental extremists" or the "chemically sensitive." It is for people who are healthy and want to stay that way. *The Safe Shopper's Bible* is for people who consider themselves smart shoppers; they have decided to take an active, holistic, and natural approach to protecting their health, and they simply want good quality in all aspects of their lives. *The Safe Shopper's Bible* is also for people with everyday complaints, ranging from rashes and dermatitis to headaches and asthma, who may not have realized that their symptoms are caused by the cosmetics and household products they use daily.

What's more, if you have children, there is another reason for knowing more about the products you buy: toxic ingredients in common household products present a real and immediate danger, especially to infants and children. In 1990, more than four thousand toddlers under age four were admitted to hospital emergency rooms because of household cleaner–related poisonings. That same year, nearly eighteen thousand pesticide-related hospital emergency room admissions were reported, and 74 percent of them were for children age fourteen and under. Of greater concern is the risk of cancer and long-term nervous system damage following prolonged exposure to unlabeled industrial chemicals or pesticides in household products, cosmetics, and foods.

Now don't panic and toss out all your cosmetics, household products, or foods and beverages. This is not a scare-of-the-week book.

While the concerns we have expressed in *The Safe Shopper's Bible* are real and do affect your health, do not start thinking *everything* is poisoned, that *everything* causes cancer, and that there is nothing you can do once you are in the supermarket and confronted by so many brand labels calling out for your consumer dollars. We have discovered *many* excellent brands and some fairly good ones. They are safe *and* effective, and they are just waiting to be discovered by *you*. The shopping charts that follow detail them.

Furthermore, we recognize that many products with the harshest ingredients—especially those used around the home for cleaning—perform their tasks most effectively; in addition, many hazards associated with these products are admittedly small and minor; often these hazards can be minimized through safe handling and use of the product.

On the other hand, rashes, eye and skin irritation, and allergies are, nevertheless, unwelcome health effects. Furthermore, *no* food or any other consumer product should contain ingredients or contaminants that cause an increased risk of cancer, nervous system damage, or birth defects, and all foods and products that contain such harmful ingredients should be immediately labeled and subsequently removed from the marketplace *especially when safer alternatives are available.*

The Safe Shopper's Bible would not be necessary if government and industry were fulfilling a basic and essential consumer right—the fundamental right to be informed by full label disclosure of toxic chemicals contained in consumer products or applied to foods—or preferably banning the use of such substances. But, in our view, government and most members of industry are neglecting their responsibility. We hope this book will make them more responsive to the health concerns that accompany many goods. But until that day, use this book as your shopping bible. It will pay off in healthy dividends!

ARE GOVERNMENT AND INDUSTRY NOT TELLING US WHAT WE NEED TO KNOW TO MAKE INFORMED PURCHASES?

Consumers today want to make intelligent, informed shopping decisions. Until now, however, most have been shopping in the dark. They receive little guidance from food producers and product manufacturers, whose advertising and labeling are too often misleading and not objective sources of information. Government also offers little guidance. Indeed, while many local, state, and federal government agencies are entrusted with protection of the public health, most have failed to assure consumers they are being adequately protected, or that they are being provided with full, if any, label disclosure of carcinogenic (i.e., cancer-causing), neurotoxic (i.e., causing damage to the nervous system), and reproductive effects, including teratogenic (i.e., birth defect–causing) chemicals in their foods and household products.

Let us look at the main players (other than yourself!) responsible for protecting your health.

Food and Drug Administration

The U.S. Food and Drug Administration (FDA) is part of the Department of Health and Human Services. It is responsible for ensuring the safety of foods, cosmetics, prescription, and over-the-counter drugs. Yet, FDA officials have consistently trivialized the risk of pesticides, industrial chemicals, food additives, and animal drugs added to the food supply, and its enforcement record has been strongly criticized. Furthermore, while the FDA has initiated label disclosure of the nutritional content of foods, it has completely failed to put into place any program that would disclose chemicals applied to foods that cause cancer, nervous system damage, and birth defects. Put another way, the FDA insists on labeling foods for cholesterol, but not for carcinogens.

Department of Agriculture

The U.S. Department of Agriculture (USDA) is responsible for the safety of the nation's meat supply. Yet its history is replete with incidences of allowing the food supply to be dangerously contaminated with bacteria as well as carcinogenic animal drugs, growth stimulants, and hormones. The deadly outbreak of E. coli poisoning that struck hundreds of people in the Pacific Northwest in 1993 is only the most recent example of the USDA's inadequate protection of the public health. So poorly has USDA monitored the safety of the nation's meat supply that in October 1993 a new labeling law went into effect requiring meat packers to warn consumers of the bacterial contamination of their products. An extensive review of government reports on the antibiotic and sulfa drug residues in meat allowed to be sold to the public indicates that edible portions are contaminated by an array of drugs, including penicillin, streptomycin, tetracycline, neomycin, oxytetracycline, gentamycin, sulfamethazine, sulfathiazole, and sulfaquinoxaline. Other unsafe drugs used regularly in livestock include dimetridazole, ipronidazole, and carbadox, each of which is carcinogenic and may leave residues in edible portions. Bite into a piece of nonorganic beef today and you are getting a taste of the rancher's modern pharmacy. Men whose bodies are built on testosterone end up dosing themselves with estrogen; women also end up ingesting estrogen, which causes breast cancer—thanks to the beef industry's use of hormonal implants for fattening up nonorganically raised beef. Some of the other drugs mentioned cause cancer at other sites in the human body; all represent consumer health hazards.

Environmental Protection Agency

The U.S. Environmental Protection Agency (EPA) is responsible for protection of the public from the effects of pesticides applied to crops and other industrial contaminants (such as dioxin and polychlorinated biphenyls) found in foods and beverages, as well as environmental hazards that threaten your health. Yet instead of calling for labeling and phasing out of all carcinogenic, neurotoxic, and teratogenic chemicals, thus implementing a policy of cancer prevention, the agency tries to "manage" consumer risks, allowing widespread exposure to such chemicals. In deliberate violation of the 1958 Delaney law's banning residues of carcinogenic chemicals in processed foods, the EPA has tried to shirk its responsibility by adopting a new standard allowing "negligible risk" of "acceptable" tolerances for all carcinogenic pesticides on foods.

The agency's present negligible risk policy, based on highly questionable estimates, allows one or more additional cancers per 100,000 people for one pesticide on one food item, which it alleges is equivalent to at least thirty-five excess cancers annually in the U.S. population. However, based on the EPA's own estimates, residues of sixty carcinogenic pesticides on thirty foods that may be eaten in just one day would result in about sixty-four thousand excess cancers a year, more than 10 percent of all current cancer deaths. Furthermore, the EPA's estimates ignore the following exposures: undisclosed inert carcinogenic pesticide ingredients; other carcinogens in food, notably color additives; residues of hormonal animal feed additives in beef; even higher risks for children; and other chemical and radioactive carcinogens not only in food, but also in air, water, and the workplace. EPA estimates also ignore unpredictable synergistic interactions from these multiple exposures, especially the cancer-accelerating effects among radiation, pesticides, and hormones.

National Cancer Institute

The National Cancer Institute (NCI) is responsible for directing the nation's "war" on cancer. Even so, from 1950 to 1989, the overall incidence of cancer in the United States (adjusted for the aging population) rose by approximately 44 percent, with lung cancer because of smoking accounting for less than a quarter of this increase. Age-adjusted incidence rates for breast cancer and male colon cancer for the general U.S. population have increased by over 50 percent, whereas the rates for some less common cancers, such as malignant melanoma, certain lymphomas, and male kidney cancer have increased by over 100 percent. Childhood cancer has also increased by about 20 percent. Higher cancer rates still are seen for people living in highly urbanized and industrialized counties (in the vicinity of petrochemical, mining, smelting, and nuclear weapons plants), and for workers in these industries. Today, more than one in three Americans will be stricken with cancer in their lifetime and more than one in four will die. Cancer has overtaken heart disease as the leading killer of middle-aged Americans, *and the baby boom genera-tion is at a far higher cancer risk than its grandparents' generation.*

NCI has taken a decidedly indifferent, if not hostile, view toward prevention despite the fact that the war on cancer is clearly being lost. It continues to lead the public and Congress into believing that "we are winning the war against cancer," with "victory" possible only given more time and money. The NCI and the American Cancer Society (ACS) also insist that there have been major advances in the treatment and cure of cancer, that there has been no increase in cancer rates (except for lung cancer, which is attributed exclusively to smoking). Yet, the facts show just the contrary. For example, a recent Swedish study found that baby boomers face a higher risk of cancer than did their great-grandparents. The study of nearly 840,000 cases in all groups reported to the Swedish government since 1958 revealed that the risk of developing cancer was almost three times higher in men born in the 1950s than in those born in the 1880s, and for women, the risk was twice as high. These differences held true even after accounting for smoking-related cancer. Despite growing evidence that cancer is caused by exposure to environmental carcinogens, NCI—which could direct millions of dollars into truly effective cancer-prevention programs that would focus on providing important information on cancer hazards in the environment and removing the environmental causes of this disease—continues its unsubstantiated claims that "victory" is only a "cure" away.

More recently, according to a September 1994 NCI report *Cancer at the Cross-roads,* Dr. Paul Calabresi, chairman of the National Cancer Advisory Board, admitted that the war against cancer has stalled and that new direction is urgently needed. But instead of seeking to direct its own massive funding into eliminating preventable causes of the disease, NCI requested still more money for moving "cures" for the disease from the laboratory to the doctor's office, and also requested appointment of a Cabinet-level official to coordinate a national effort to win the war against cancer. In effect, NCI used the ploy of shifting the blame for its fail-ing policies to Congress, arguing that if the war continues on its losing course, it would now be the "burden" of Congress for its failure to provide additional and massive funding.

Consumer Product Safety Commission

The Consumer Product Safety Commission (CPSC), an independent regulatory agency created in 1972, is charged with ensuring that common consumer household products are safe from unreasonable risk of injury and death. The CPSC has jurisdiction over more than fifteen thousand consumer products. Yet manufacturers of household products are required by law to disclose only a minuscule number of the hazardous ingredients used in their products. Federal regulations *do* require manufacturers to provide minimal label information (e.g., the presence of acutely poisonous, irritating, caustic, or flammable ingredients), but not for carcinogenicity, neurotoxicity, or reproductive effects, which hardly constitutes adequate disclosure. Although new labeling regulations have been proposed by the CPSC, disclosure of harmful ingredients will remain minimal as long as responsibility for disclosure rests with manufacturers and government oversight remains minimal.

Industry

Quite apart from government, industry perhaps plays the most key role in ensuring the safety of foods and consumer products. Indeed, making foods and consumer products safer will be difficult, if not impossible, without the cooperation and leadership of responsible industry.

Our goal is to encourage industry to provide consumers more information and to produce safer foods and products by reducing reliance on toxic chemicals. In fact, many major corporations are now moving toward responsible production of foods and consumer products. Some 15 percent of all new products marketed in 1992 were advertised as being environmentally friendly. Furthermore, to ensure the integrity of such claims, many leading retailers, including Home Depot, are now requiring that such claims be scientifically screened by certification groups such as Green Seal or Scientific Certification Systems. Meanwhile the largest organic farmer in the United States is now Gallo Wine Company. The firm that fought the United Farm Workers in the 1960s now has six thousand acres of vineyards under organic cultivation. Major fashion manufacturers such as Esprit are producing clothing made with organic cotton and environmentally friendly zippers and snaps. And JCPenney is now offering a wholly natural line of nonpetrochemical cosmetics and personal care products known as Earth Preserv. These changes are only the beginning. They signify the changing attitudes of industry toward the environment and consumer safety. After all, consumer confidence and taking care of the environment makes good business sense.

Consumers' Right to Know

Consumers have an inalienable right to know what ingredients are in products they use daily, and to be certain that chemicals posing chronic health risks will be phased out when alternatives are available. These are rights regardless of one's perception of the risk of the ingredient. Yet walk down the aisle of any supermarket and you will quickly see how minimal regulation has led to grossly inadequate labeling.

How bad is the situation? Some leading household products do not disclose to the consumer that they contain carcinogens, such as crystalline silica and trisodium nitrilotriacetate; neurotoxins, such as formaldehyde; or other hazardous substances. Shoppers may choose these products anyway and may want to continue using them but deserve complete labeling information to make an informed choice.

As for cosmetics, while consumers are told what ingredients have been intentionally added to products, they are not provided with information that would alert them, for example, to carcinogenic contaminants or preservatives that release formaldehyde; nor are they told about ingredients in hair color products likely to be associated with cancer, or substances in fragrances that are potentially neurotoxic or teratogenic. Not a single cosmetic company warns consumers of the presence of carcinogens in its products—despite the fact that several common cosmetic ingredients or their contaminants are carcinogenic themselves or are carcinogenic precursors.

And with regard to foods and beverages, when was the last time your supermarket or seafood shop told you which fish or other food item has chemicals that cause cancer or birth defects? For women who are pregnant or intend to have children and for parents who wish to minimize their children's exposure to such toxins, this information is essential. It is also important to know about other food hazards. For example, children who eat hot dogs containing nitrite preservatives (which are precursors of carcinogenic nitrosamines) about a dozen times a month are at a risk nine times higher than normal for leukemia. But parents also need to know that, by becoming informed, selective shoppers, they can conveniently buy hot dogs that do not present this hazard. This is *essential* health information.

Government and industry have failed abysmally to protect consumer health adequately; at the very least, they have failed to inform consumers fully of the hazardous ingredients used in household products, cosmetics, and foods. This glaring void leaves consumers at peril, uninformed, and feeling powerless and frightened by the lack of information. One of the major reasons for our publishing *The Safe Shopper's Bible* is to empower you to transform your lifestyle into one that is healthier, more natural, and in greater harmony with the health of our environment.

HOW WILL *THE SAFE SHOPPER'S BIBLE* HELP ME?

The major dilemma for consumers anxious to find safe foods and products is that they do not know where to turn for information. The only consumer guides available today stress homemade alternatives to household products or point up *only* those often more expensively priced brands available through health food markets and mail order. But most people today are so busy making a living, taking care of their children, and doing other daily chores that they do not have the time or patience to mix their own household cleaners or make their own laundry soap and cosmetics. Furthermore, health food markets are not always conveniently situated, nor are they the best source for affordable foods and products. The fact is that most consumers buy from mainstream supermarkets.

The Safe Shopper's Bible is designed as a tool to help shoppers find the safest foods and consumer products, whether major or alternative brands. Several thousand foods and brands of consumer products have been evaluated.

The Safe Shopper's Bible is narrowly focused and easy to use. Its shopping charts and written summaries at the beginning of each food and product category address potential health hazards, point up the safest leading and alternative foods and consumer brands, and report recent product developments. It also provides information about protective clothing, safety equipment, and other methods of self-protection for the safe use and handling of hazardous household products.

Shoppers will also find that the safest foods and products are often competitively priced with those that are most hazardous.

In every food and product category, some brands have been designated as our recommendations. These are the foods and brands presenting the fewest health hazards and containing the fewest hazardous chemicals. We have made sure to recommend enough brands to give you choices at almost any store.

Occasionally, however, recommended brands are available only at health food stores or through mail-order catalogs that specialize in environmentally safe products. You may find yourself becoming a dual-market shopper, using both health food markets and supermarkets, and sometimes even catalogs. But simply shopping in a health food store is no guarantee of buying the safest products or foods. Many health food stores sell foods grown with pesticides and consumer products that are no safer (and often more expensive) than those found in your favorite major supermarket. Furthermore, many of their health products make false or misleading claims.

HOW WE OBTAINED INFORMATION TO
EVALUATE PRODUCTS, FOODS, AND BEVERAGES

Household Products

Obtaining information on household products for *The Safe Shopper's Bible* was not always easy. At first we began by telephoning major manufacturers and explaining that a consumer who used their products wanted additional information contained in Material Safety Data Sheets (MSDSs). The Department of Labor's Occupational Safety and Health Administration (OSHA) requires manufacturers to make available MSDSs for all workers including those employed in the production of consumer as well as other products.

MSDSs are supposed to disclose potentially hazardous chemicals added to the formulations in amounts above 1 percent, but otherwise they provide minimal information about a product's health hazards and recommendations for safe-handling procedures. Typically, they vary in length from one to eight pages. MSDSs are one of the most convenient avenues available to shoppers to learn about potential health hazards associated with a product.

Information contained in MSDSs is very far from perfect. Some data are misleading or simply just missing. For example, although federal regulations require manufacturers to list only those hazardous chemicals above 1 percent of the formulation, 1 percent or less of a carcinogenic, neurotoxic, or teratogenic chemical can constitute an extremely high-level exposure. Furthermore, workers employed in manufacturing are usually healthy, receive training in the handling of hazardous chemicals, are provided with protective clothing, and are exposed for eight hours or less each day. Homemakers, including pregnant women and children, on the other hand, receive no warning about hazardous ingredients or training in handling products containing hazardous substances, are not provided with protective clothing, and may be exposed to the products for up to twenty-four hours a day.

Criticisms notwithstanding, MSDSs are one of the few information sources available—short of running every product through a toxicological analysis. To complement the MSDSs, however, we also interviewed government officials, independent scientists, and manufacturers' representatives; reviewed standard toxicological and industry publications; consulted publications from the World Health Organization's International Agency for Research on Cancer (IARC), the National Toxicology Program, and the EPA; and consulted consumer activists and organizations. Finally, we relied on our own experience and knowledge of the extensive scientific literature.

Cosmetics and Personal Care Products

Gathering information on cosmetics and personal care products posed a different challenge. The cosmetic and personal care product industry discloses most ingredients on labels (with the notable exception of carcinogenic contaminants and ingredients used in formulating fragrances and perfumes). However, the industry provides no information whatsoever on their health hazards. To evaluate the health hazards posed by cosmetic ingredients, we reviewed standard industry and consumer publications as well as toxicological reports in medical journals; consulted government health officials, independent scientists, industry experts, and consumer activists; and sought out senior FDA officials, who were interviewed extensively and asked to provide their assistance, when necessary, in evaluating products. However, it should be made clear that all evaluations of cosmetics and personal care products are those of the authors.

Foods and Beverages

We acquired much of the information used for the evaluations of foods and beverages through use of the federal Freedom of Information Act (FOIA). This important piece of federal legislation enables citizens to obtain government documents that are not ordinarily made available to the public. Through FOIA and other more routine requests, we obtained data on ingredients and chemical contaminants from the USDA, FDA, EPA, and Bureau of Alcohol, Tobacco, and Firearms. We also consulted World Health Organization reports, particularly those from the IARC. The data that we reviewed generally listed a commodity (e.g., grapes, pasta, lamb, orange roughy); pesticides; or other hazardous chemicals identified in the product; the amount; where the food came from; and date gathered. Information we obtained ran from approximately 1969 to the present, although we relied primarily on data from the last few years.

Most of the data we gathered were concerned with carcinogens. Cancer is the most important, rapidly increasing disease today for which specific national information on trends and incidences is available, and many of the cancer-causing chemicals found in foods have been indexed by the EPA for their relative potency. Also, it must be emphasized that most carcinogens also pose other serious chronic health hazards, including neurotoxicity and reproductive effects. This emphasis on the evaluation of foods for their carcinogenic contaminants should not be construed as neglecting the risk from exposure to neurotoxic or teratogenic chemicals. It is simply a reflection of the relative lack of information available for assessing chemicals for neurotoxic and reproductive risks, and of our view that the presence of carcinogens in consumer products and in our food supply is one of the most serious risks facing America today.

OVERVIEW OF EVALUATIONS AND HEALTH ADVISORIES

In our charts, we evaluated household products, cosmetics, and foods and beverages for their risks based on three categories as explained below. These risks are based on information on the toxic effects of ingredients or contaminants subsequently numerically identified in tables at the beginning of each section, on pages 25, 198, and 306. The ingredients or contaminants in each product or food are further identified in the shopping charts by number corresponding to the same numbers in the table.

Little to No Risk

(⊞) Products or foods that are safest are rated with this symbol. For most people such products are likely to cause few, if any, health problems, although chemically sensitive people could have problems, as they might with any product.

Minimal Risk

(⊞) Products or foods that pose minimal risk for health hazards are rated with this symbol. The difference between those products posing a minimal risk and those posing little to no risk for hazards may be negligible. Also, these evaluations are meant only as guidelines and they cannot express gradations as subtly as we sometimes needed. A product rated for minimal risk, such as some laundry detergents, may cause irritation only on prolonged, direct contact with the eyes or skin. Many other products, which are otherwise acceptable, pose small fire hazards. Another example: household cleaning products are sometimes necessarily harsh because of the tasks they must perform, such as whitening porcelain dish basins. Yet, if you are aware of their *potential* hazards and you take proper precautions for safe handling, then you can use these products with complete safety.

A product rated minimal risk for flammability, causticity, irritancy, allergy, and sensitization is usually a safe product. It may be acceptable for long-term use, depending on your use of safety guidelines and your personal judgment of how it affects your health. You will need to try a product and see how you feel about its use. By following safe use guidelines and label directions, you may well find that you can use these products with a great degree of confidence in their safety. Thus, if household products are rated for minimal risk in the categories of flammability, causticity, irritancy, or allergenicity, you should follow label directions and safe use guidelines should you choose to continue to use them. Of course, all bets are off if you are one of the 15 percent of Americans who are chemically sensitive. In that case you may well want to select products rated as posing little to no risk.

On the other hand, if the household product, cosmetic, or food is rated for minimal risk in the categories of carcinogenicity, neurotoxicity, or reproductive effects, then you may well want to avoid their use completely. In spite of the warnings, if you decide to use these household products, then you should take extra precautions, including wearing proper protective clothing such as impermeable gloves (see page 23).

Caution

⊞ Products and foods that deserve caution are rated with this symbol. *In many cases, you should find alternatives immediately if they are available.* Once again, however, we stress that, in some instances, advisories concern *potential* health problems. Take household ammonia or bleach, for example, which under some categories in the acute health advisory are rated for caution; this is because if such products are used carelessly, so that some of the liquid is swallowed or splashed into the eyes or on the skin, it can cause real damage. Yet, following label directions and guidelines for safe use and storage will protect most people (although the chemically sensitive may not be adequately protected). Or take another example: You may have to run to the store on the spur of the moment to buy paint. Your store may not have a recommended brand. By knowing about the potential health hazards of paint and by having the proper safety equipment, you can still protect yourself by wearing appropriate clothing, especially nonpermeable gloves and an inexpensive respirator. In the area of acute toxicity, there is ample opportunity to reduce your exposure to harmful chemicals—if you are aware of their presence. On the other hand, it is our view that if products are rated for caution under the categories of carcinogenicity, neurotoxicity, or reproductive effects, then, in most cases, you should not use them. We do not believe that the use or convenience of any consumer product or food warrants the risk involved in exposure to carcinogenic, neurotoxic, or teratogenic substances. We recognize that in some instances our views are more conservative than the government's. As noted, we wish the government were more responsive to the concerns we identify.

Recommendations and Recommended Alternatives

✓ Every food and product category contains our recommendations—foods and brands that present the fewest, if any, health hazards and contain the fewest, if any, hazardous chemicals. Our recommended products are not always absolutely perfect; still, they are the best of what is available now.

For household products, we have also gone to some of the nation's leading experts to show you how you can make your own alternative solutions from basic supplies like baking soda, borax, distilled white vinegar, lemon juice, and washing soda. In many cases, recommended alternatives are not only safer and less irritating, but are also more effective!

PART I

HOUSEHOLD PRODUCTS

Homemaking Can
Be a Dangerous Job!

Household products have changed radically since the post–World War II "petro-chemical" revolution when industry discovered that a wide range of new chemicals could be synthesized from petroleum. Whereas Grandma could rely on fairly effective and safe all-around cleaners made with vinegar, borax, and lemon juice and Grandpa used milk paints similar to those Tom Sawyer whitewashed Aunt Polly's fence with, today the synthetic, industrial chemicals in use by consumers are far more varied and numerous. Production rates for synthetic petrochemicals have burgeoned from 1 billion pounds per year in 1940 to over 400 billion pounds per year in the 1980s. Since 1965 more than four million distinct chemical compounds have been reported in the scientific literature—some six thousand per week. Of these, about seventy thousand are now in commercial production; many accumulate in the human body and cause cancer and other diseases, yet have been inadequately tested or remain completely untested for their safety, raising concern for their hazards. However, only about six hundred of these chemicals are known to cause cancer, making the task of labeling their presence in products much easier.

Furthermore, many chemicals used in household products are volatile. That means they become gaseous at room temperature or are sprayed from an aerosol can or hand pump and thus take the form of microscopic particles that are easily inhaled. In either case, they can cause damage to the lungs or other organs as they are taken into the bloodstream. Because indoor pollutants are not as easily dispersed or diluted as outdoor pollutants, concentrations of toxic chemicals may be much greater indoors than outdoors. Peak concentrations of twenty toxic compounds—some linked with cancer and birth defects—were two hundred to five hundred times higher inside some homes than outdoors, according to a five-year EPA study that surveyed six hundred individuals in six cities to find out what their exposure was to common air pollutants. Not surprisingly, EPA experts say that indoor air pollution is one of the nation's most pressing personal health concerns. "If we measured outdoors what we are measuring indoors," says EPA indoor air specialist Lance Wallace, "there would be a tremendous hue and cry to clean up outdoor air."

In the last few years consumers have discovered that some of the chemicals in household products whose safety was taken for granted are hazardous. For instance, methylene chloride (also known as dichloromethane), the propellant used in many aerosol products, is carcinogenic. Although some products containing methylene chloride have been pulled from the market, thanks to belated government regulations, this carcinogen continues to be found in many consumer products such as spray paint and stripper.

More recently, a limited number of shoppers learned that indoor latex paints used widely for decades contained highly neurotoxic mercury-based fungicides. But it was not until 1990 that manufacturers finally removed most of these potent neurotoxins.

The bottom line is that millions of people suffer from the effects of indoor air pollution, and that household products are important contributors to unhealthy indoor air. Symptoms such as a runny nose, itchy eyes, a scratchy throat, headaches, fatigue, dizziness, skin rash, and respiratory infections are all common reactions to indoor air pollution. Long-term exposure to indoor pollution can result in lung cancer, or damage to the liver, kidneys, and central nervous system. Young children are especially vulnerable to impaired lung function and respiratory infection.

Your home should be a place of refuge where your body can heal and regroup from the stresses of the outside world. With a polluted home, just the opposite is true. Your body may continually be under siege by indoor airborne toxins. That is why you should be careful that the products you use in your home contain the safest ingredients available.

HOW WE EVALUATED HOUSEHOLD PRODUCTS

Household products were evaluated for two classes of hazards—short-term (*acute*) and delayed or long-term (*chronic*). For almost every evaluation, we consulted manufacturers' MSDSs as part of the product's hazard evaluation.

Acute Hazards

Flammability

Some household products—especially aerosols—can easily ignite or explode when exposed to intense heat. Others contain flammable solvents. All products with a minimal risk or caution rating should be handled carefully.

Causticity

Found primarily in household products used for cleaning, caustic chemicals can burn the skin, eyes, or even internal organs if accidentally ingested or inhaled. Examples of these products include bleaches, drain openers, and oven cleaners. Another term we have sometimes used synonymously with causticity is corrosive.

Irritants

Direct contact with strong alkalies, acids, and defatting substances such as solvents often irritates the eyes, skin, and respiratory tract. Many household products pose a hazard for irritation—especially on contact with the eyes. The real issue is which products pose the greatest hazard; the degree of hazard is often determined by the concentration of a chemical in a product and how it is used.

Furthermore, most aerosol products evaluated in *The Safe Shopper's Bible* have been rated for caution in the irritation category. Although manufacturers have made progress in increasing the safety of aerosol products, aerosol mists nevertheless continue to contain a small percentage of easily inhaled fine particles that cause immediate injury to lung tissue as well as additional harm when absorbed into the bloodstream. Furthermore, aerosol sprays not only saturate their target, but also form an extensive cloudy mist surrounding the user, who ends up breathing these particles. Pump products are a better choice. They provide more control, have larger droplets, and are more liquid. Prefer pumps with highly liquefied streams to those with fine mists, and always use them in well-ventilated areas. However, our bottom-line recommendation is not to use either—certainly not aerosols, and, when possible, not pumps.

Allergens and Strong Sensitizers

An allergic reaction is an abnormal reaction of the human immune system. Allergies such as asthma are often characterized by an excessive reaction to a relatively small amount of a substance. Other chemicals can *sensitize* a person, meaning that repeated contact with that chemical or similar chemicals, even in minute amounts, will produce a strong reaction. People who have been "sensitized" are especially vulnerable to very low-level or short-term exposures to the same or related substances, which can trigger extreme allergic reactions. For this reason, some people can be stricken by biological or chemical exposures that affect no one else. Any ingredient can cause an allergic reaction in *somebody*. It is impossible to accurately predict *all* the chemicals that can cause allergic reactions or sensitization. The goal of discussing such substances is to alert consumers to products with ingredients that pose the greatest hazard.

Chronic Hazards

Carcinogens

Chemicals that cause cancer are called *carcinogens*. In the evaluation of such chemicals, we considered the weight of the evidence for the carcinogenicity of each chemical, largely based on recommendations from the IARC, NTP, and EPA, as well as information derived from the scientific literature and manufacturers' MSDSs. We have rated all carcinogenic chemicals for caution. Chemicals for which data are inadequate or limited are rated for minimal risk. We have also rated for minimal risk those chemicals in products, such as nitrites, whose presence causes a reaction that leads to the formation of new substances that are carcinogenic.

The evaluations used in *The Safe Shopper's Bible* are much less relaxed than those used by government and industry. In regulating carcinogens, federal agencies examine the amount of the consumer's exposure to a chemical before declaring a product poses a hazard. For example, certain cleansers and many brands of cat litter contain the carcinogen crystalline silica, while many other products, especially those used for cleaning your car, contain formaldehyde. The CPSC alleges that consumer exposure to these chemicals is minimal, and that the hazard therefore is also minimal. This follows the highly misleading axiom that the dose equals the poison. In fact, the overwhelming consensus in the independent scientific community is that no safe exposure threshold to a carcinogen exists. Furthermore, there is also no reason for the consumer to be exposed to chemicals that have been inadequately tested for carcinogenicity. A chemical should be proven safe before consumers are exposed to it. Generally, when different bodies of equally credible experts have differed in their evaluation of a chemical's carcinogenicity, we have used the most cautious.

The policy of *The Safe Shopper's Bible* is to alert consumers whenever carcinogenic chemicals, or those that are inadequately tested or are carcinogen precursors, are known to be present in household products. In our view, in almost all cases you should avoid those products for which a rating of caution is given. In a few cases, some products that pose minimal risk for carcinogenicity have been recommended, if they are clearly superior to their competitors. For example, Perma-Guard Diacide, which contains talc, is recommended even though talc has shown evidence of carcinogenicity; it is a better product than its competitors, which contain far more toxic and volatile pesticides. Also, some products with artificial colors have been recommended without necessarily disclosing their presence. The use of artificial colors is certainly not natural and not an ideal situation. Despite this shortcoming, some products containing artificial colors nevertheless are better than their competitors, and one of the important aspects of *The Safe Shopper's Bible* is to provide an adequate range of choices for a variety of consumers.

Neurotoxins

Chemicals that adversely affect the nervous system, reducing emotional well-being, mental alertness, coordination, and other functions associated with intelligence, are called *neurotoxins*. In everyday terms, the acute effects of neurotoxins include feeling drunk, dumb, angry, tired, confused, fatigued, irritable; experiencing personality changes; being unable to think clearly; or feeling depressed for no apparent reason. Long-term effects include behavioral changes, memory loss, emotional disturbances, and organic brain damage that can even proceed to dementia (organic brain syndrome). These chemicals have the capacity to cause subtle and possibly cumulative damage to the nervous system over months or years without your being aware of the effects until it is too late, and the harm is both serious and irreversible. Exacerbating this problem is that many consumer products containing neurotoxins are aerosolized or highly volatile (i.e., they become gaseous at room temperature). That means exposure occurs not only through skin absorption, but also through inhalation, and the exposure can continue for an extended duration. Even seemingly innocuous products such as correction fluid, flea foggers, furniture polish, and spot removers contain neurotoxins.

Reproductive Effects

Occasionally a product contains a chemical that can cause harm to the unborn—including miscarriages, pregnancy complications, birth defects—or reproductive harm to men and women such as sterility and infertility. Such chemicals are called reproductive toxins. A substance that specifically causes birth defects is called a *teratogen*. In general, these are chemicals that men and women who intend to have children should avoid.

SAFE USE RECOMMENDATIONS

Buying and Handling Products

Before you buy any product, consider the following suggestions:

- Do I really need this product?
- Does this product require safety equipment?
- Am I buying more than I need?
- Is there a safer, gentler alternative?
- Have I made sure this product is free of ingredients that can cause serious acute effects, cancer, neurotoxicity, or birth defects?
- Can I safely dispose of the excess or does it require a household hazardous waste collection?
- Can I safely store this product in my home?

You will find the following general guidelines helpful in handling most household products:

- Read all labels carefully before using products. Be aware of their uses and dangers.
- Leave products in their original container with the label that clearly identifies the contents.
- Never put household products in food or beverage containers.
- Do not mix products unless the label directs you to do so. This can cause explosive or poisonous chemical reactions. Even different brands of the same product may contain incompatible ingredients.
- Use only what is needed. Twice as much does not mean twice the results. Follow label directions.
- If pregnant, avoid toxic chemical exposure as much as possible. Many toxic products have not been adequately tested for their effects on the unborn.
- Use products in well-ventilated areas to avoid inhaling fumes. Work outdoors whenever possible. When working indoors, open windows and use an exhaust fan, making sure air is exiting outside rather than being recirculated indoors. Take plenty of fresh air breaks. Be sure to use adequate skin, eye, and respiratory protection.
- Do not eat, drink, or smoke while using hazardous products. Traces of hazardous chemicals can be carried from hand to mouth. Smoking can start a fire if the products are flammable.
- Clean up after using hazardous products. Carefully seal containers. Properly refasten all childproof caps.
- Substitute safer alternatives.

Eye Protection

Eyes are particularly vulnerable to injury from hazardous products through either use of aerosols, splashing, or diffusion of volatile chemicals. It is vitally important to protect your eyes when using household products containing hazardous ingredients. Many hazardous products such as oven cleaners, drain openers, and paint thinners may cause severe and permanent eye damage if splashed into the eye. Other potentially dangerous substances include caustic chemicals, pesticides, strippers, and solvents. Standard eyeglasses do not provide adequate protection.

Wear wraparound safety goggles to protect the eyes from chemical splashes, mists, vapors, and scratches from particulate materials such as paints and solvents, garden chemicals, and hobby products, including photographic solutions, particulates from sanding or grinding, swimming pool chemicals, and welding, as well as cleaners with ammonia, aluminum cleaners, disinfectants, drain cleaners and openers, oven cleaners, and septic tank cleaners. Safety goggles are inexpensive; they cost less than $10 and can be bought from safety equipment stores, hardware stores, automobile supply stores, and farm equipment stores.

Do not wear contact lenses—especially soft lenses—when working with hazardous products. The hazardous vapors or mists may be absorbed by the lenses, holding the irritant against your eye and increasing the potential for damage.

Skin Protection

Wear protective (impermeable) clothing other than your everyday clothes when working with highly volatile, hazardous products. If you really intend to get serious, you will probably end up buying protective clothing made from a variety of impermeable rubber and plastic materials matched to your needs. Be aware that no one single material is resistant to all chemicals. Your needs will be based on what parts of your body are being exposed to the toxic chemicals with which you work. The clothing will protect your body from contact with the toxic chemicals, preventing absorption through your skin. Also, hazardous products may stain or discolor your clothing. Replacing or cleaning them may cost a bundle.

To keep the toxic chemical from spreading to other clothing, wash work clothes separately in a washing machine with a full water level of hot water and detergent. Rinse the machine thoroughly after laundering contaminated clothes.

Line dry the work clothes rather than putting them in a dryer because the high heat of the dryer can ignite any flammable vapors remaining in the clothing.

The skin of the hands and fingers is the area most exposed to hazardous products. Because so many chemicals permeate into the bloodstream through the skin, it is important to wear gloves. To protect your hands, wear the right type of glove for the product you are using. Different materials resist different types of toxic chemicals. Latex gloves are all right for doing dishes, but you will also want a stronger, more durable pair of gloves for more hazardous chemicals such as solvents. *Nitrile* and *neoprene* gloves are effective protection against most household products.

Your gloves will last longer and help you handle the hazardous product better if they fit properly. The life of your gloves can be extended by washing them with warm water and soap and then allowing them to air-dry before using them again.

Ventilation and Respirators

Good ventilation is essential when using volatile or dusty chemicals. If possible, work outside. If you work inside, use fans to direct air away from the work area to open windows. Be sure you are not directing the toxic chemicals to others who may also be working inside. Artists and other people who regularly use hazardous chemicals should fit their work area with both fans and local exhaust ventilation to the outside. Preferably the artist or other user of volatile or dusty substances should have a work space separate from the living area and away from areas other people frequent regularly.

Air conditioners do not remove contaminants from the air. Nor do they provide sufficient ventilation because they recirculate air, even when they are on vent. If you can smell a toxic chemical (although not all harmful chemicals have an odor), your ventilation is not sufficient, and you probably need a mask or respirator for self-protection.

Respirators are as important to the home hobbyist and homemaker as they are to the man or woman in an occupational setting. We highly recommend that consumers get in the habit of using respirators when working with volatile or dusty chemicals in products like paints, strippers, and pesticides. We are not speaking of respirators connected to air supplies that cost a lot of money, but of those half face masks or full face masks that simply filter the air before you inhale.

There are different types of masks and respirators to protect you from specific toxic materials. Whatever brand you choose should be approved by the National Institute for Occupational Safety and Health (NIOSH) for the particular contaminant to which you will be exposed (see table 1 on page 25).

The cheapest protection is called a particle mask. It is inexpensive and provides minimal protection from dusts. But it is wholly inadequate for use with products that produce vapors, fumes, or mists.

Two types of respirators provide more complete protection, *maintenance-free respirators* and *reusable gas and vapor respirators.*

Maintenance-free respirators are filtering devices that contain fibers to trap particles, or absorbent materials that trap and hold gases and vapors. When a maintenance-free respirator becomes clogged or you can smell the toxic chemical, you throw the respirator away. Maintenance-free respirators cost between $8 and $20.

Reusable gas and vapor respirators are used with *cartridges* and *prefilters* that provide protection. Prefilters trap the airborne particles in a fibrous filtering material. Cartridges contain activated carbon or other substances that absorb—and in some cases neutralize—the chemicals in vapors, fumes, or mists.

Reusable gas and vapor respirators cost more than particle masks and maintenance-free respirators—usually around $25 to $35—but they are worth every dollar, and they are far less expensive over the long run. They can be bought at safety equipment stores, hardware stores, automobile supply stores, and farm equipment stores.

Correct fit is essential. The reusable gas and vapor respirator should be comfortable and fit correctly so that it is leak-proof. Different people have different face sizes, so try on respirators until you find the right one. To test the fit, cover the cartridge or prefilter inlets with the palms of your hands (or put on their seals), inhale gently until the respirator collapses slightly, and hold your breath for ten seconds. If the fit is not adequate, the respirator will resume its normal shape because air leaked in. In addition, test the fit by blocking the exhalation valve and gently breathing out. These actions should cause the mask to expand. If air leaks passed the edge of the mask, the mask will collapse to its normal shape. If the respirator fails any of these tests, try adjusting the straps and face piece.

Replacement of cartridges and prefilters is important. The prefilters and cartridges of reusable respirators have to be replaced regularly. When it is difficult to breathe through a respirator, the prefilter is probably clogged and needs to be replaced. If you can smell the toxic chemical through the respirator, the purifying chemicals are used up and the cartridge needs to be replaced. Replacement cartridges and prefilters cost $4 to $6.50. Buy an extra set when you first buy your respirator.

Change cartridges after about eight hours of cumulative use or if you can smell the contaminant. If you rely on the odor as a cue to replace the cartridge, be sure the material is odor producing. Chemicals that do not produce odors include methanol (methyl alcohol) and carbon monoxide.

To prolong the life of the cartridge, store your respirator in an airtight, resealable plastic bag.

Always be sure to match your job with the proper cartridge and filter. The label of the respirator or the replacement cartridge and filter will tell you what jobs it was designed to perform. Table 1 will help you to make the right choice.

Table 1. Types of Cartridges and Prefilters

Product	Cartridge Required	Prefilter Required
Paints and Solvents		
Aerosol Spray Paints	Organic Vapor	Paint Spray
Lacquer Thinner	Organic Vapor	Paint Spray
Paint and Varnish Removers	Organic Vapor	Paint Spray
Turpentine	Organic Vapor	Paint Spray
Varnishes	Organic Vapor	Paint Spray
Garden		
Pesticides, Dust	Pesticide	Pesticide
Pesticides, Spray	Pesticide	Pesticide
Flea Powder	Pesticide	Pesticide

Product	Cartridge Required	Prefilter Required
Hobbies		
Dusts (from wood, stone, pigment, clay, fiber, shell, and bone)	None	Dust and/or Mist
Photography Solvents	Organic Vapor	None
Printmaking Solvents	Organic Vapor	None
Soldering, Welding	High Efficiency	Dust, Mist, and Fumes
Cleaners		
Aluminum Cleaner (with hydrofluoric acid)	Acid Gas	None
Ammonia and Amine Gas	Ammonia	None
Lye	Organic Vapor	None
Oven Cleaner	Organic Vapor	None
Septic Tank Cleaner	Organic Vapor	None

WHERE TO OBTAIN INGREDIENTS FOR RECOMMENDED HOMEMADE ALTERNATIVES

We have included suggestions for homemade alternatives to many commercial household products. These alternatives are based on the work of leading nontoxic-cleaning experts, such as Annie Berthold-Bond, author of *Clean and Green,* and Debra Lynn Dadd, author of *Nontoxic, Natural and Earthwise* and *The Nontoxic Home & Office.*

You may obtain the ingredients from health food stores, supermarkets, and occasionally hardware stores and chemical supply shops.

Among least toxic alternative ingredients are the following:

- *Baking Soda.* An excellent cleaner and deodorizer, baking soda is available in supermarkets and health food stores.
- *Beeswax.* Made from honeybee wax, beeswax is available from art stores, furniture repair shops, and some hardware stores.
- *Borax.* An excellent disinfectant, borax is available in supermarkets and health food stores.
- *Distilled white vinegar.* An excellent cleaner, distilled white vinegar is available in both supermarkets and health food stores.
- *Essential oils.* Essences distilled from plant oils, essential oils are less allergenic than synthetic fragrances and they are available at health food stores. They add a pleasing fragrance to your cleaning formulas.

- *Hydrogen peroxide.* An alternative to bleach, hydrogen peroxide is available at supermarkets and drugstores.
- *Lemon juice.* Available in both health food stores and supermarkets, or squeeze fresh lemons and make your own. Lemon juice is an excellent cleaner.
- *Liquid soaps.* An alternative to harsher detergents and other cleaning agents, liquid soaps can be bought in health food stores and supermarkets in either the cosmetic or dishwashing sections.
- *Pumice stone.* Excellent as a stain remover, pumice stones are available in health food stores, drugstores, and supermarkets.
- *Sodium perborate.* An alternative to standard bleaches made with sodium hypochlorite, sodium perborate is available from chemical supply companies.
- *Sodium percarbonate.* An alternative to standard bleaches made with sodium hypochlorite, sodium percarbonate is available from chemical supply companies.
- *Trisodium phosphate (TSP).* A powerful cleaning material, TSP can be irritating and caustic; it does not pose long-term health hazards such as carcinogenicity, neurotoxicity, or reproductive effects. Trisodium phosphate is available at supermarkets, drugstores, and hardware stores. Be aware that some products with the name TSP on their container do not actually contain trisodium phosphate. Read the label to make sure the product you buy contains trisodium phosphate.
- *Washing soda (also known as sodium carbonate, soda ash, and sal soda).* A strong cleaner, washing soda is available in supermarkets and health food stores.
- *Zeolite.* This naturally occurring mineral is an excellent deodorizer and available from G&W Supply, 1441 W. 46th Avenue #31, Denver, CO 80211 (303) 455-8834.

HOW TO USE THE SHOPPING CHARTS

You can determine the safety of your present brand or any brand that you are thinking of buying by checking its evaluation in the shopping charts under each category. In the chart excerpt below, for example, the first column lists various cleansers in alphabetical order and includes numbers representing their hazardous ingredients.

A table of hazardous ingredients appears on pages 28–38. While we have not listed every product's hazardous ingredients (primarily because of the lack of such information on some MSDSs), for most you can determine the major hazardous ingredients in the product by referring to column one and comparing the numbers listed alongside the name with the table that follows.

Under column two, the product is rated for its immediate (i.e., acute) hazards and under column three for its delayed (i.e., chronic) hazards. In the chart excerpt, you can see that the two AFM products and Bon Ami's cleaning powder are safer than Ajax. Table 2 also tells you that Ajax contains crystalline silica (33), an irritant and carcinogen; sodium hypochlorite (132), an irritant and sensitizer; and washing soda (159), which is caustic (but poses little to no risk in this product).

All-Purpose Cleaners

	Column One				Column Two				Column Three		
	Product				Acute Health Advisory				Chronic Health Advisory		
	🛒 Little to No Risk	🛒 Minimal Risk	🛒 Caution	✓ Recommended	Flammability	Causticity	Irritants	Allergens and Strong Sensitizers	Carcinogens	Neurotoxins	Reproductive Effects
AFM Enterprises Super Clean ✓					🛒	🛒	🛒	🛒	🛒	🛒	🛒
AFM Enterprises Safety Clean ✓					🛒	🛒	🛒	🛒	🛒	🛒	🛒
Ajax Cleanser 33, 132, 159					🛒	🛒	🛒	🛒	⬤	🛒	🛒
Bon Ami Cleaning Powder ✓ 57					🛒	🛒	🛒	🛒	🛒	🛒	🛒

To determine the hazards of various ingredients, we consulted primarily EPA, NTP, and IARC; manufacturers' MSDSs; standard texts, including the *Hazardous Chemicals Desk Reference* by N. Irving Sax and Richard J. Lewis, Sr., and the *Basic Guide to Pesticides* by Shirley A. Briggs and the Rachel Carson Council; and health experts from government, industry, and consumer groups.

TABLE 2. HAZARDOUS INGREDIENTS
IN HOUSEHOLD PRODUCTS *

1. **Acetone:** Skin and eye irritant. Neurotoxic. Used in some adhesives, art products, and paint removers and strippers.
2. **Acetoxyphenylmercury:** Neurotoxic. Teratogenic. Used in some paints.
3. **Acid blue 9:** Carcinogenic. Used in some toilet bowl cleaners and deodorizers.

---

* Although some chemicals' names may seem similar to others, each listing in this chart represents a manufacturer's specific chemical formulation. Furthermore, additional pesticides not listed in this chart are discussed elsewhere in the section on Home and Garden Pesticides (pages 107–19).

4. **Alcohol, Denatured:** Dangerous fire hazard. Irritant. Acutely poisonous.

5. **Aliphatic hydrocarbons:** Prolonged exposure and inhalation may cause irritation to skin, digestive system, throat, and lungs. Neurotoxic. Used in some car waxes.

6. **Aliphatic naphtha:** Eye irritant. Neurotoxic. Used in some furniture polishes.

7. **Aliphatic petroleum distillate:** Flammable. Eye and skin irritant. Neurotoxic. Used in some car cleaning products.

8. **Aliphatic petroleum solvent:** Moderately irritating to skin on prolonged contact. Neurotoxic. Used in some carpet cleaners.

9. **Alkaline bacillus:** Allergen. Used in some laundry soil and stain removers.

10. **Alkylphenol:** Eye irritant. May cause skin sensitization. May act on the body with weak estrogenic effects. Used in some adhesives.

11. **Allethrin:** Eye and skin irritant. Can cause sudden swelling of face, eyelids, lips, mouth, and throat tissues, as well as hay fever–like symptoms. Neurotoxic. Damaging to the immune system. Highly toxic. Used in some pet flea-control products.

12. **Aluminum:** Inhalation of powder has been reported as a cause of lung disease. May be implicated as one of the factors in the onset or exacerbation of Alzheimer's disease. Used in some drain openers.

13. **Aluminum silicate:** Suggestive evidence of carcinogenicity; its hazard is in the dry state (e.g., when sanding or scraping). Used in some paints.

14. **Ammonia:** Undiluted, a powerful eye and systemic irritant that may cause severe burning pain and corrosive damage, including chemical burns, cataracts, and corneal damage. Mild exposure to vapors may cause respiratory irritation. Repeated or prolonged exposure to vapors may cause irritation, bronchitis, and pneumonia. Used in a wide range of household cleaning and auto products.

15. **Ammonium chloride:** Corrosive to the eyes; can cause permanent damage. Used in some toilet bowl cleaners and deodorizers.

16. **Ammonium hydroxide:** Eye irritant. Safe when highly diluted as in most household products. Used in some air fresheners.

17. **Amorphous fumed silica:** Eye, skin, and respiratory irritant. Poses little to no risk when used, as it commonly is, in fragrance pottery.

18. **Aromatic hydrocarbon:** Highly flammable. Heating may cause pressure buildup and possible rupture of the container. Eye and skin irritant. May contain traces of benzene, which is carcinogenic. Neurotoxic. Used in some adhesives.

19. **Barium:** Moderate eye, skin, and respiratory irritant. Used in some artist's oil colors.

20. **Bendiocarb:** Eye and skin irritant. Allergenic. Sensitizer. Neurotoxic. Used in some home and garden pesticides.

21. **Butane:** Flammable. Neurotoxic at very high concentrations. Used as a propellant in a wide range of consumer aerosol products.

22. **Butyl acetate:** Flammable. Skin and eye irritant. Mild allergen. Neurotoxic. Used in shoe products.

23. **Butyl cellosolve (also known as 2-butoxy-1-ethanol or ethylene glycol monobutyl ether):** Mild skin and eye irritant. Damages blood and body's ability to make blood, central nervous system, kidneys, and liver. Readily absorbed through the skin. Neurotoxic. Used in some all-purpose cleaners, window cleaners, and a wide range of other household cleaning products.

24. **Cadmium:** Inhalation affects respiratory system and kidneys. Carcinogenic. Teratogenic. Used in some artist's oil colors.

25. **Calcium carbonate:** Moderate to severe eye irritant. Used in some all-purpose cleaners.

26. **Calcium hypochlorite:** Can cause severe irritation of skin and mucous membranes. Used as a disinfectant for pool chlorine.

27. **Calcium oxide:** Characterized as a powerful caustic to living tissue. Used in some home and garden pesticides.

28. **Carbaryl (Sevin):** Eye and skin irritant. Allergenic. Sensitizer. Highly neurotoxic; symptoms include increased salivation, coughing, difficult breathing, and phlegm. Associated with birth defects. Used in a wide range of pet flea-control products.

29. **Chlorpyrifos (Dursban):** Severe eye, skin, and respiratory irritant. Allergenic. Sensitizer. Highly neurotoxic. Significant reproductive effects. Commonly used by home exterminators, for lawn care, and in pesticide products sold in stores. Poses acute and chronic hazards to both pets and owners.

30. **Cobalt:** Carcinogenic. Used in some artist's oil paints.

31. **Cocodiethanolamide:** Mild eye and skin irritant. Used in some interior and exterior cleaners and protectants.

32. **Concentrated perfume oil:** Mild eye irritant. Used in some air fresheners.

33. **Crystalline silica:** Eye, skin, and lung irritant. Carcinogenic. Its hazard occurs when it is in the dry, not liquid, state. Used in some highly popular brands of cleanser, cat litter, paints, and some powdered flea-control products for pets.

34. **Cyanoacrylate ester:** Combustible. Vapors can irritate the skin and eyes, as well as mucous membranes. Used in some adhesives.

35. **Cyclohexane:** Flammable. Moderate eye, skin, respiratory irritant. Used in some adhesives.

36. Cyfluthrin: Eye and skin irritant. Can cause sudden swelling of face, eyelids, lips, mouth, and throat tissues, as well as hay fever–like symptoms. Neurotoxic. Used in some pet flea-control products.

37. D-cis trans allethrin: Eye and skin irritant. Can cause sudden swelling of face, eyelids, lips, mouth, and throat tissues, as well as hay fever–like symptoms. Neurotoxic. Used in some home and garden pesticides.

38. DEET: Eye and skin irritant. Sensitizer. Neurotoxic. Readily absorbed into skin. Used in some mosquito and insect repellents, as well as pet flea-control products.

39. Detergents and soaps (uncharacterized): Can cause temporary respiratory tract irritation when in powder form (as in the case of laundry detergents) and mild to severe irritation of the eyes in both powder and liquid form (as with dishwashing liquids or other, harsher liquid cleaning products). Symptoms of respiratory distress include coughing, sore throat, wheezing, and temporary shortness of breath. Eye-related symptoms include stinging, tearing, itching, swelling, or redness. Used in some carpet cleaners, dishwashing products, laundry detergents, and a wide range of other household cleaning products.

40. Diazinon: Combustible. Corrosive to eyes. Severe eye and skin irritant. Allergenic. Sensitizer. Highly neurotoxic. Toxic to the fetus. Toxic to birds. Used in lawn pesticides and flea collars, as well as by home exterminators and lawn care companies.

41. 1,4-Dichlorobenzene (para-dichlorobenzene): Carcinogenic. Highly volatile. Causes liver and kidney damage. Used in moth repellents and toilet deodorizers.

42. Dichlorodifluoromethane: Eye irritant. Neurotoxic. Used in some drain openers.

43. Dichlorvos (DDVP): Eye and skin irritant. Allergenic. Sensitizer. Carcinogenic. Highly neurotoxic. Teratogenic: causes sperm and other reproductive abnormalities. Used in some no-pest strips, flea collars, and other pet flea-control products.

44. Diethanolamine (DEA): Mild skin and severe eye irritant. Reacts with nitrites (added as undisclosed preservatives to some products or their raw materials or present as contaminants) to form highly potent carcinogenic nitrosamines. Nitrosamines have been shown to readily penetrate the skin. Used in a wide range of household cleaning products.

45. D-limonene: Eye and skin irritant. Sensitizer. Suggestive evidence of carcinogenicity. Neurotoxic. Teratogenic. Used in some paints and pet flea-control products and passed off as safe. Its safety is suspect.

46. Dimethylbenzyl ammonium chloride: Severe eye and skin irritants. Used in some bathroom cleaners and toilet bowl cleaners and deodorizers.

47. **Dimethyl ethylbenzyl ammonium chloride:** Severe eye and skin irritants. Used in some bathroom cleaners.
48. **Dioctyl phthalate (di [2-ethylhexyl] phthalate):** Skin and severe eye irritant. Carcinogenic. Reproductive toxin. Used in adhesives and correction fluid.
49. **Dipropylene glycol methyl ether:** Eye and skin irritant. Used in some laundry soil and stain removers, car interior and exterior cleaners and protectants, and shoe products.
50. **D-trans allethrin:** Eye and skin irritant. Can cause sudden swelling of face, eyelids, lips, mouth, and throat tissues, as well as hay fever–like symptoms. Neurotoxic. Used in some pet flea-control products.
51. **Ethoxylated alcohols:** May be contaminated with 1,4-dioxane, which is carcinogenic and rapidly penetrates the skin.
52. **Ethoxylated nonyl phenol:** Eye and skin irritant. Used in some car bug, insect, and tar removers.
53. **Ethyl alcohol:** Mild eye, skin, respiratory tract irritant. Used in air fresheners, pet flea-control products, and a wide range of other household cleaning products.
54. **Ethyl benzene:** Neurotoxic. Used in some art products.
55. **Ethylene glycol:** Flammable. Eye, skin, respiratory irritant. Excessive exposure may cause kidney, blood, and possibly liver damage. Neurotoxic. Reproductive toxin. Absorbed through the skin. Used in antifreeze, metal polishes, stains, car waxes, and shoe products.
56. **Ethylene glycol propyl ether:** Eye and skin irritant. Neurotoxic. Used in some paints.
57. **Feldspar:** Mild respiratory irritant. Used in some all-purpose cleaners.
58. **Fenvalerate:** Highly neurotoxic to humans and pets. Can cause tingling and burning sensation of the hands and face. Sweden has discontinued its use among forestry workers. Used in some home and garden pesticides, as well as pet flea-control products.
59. **Formaldehyde:** Poisonous irritant to the skin, eyes, and mucous membranes. A sensitizer. Carcinogenic. Neurotoxic. Used in some furniture polishes, car cleaners and waxes, and a wide range of other consumer items, especially paints and related products.
60. **Glycol ether:** Eye irritant. Used in some household cleaning products.
61. **Heptane:** Flammable. Neurotoxic. Used in some shoe products.
62. **Hexachlorobenzene (HCB):** Eye and skin irritant. Sensitizer. Carcinogenic. Neurotoxic. Teratogenic. Used in some artist's oil colors.
63. **Hexane:** Flammable. Eye, skin, and respiratory tract irritant. Neurotoxin. Used in some adhesives and art products.
64. **Hydramethylnon:** Carcinogenic. Used in some home and garden pesticides.

65. **Hydrocarbon solvent:** Slight to moderate skin irritant. Neurotoxic. Used in some furniture polishes and a wide range of other consumer products.

66. **Hydrochloric acid:** Corrosive. Severe eye, skin, and mucous membrane irritant; highly toxic if inhaled with unknown systemic effects. Inhalation of vapors may cause severe irritation of the respiratory system, coughing, and difficulty breathing. Used in some toilet bowl cleaners and deodorizers.

67. **Iodine:** Can cause stinging and burning of eyes and conjunctivitis. Skin irritant. Used in some toilet bowl cleaners and deodorizers.

68. **Isobutane:** Flammable. Neurotoxic at very high concentrations. Used as a propellant in aerosols.

69. **Isobutyl acetate:** Flammable. Skin and eye irritant. Used in some adhesives.

70. **Isoparaffinic hydrocarbon:** Moderate eye and skin irritant. Used in a wide range of household cleaning products, including air fresheners and car waxes.

71. **Isopropyl alcohol:** Combustible. Can be a moderate eye irritant. Neurotoxic at high concentration. Used in some carpet cleaners and car waxes.

72. **Kerosene:** Flammable. Slight to moderate eye and skin irritant. May contain traces of benzene, which is carcinogenic. Neurotoxic. Used in some furniture polishes and car waxes.

73. **Lead:** Carcinogenic. Neurotoxic. Reproductive effects. Used in some artist's oil paints.

74. **Light petroleum distillates:** Eye, skin, and respiratory irritant. Can cause rashes of the skin. Neurotoxic. Repeated exposure has caused kidney disorders and damage in experimental animals. Used in some spot removers.

75. **Limonene fraction terpenes:** Eye, skin, and respiratory irritant. Used in some spot removers.

76. **Medium aliphatic hydrocarbons:** Suggestive evidence of carcinogenicity. Used in some car waxes.

77. **Medium aliphatic solvent naphtha:** Eye and skin irritant. Neurotoxic. Used in some auto products.

78. **Methanol (methyl alcohol):** Severe eye and skin irritant. Can cause permanent blindness. Neurotoxic. Used in some paint removers and strippers and art products.

79. **Methoxychlor:** Eye and skin irritant. Sensitizer. Limited evidence of carcinogenicity. Reproductive toxin. Weak estrogen-like effects. Used in some pet flea-control products.

80. **Methyl ethyl ketone:** Eye, skin, and respiratory irritant. Neurotoxic. Reproductive toxin. Used in some thinners and adhesives.

81. **Methylene chloride (dichloromethane):** Severe skin and moderate eye irritant. Can cause irregular heartbeat, even heart attack, when inhaled. Carcinogenic. Neurotoxic. Used in some paint strippers and spray paints.

82. **Mineral seal oil:** Eye and skin irritant. Can cause dermatitis. Used in some furniture polishes.

83. Mineral spirits: Severe eye and skin irritant. Neurotoxic. Used in some floor cleaners, waxes, polishes, and many paints and related products.

84. Monethanolamine: Moderate skin, severe eye irritant. Used in some paint removers and strippers.

85. Morpholine: Moderate to severe eye, skin, and mucous membrane irritant. Reacts with nitrites (added as undisclosed preservatives to some products or their raw materials or present as contaminants) to form carcinogenic nitrosamines. Can cause kidney damage. Used in some furniture polishes and car waxes.

86. Naled: Eye and skin irritant. Neurotoxic. Transformation product includes dichlorvos, which is carcinogenic and a reproductive toxin. Used in some pet flea-control products.

87. Naphthalene: Combustible. Eye and skin irritant. Can cause corneal damage and cataracts. Neurotoxic. Reproductive toxin: transported across the placenta and can cause blood damage. Used in some moth repellents and car waxes.

88. N-octyl bicycloheptene dicarboximide: Eye and respiratory tract irritant. Used in some household and garden pesticides, as well as pet flea-control products.

89. Nonionic surfactants: Eye irritant. Used in some toilet bowl cleaners and deodorizers.

90. Nonoxynol 4: Eye and skin irritant. Used in some laundry soil and stain removers.

91. Nonylphenol ethoxylate: Mild eye irritant. Used in some air fresheners.

92. Nonylphenol polyethylene oxide: Eye, skin, and respiratory tract irritant. Used in some spot removers.

93. Nonylphenol resin: Skin and eye irritant. May cause skin sensitization. Used in some adhesives.

94. Oil of orange: Skin irritant. Carcinogenic. Used in some all-purpose cleaners, furniture polishes, and spot removers.

95. Oleic diethanol amide: Eye and skin irritant. Used in some car waxes.

96. Ortho phenylphenol: Severe eye and skin irritant. IARC says the evidence is inadequate to assess its carcinogenicity. EPA says it is probably carcinogenic to humans. (As is our general policy, we have used the higher ranking.) Used in some air fresheners and disinfectants.

97. Oxalic acid dihydrate: Moderate eye and skin irritant. Can be allergenic. Used in some cleansers.

98. Parabens (methyl, propyl): Allergenic. Used as preservatives in some household products.

99. Permethrin: Eye and skin irritant. Can cause sudden swelling of face, eyelids, lips, mouth, and throat tissues, as well as hay fever–like symptoms.

Carcinogenic. Neurotoxic. Used in some household and garden pesticides, and pet flea-control products.

100. **Petroleum distillates:** Fire hazard. Eye, skin, and respiratory irritant. Can cause conjunctivitis and dermatitis. May contain traces of benzene, which is carcinogenic. Mild to significant neurotoxic effects leading to organic brain damage, depending on concentration and duration of exposure. Used in a wide range of products, including heavy-duty cleaners, laundry stain removers, home and garden pesticides, pet flea-control products, and car waxes.

101. **Petroleum hydrocarbons:** Eye, skin, and respiratory irritant. May contain traces of benzene, which is carcinogenic. Neurotoxic. Used in some furniture polishes.

102. **Petroleum process oil:** Eye, skin, and respiratory tract irritant. May contain traces of benzene, which is carcinogenic. Neurotoxic. Used in some furniture polishes.

103. **Petroleum solvents:** Severe eye, skin, and respiratory irritant. May contain traces of benzene, which is carcinogenic. Significant neurotoxic effects. Used in some floor cleaners, waxes, and polishes.

104. **Petroleum spirits:** Eye, skin, and respiratory irritant. May contain traces of benzene, which is carcinogenic. Neurotoxic. Used in some spot removers.

105. **Phenothrin (sumithrin):** Eye and skin irritant. Can cause sudden swelling of face, eyelids, lips, mouth, and throat tissues, as well as hay fever–like symptoms. Neurotoxic. Used in some pet flea-control products.

106. **Phosphoric acid:** Corrosive. Severe eye, skin, respiratory irritant. Breathing vapors can make lungs ache. Used in some bathroom cleaning products, especially those that remove lime and mildew, metal polishes

107. **Pine oil:** Weak allergen. Very large doses cause central nervous system depression. Used in a wide range of household cleaning products.

108. **Polychlorinated biphenyls (PCBs):** Cause dermatitis. Carcinogenic. Neurotoxic. Teratogenic. Used in some artist's oil paints.

109. **Poly (methyl methacrylate):** Skin, eye, and respiratory irritant. Limited evidence of carcinogenicity. Used in some adhesives.

110. **Polyoxyethylene oleyl ether:** Moderate eye and skin irritant. Used in some air fresheners.

111. **Polystyrene resin solution:** Flammable. Eye and skin irritant. Used in some adhesives.

112. **Propane:** Flammable. Neurotoxic at high concentrations. An aerosol propellant used in a wide range of consumer products.

113. **Propoxur:** Carcinogenic. Neurotoxic. Used in some home and garden pesticides.

114. **Propylene glycol methyl ether:** Mild to moderate eye, skin, and respiratory irritant. Used in some carpet and car cleaning products.

115. **Propylene oxide:** Flammable. Skin and eye irritant. Carcinogenic. Neuro-toxic. Used in some adhesives.

116. **Proteinase:** Allergenic. Used in laundry soil and stain removers.

117. **Proteolytic enzymes:** Mild eye irritant. May cause sensitization with symptoms ranging from mild hay fever and asthma to dermatitis. Used in some laundry soil and stain removers.

118. **Pyrethrins:** Allergenic. Neurotoxic. Used in some household and garden pesticides, as well as pet flea-control products.

119. **Quaternary ammonium compound:** Eye and skin irritant. Used in some all-purpose cleaners and laundry fabric softeners.

120. **Quaternary Dicco:** Slight fire hazard. Moderate to severe skin and eye irritant; in some cases may cause skin burns and corneal damage to the eye. Used in some car interior and exterior cleaners and protectants.

121. **Quaternium 15:** Eye and skin irritant. Allergen. Can release formaldehyde. Used in some hand and automatic dishwashing products.

122. **Resmethrin:** Can cause sudden swelling of face, eyelids, lips, mouth, and throat tissues, as well as hay fever–like symptoms. Neurotoxic. Used in some pet flea-control products.

123. **Rotenone:** Skin irritant. Carcinogenic. Neurotoxic. Tetrogenic. Used in some pet flea-control products.

124. **Silicon dioxide:** Eye and skin irritant. Used in some auto products.

125. **Silicone emulsion:** Slight fire risk. Used in some interior and exterior car cleaners and protectants.

126. **Sodium bisulfate:** Corrosive and damaging to the eyes, skin, and internal tissues if ingested. Can cause asthma attacks. Used in some toilet bowl cleaners and deodorizers.

127. **Sodium dichloroisocyanurate dihydrate:** Corrosive. Severe eye, skin, and respiratory irritant. Can form chlorine gas that can cause burning and watering of the eyes, as well as burning of the nose and mouth. Used in some toilet bowl cleaners and deodorizers.

128. **Sodium 2,4-dichlorophenoxyacetate (2,4-D):** Irritant. Sensitizer. Carcinogenic. Neurotoxic. Teratogenic. Used as a herbicide in lawn care products.

129. **Sodium dithionate:** Eye, skin, and respiratory irritant. Used in some spot removers.

130. **Sodium dodecylbenzene sulfonate:** Eye and skin irritant. Used in some laundry soil and stain removers.

131. **Sodium hydroxide:** Corrosive. Eye, skin, and respiratory irritant. When highly concentrated as used in some drain openers and oven cleaners, it can burn eyes, skin, and internal organs. Can be fatal if swallowed. Used in a wide range of household cleaners.

132. **Sodium hypochlorite (bleach):** Corrosive. Eye, skin, and respiratory irritant. Sensitizer. Can be fatal if swallowed. Especially hazardous to people with heart conditions or asthma. Used in a wide range of household cleaners.

133. **Sodium metasilicate:** Corrosive. Severe eye, skin, and respiratory irritant. Inhalation of dust can cause throat and lung damage. Used in some driveway and garage floor cleaners.

134. **Sodium ortho-phenylphenol:** Eye and skin irritant. Carcinogenic. Used in some bathroom cleaners.

135. **Sodium silicate:** Can be corrosive. Can cause burns to the eyes and tissue damage to the skin, as well as cause burns to mouth, throat, and stomach if swallowed. Used in some automatic dishwashing detergents and car interior and exterior cleaners and protectants.

136. **Sodium sulfate:** Corrosive. Severe eye, skin, and respiratory irritant. Can cause asthma attacks. Used in some toilet bowl cleaners and deodorizers.

137. **Solvents (uncharacterized):** Eye, skin, and respiratory irritant. Neurotoxic. Used in some paint removers and strippers.

138. **Solvent orange 3 dye/solvent red 49 dye:** Carcinogenic. Used in some shoe polishes.

139. **Starch:** Allergenic. Used in some laundry starches.

140. **Stoddard solvent:** Slight fire hazard. Eye and mucous membrane irritant. Neurotoxic. Used in some auto, floor wax, and shoe products.

141. **Sulfur:** Poses minimal risk for eye, skin, and respiratory irritation, as well as nausea and allergic sensitization. Frequently used in least-toxic pesticides, especially for organic gardening, sulfur products are some of the safest chemicals available for use—for both people and the environment.

142. **Surfactants (uncharacterized):** Eye irritant. Used in a wide range of household cleaning products.

143. **Talc:** Carcinogenic when inhaled. Used in some home and garden pesticides.

144. **Tetrachloroethylene (perchloroethylene):** Eye, skin, and respiratory irritant. Carcinogenic. Neurotoxic. Used in some spot removers.

145. **Tetrachlorvinphos:** Eye and skin irritant. Carcinogenic. Used in some pet flea-control products.

146. **Tetrahydrofuran:** Irritant to eyes and mucous membranes. Neurotoxic. Can cause injury to liver and kidneys. Used in some adhesive products.

147. **Tetramethrin:** Eye and skin irritant. Can cause sudden swelling of face, eyelids, lips, mouth, and throat tissues, as well as hay fever–like symptoms. Neurotoxic. Used in some pet flea-control products.

148. **Tetrasodium EDTA:** Eye irritant. Used in some bathroom cleaners.

149. **Titanium dioxide: Limited evidence of carcinogencity:** Hazardous, not as a liquid, but as a dust (as when paint containing titanium dioxide is being sanded or scraped). Used in some paints and shoe polishes.

150. **Toluene:** Eye and skin irritant. Can cause cardiac sensitization. Neurotoxic. Reproductive effects. Used in some spot removers and art products.

151. **1,1,1-trichloroethane:** Moderate skin and severe eye irritant. Can sensitize the heart, cause cardiac arrest. Inadequate evidence to determine its noncarcinogenicity. Significant neurotoxic effects. Used in some metal polishes, spot removers, household pesticides, and a wide range of other consumer products.

152. **Tri (dimethylaminomethyl) phenol:** Eye and skin irritant. May cause skin sensitization. Used in some adhesives.

153. **Triethanolamine (TEA):** Eye and skin irritant. Can react with nitrites (added as undisclosed preservatives to some products or their raw materials or present as contaminants) to form carcinogenic nitrosamines. Nitrosamines have been shown to readily penetrate the skin. Used in some liquid all-purpose cleaning products, metal polishes, spot removers, and other household cleaning products.

154. **Tripropylene glycol monomethyl ether:** Prolonged and repeated skin exposure to large doses can result in narcosis and kidney injury. Used in some floor cleaners, waxes, and polishes.

155. **Trisodium nitrilotriacetate:** Carcinogenic. Used in some bathroom cleaning products.

156. **Turpentine:** Flammable. Eye irritant. Can cause allergenic sensitization. Neurotoxic. Can cause serious irritation of the kidneys. Used in some furniture polishes, auto, art, and shoe products.

157. **Urea:** Skin irritant. Allergen. Used in some laundry soil and stain removers.

158. **VM&P naphtha:** Eye and skin irritant. Neurotoxic. Used in some furniture polishes.

159. **Washing soda:** Caustic. Can cause eye burns with potential injury on prolonged contact. Used in some laundry detergents.

160. **White mineral oil:** Eye and skin irritant. Neurotoxic. Used in some furniture polishes.

161. **Xylene:** Severe eye and moderate skin irritant. Significant neurotoxic effects. Reproductive effects. Used in some spot removers, car cleaners, paints, and other consumer products.

CHAPTER 1

Cleaning Products

AIR FRESHENERS, DEODORIZERS, AND ODOR REMOVERS

Product Types

Aerosol; diffuser (fragrance jar and plug-in); dried botanical matter; pump.

Health Advisory

We recommend against the use of aerosol air fresheners. Spraying them puts many tiny particles in the air that you will end up inhaling. Quite apart from tissue irritation, the impurities attached to these particles also go into your lungs.

Recommended Alternatives

You can find a wide range of safe, effective brands in both mainstream supermarkets and health food stores. Fragrance jars and dried botanicals are among the safest. You will also find some safe nonaerosol pumps.

You also can make your home, work area, and other spaces fresh through a variety of natural, inexpensive alternatives.

For example:

- Several common house plants are known for their use in the removal of contaminants from indoor air. See page 154.
- Place fragrant flowers and herbs, such as roses, lemon verbena, or lavender, or bowls of petals of fragrant flowers and herbs in various rooms. You can also buy flower sachets and place them in various areas of the room.

- Baking soda is an excellent, inexpensive odor remover. Place a box of baking soda in closets and other enclosed areas to absorb odors.
- Open windows and turn on a fan if you live in an area with good air quality. Contaminants in the air, including molds and bacteria, become trapped in poorly ventilated rooms. Sunshine is a natural disinfectant.
- Empty garbage frequently. Never leave table scraps indoors in the trash.
- Vacuum frequently.
- Dust frequently.
- Never leave unwashed plates in the sink.
- Keep moldy areas dry and light; use small bags of silica gel (available from camera stores) to absorb moisture.
- A more expensive alternative but worthy of consideration is to buy a good quality two-stage air purifier that combines a high-efficiency particle air (HEPA) filter with a carbon filter. Models can also be bought for automobiles. See *Air Filters*, page 153.

Air Fresheners, Deodorizers, and Odor Removers

Legend: 🛒 Little to No Risk | 🛒 Minimal Risk | 🛒 Caution | ✓ Recommended

Product	Acute Health Advisory				Chronic Health Advisory		
	Flammability	Causticity	Irritants	Allergens and Strong Sensitizers	Carcinogens	Neurotoxins	Reproductive Effects
Airwick Stick Ups ✓	🛒	🛒	🛒	🛒	🛒	🛒	🛒
Arm & Hammer Deodorizing Air Freshener Aerosol (all scents) 16, 68, 112	🛒	🛒	●	🛒	🛒	🛒	🛒
Citrus Magic ✓	🛒	🛒	🛒	🛒	🛒	🛒	🛒
Crystalaire Air Freshener (all scents) 53, 91	🛒	🛒	🛒	🛒	🛒	🛒	🛒
Dasun Liquid Odor Degrader ✓	🛒	🛒	🛒	🛒	🛒	🛒	🛒
Dr. Harvey's Fresh Air ✓	🛒	🛒	🛒	🛒	🛒	🛒	🛒
Ecco Bella Citrus Air Purifying Mist ✓	🛒	🛒	🛒	🛒	🛒	🛒	🛒
Glade Aerosols (all scents) 68, 112	●	🛒	●	🛒	🛒	🛒	🛒
Glade Aerosols with Chlorophyll (all scents) 21, 68, 112	●	🛒	●	🛒	🛒	🛒	🛒
Glade Country Dried Botanical (all scents) ✓	🛒	🛒	🛒	🛒	🛒	🛒	🛒

Product	Acute Health Advisory				Chronic Health Advisory		
	Flammability	Causticity	Irritants	Allergens and Strong Sensitizers	Carcinogens	Neurotoxins	Reproductive Effects
Glade Country Pottery (all scents) ✓ *17*	Little to No Risk	Minimal	Minimal	Minimal	Minimal	Minimal	Minimal
Glade Plug-Ins (all scents) 17, 70	Minimal	Minimal	Caution	Minimal	Minimal	Minimal	Minimal
Glade II (all scents) ✓	Little to No Risk	Minimal	Caution	Minimal	Minimal	Minimal	Minimal
Glade Potpourri Aerosol (all scents) 21, 68, 112	Caution	Minimal	Caution	Minimal	Minimal	Minimal	Minimal
Glade Pump Air Freshener (all scents) 53, 110	Little to No Risk	Minimal	Little to No Risk	Minimal	Minimal	Minimal	Minimal
Glade Spray Disinfectant Aerosol 21, 53, 112	Caution	Minimal	Caution	Minimal	Minimal	Minimal	Minimal
Head Air Deodorizer ✓ *71*	Minimal	Minimal	Minimal	Minimal	Minimal	Minimal	Minimal
Lysol Disinfectant (all scents) 53, 96	Caution	Minimal	Caution	Minimal	Caution	Minimal	Minimal
Magic Mushroom (all scents) ✓ *53*	Minimal	Minimal	Minimal	Minimal	Minimal	Minimal	Minimal
Mia Rose Air Therapy (all non-aerosol scents) ✓	Minimal	Minimal	Minimal	Minimal	Minimal	Minimal	Minimal
Mia Rose Pet Air Aerosol	Minimal	Minimal	Caution	Minimal	Minimal	Minimal	Minimal
Natural Chemistry for Litter and Cage ✓	Minimal	Minimal	Minimal	Minimal	Minimal	Minimal	Minimal
Natural Chemistry for Smells and Stains ✓	Minimal	Minimal	Minimal	Minimal	Minimal	Minimal	Minimal
NonScents from Dasun (all products) ✓	Minimal	Minimal	Minimal	Minimal	Minimal	Minimal	Minimal
Power 90 Spray ✓	Minimal	Minimal	Minimal	Minimal	Minimal	Minimal	Minimal
Prevail Aerosol Air Freshener 21, 112	Caution	Minimal	Caution	Minimal	Minimal	Minimal	Minimal
Renuzit Adjustable Air Freshener ✓	Minimal	Minimal	Minimal	Minimal	Minimal	Minimal	Minimal
Renuzit Air Deodorizer 21, 83, 112	Caution	Minimal	Caution	Minimal	Minimal	Little to No Risk	Minimal
Renuzit Fragrance Jars (all scents) ✓ *32*	Little to No Risk	Minimal	Little to No Risk	Minimal	Minimal	Minimal	Minimal
Renuzit Fresh 'n Dry Aerosol 21, 112	Caution	Minimal	Caution	Minimal	Minimal	Minimal	Minimal
Renuzit Freshell Long Lasting Air Freshener ✓ *71*	Little to No Risk	Minimal	Minimal	Minimal	Minimal	Minimal	Minimal

Legend: Little to No Risk · Minimal Risk · Caution · Recommended ✓

Product				Acute Health Advisory				Chronic Health Advisory		
Little to No Risk	Minimal Risk	Caution	Recommended	Flammability	Causticity	Irritants	Allergens and Strong Sensitizers	Carcinogens	Neurotoxins	Reproductive Effects
Renuzit Roommate Liquid Air Freshener ✓ 71				Minimal Risk	Caution	Caution	Caution	Caution	Caution	Caution
Wizard Aerosol Air Freshener (all scents) 21, 112				Caution	Caution	Little to No Risk	Caution	Caution	Caution	Caution

ALL-PURPOSE CLEANERS

Product Types

Aerosol; gel; pump; liquid.

Health Advisory

Chronic

All-purpose cleaners contain substances that are not carcinogenic in themselves but that interact with other chemicals to form carcinogens. Diethanolamine (DEA), morpholine, and triethanolamine (TEA), found in some all-purpose cleaners, can each react with nitrites (added as undisclosed preservatives to some products or their raw materials or present as contaminants) to form carcinogenic nitrosamines. Nitrosamines readily penetrate the skin.

Another reason for hand protection is that most colored products are dyed with artificial coal tar colors that cause cancer or contain impurities such as arsenic or lead that cause cancer.

We recommend that consumers avoid products containing butyl cellosolve. It is neurotoxic and rapidly penetrates the skin.

Safe Use Tips

- If you use chlorine cleaners or bleach, **DO NOT** mix them with ammonia, acids, or any other cleaning products. Toxic chloramine gas can be produced.
- Be sure to wear gloves when working with all-purpose cleaners to prevent skin absorption of carcinogenic contaminants that may be present, including nitrosamines, 1,4-dioxane, and coal tar colors, as well as absorption of butyl cellosolve.
- Avoid products dyed with unspecified artificial colors.

Recommended Alternatives

Fortunately, many excellent brands are widely available at both supermarkets and health food stores. You will have no problem finding just the right, safe all-purpose cleaner for your needs.

There also are many inexpensive ways of making your own all-purpose cleaners. We have used them and know that they work well.

- A disinfectant cleaner can be made with a mixture of 1 teaspoon of borax, 2 tablespoons of distilled white vinegar, $1/4$ cup liquid soap, and 2 cups of hot water in a refillable spray bottle.

- A stronger all-around household cleaner can be made with liquid soap and trisodium phosphate (TSP). Again, you will need a refillable spray bottle. Mix 1 teaspoon of liquid soap, 1 teaspoon TSP, 1 teaspoon of borax, 1 teaspoon of distilled white vinegar and 1 quart warm-to-hot water. This formula is effective against both grease and mildew. One warning: Be sure to use TSP only when it is diluted; wear latex gloves.

- You can also replace standard bleaching products, containing highly caustic sodium hypochlorite, with safer alternatives using hydrogen peroxide. Hydrogen peroxide, in a standard 3 percent solution, is less caustic and irritating than sodium hypochlorite and it is safe enough to keep on hand as a mild antiseptic and spot remover. Also try using baking soda or TSP instead of products containing ammonia and lye. Although TSP is alkaline as well, it is the least toxic cleaner in this class. Baking soda is also slightly alkaline but will not burn and is safe.

All-Purpose Cleaners

Product				Flammability	Causticity	Irritants	Allergens and Strong Sensitizers	Carcinogens	Neurotoxins	Reproductive Effects
🛒 Little to No Risk	🛒 Minimal Risk	🛒 Caution	✓ Recommended							
AFM Safety Cleaner ✓				🛒	🛒	🛒	🛒	🛒	🛒	🛒
AFM Super Clean ✓				🛒	🛒	🛒	🛒	🛒	🛒	🛒
Ajax All Purpose Liquid Cleaner Ammonia Fresh ✓ 14				🛒	🛒	🛒	🛒	🛒	🛒	🛒
Ajax All Purpose Liquid Cleaner Lemon Fresh ✓				🛒	🛒	🛒	🛒	🛒	🛒	🛒
Allen's Naturally All-Purpose Cleaner 44, 121, 148				🛒	🛒	🛒	🛒	🛒	🛒	🛒

Product				Little to No Risk / Minimal Risk / Caution / Recommended ✓

Legend: 🛒 Little to No Risk 🛒 Minimal Risk 🛒 Caution ✓ Recommended

Product	Flammability	Causticity	Irritants	Allergens and Strong Sensitizers	Carcinogens	Neurotoxins	Reproductive Effects
Aubrey Clean Up! All Purpose Household Cleaner ✓	Little	Little	Little	Little	Little	Little	Little
Aubrey Liquid Sparkle Natural Spray Cleaner ✓	Little	Little	Little	Little	Little	Little	Little
Auro Organics Plant Soap ✓	Little	Little	Little	Little	Little	Little	Little
Auro Organics Cleaning Emulsion ✓	Little	Little	Little	Little	Little	Little	Little
Bioclean ✓	Little	Little	Little	Little	Little	Little	Little
Biofa Household Cleaner ✓	Little	Little	Little	Little	Little	Little	Little
Bon Ami Cleaning Cake ✓ 57	Little	Little	Little	Little	Little	Little	Little
Bon Ami Cleaning Powder 57	Little	Little	Minimal	Little	Little	Little	Little
Bon Ami Foam Cleaner Aerosol 21, 68, 85, 112	Caution	Little	Caution	Little	Minimal	Little	Little
Cal Ben Soap Company Pure Soap ✓	Little	Little	Little	Little	Little	Little	Little
Cinch Glass and Multi-Surface Cleaner ✓ 71	Little	Little	Little	Little	Little	Little	Little
Citri-Glow ✓	Little	Little	Minimal	Little	Little	Little	Little
Citra-Solv 75, 92, 94	Minimal	Little	Caution	Little	Caution	Little	Little
Comet Liquid ✓ 132	Little	Little	Minimal	Little	Little	Little	Little
Dial Corporation 20 Mule Team Borax ✓	Little	Little	Little	Little	Little	Little	Little
Dr. Bronner's Pure Castile Soaps ✓	Little	Little	Little	Little	Little	Little	Little
Dr. Bronner's Sal Suds ✓	Little	Little	Little	Little	Little	Little	Little
Dr. Harvey's All Purpose Clean ✓	Little	Little	Little	Little	Little	Little	Little
Earth Friendly Orange Plus All-Purpose Cleaner ✓	Little	Little	Minimal	Little	Little	Little	Little
EarthRite All Purpose Cleaner ✓	Little	Little	Little	Little	Little	Little	Little
EarthRite Countertop Cleaner ✓	Little	Little	Little	Little	Little	Little	Little

Product				Acute Health Advisory				Chronic Health Advisory		

Legend:
- 🛒 Little to No Risk
- 🛒 Minimal Risk
- 🛒 Caution
- ✓ Recommended

Product	Flammability	Causticity	Irritants	Allergens and Strong Sensitizers	Carcinogens	Neurotoxins	Reproductive Effects
Ecover Cream Cleaner ✓	🛒	🛒	🛒	🛒	🛒	🛒	🛒
Fantastik All Purpose Cleaner 23	🛒	🛒	🛒	🛒	🛒	🛒	🛒
Formula 409 23	🛒	🛒	🛒	🛒	🛒	🛒	🛒
Granny's E.Z. Maid Dish & All-Purpose Liquid 51	🛒	🛒	🛒	🛒	🛒	🛒	🛒
Greenspan Healthy Kleaner ✓	🛒	🛒	🛒	🛒	🛒	🛒	🛒
Gunk Green Concentrated Cleaner 23, 71	🛒	🛒	🛒	🛒	🛒	🛒	🛒
Household Ammonia 14	🛒	🛒 (dark)	🛒 (dark)	🛒	🛒	🛒	🛒
Infinity Heavenly Horsetail All Purpose Cleaner 44	🛒	🛒	🛒	🛒	🛒	🛒	🛒
Life Tree Home-Soap All-Purpose Cleanser 44, 98, 153	🛒	🛒	🛒	🛒	🛒	🛒	🛒
Livos Avi-Soap Concentrate ✓	🛒	🛒	🛒	🛒	🛒	🛒	🛒
Livos Kiros-Alcohol Thinner ✓	🛒	🛒	🛒	🛒	🛒	🛒	🛒
Livos Latis-Soap Concentrate ✓	🛒	🛒	🛒	🛒	🛒	🛒	🛒
Mr. Clean ✓	🛒	🛒	🛒	🛒	🛒	🛒	🛒
Mr. Clean Lemon Fresh ✓	🛒	🛒	🛒	🛒	🛒	🛒	🛒
Mr. Clean Liquid Synthetic Detergent ✓	🛒	🛒	🛒	🛒	🛒	🛒	🛒
Mr. Clean with Bleach ✓ 132	🛒	🛒	🛒	🛒	🛒	🛒	🛒
Murphy Oil Soap Liquid 142, 153	🛒	🛒	🛒	🛒	🛒	🛒	🛒
Murphy Oil Soap Spray 142, 153	🛒	🛒	🛒	🛒	🛒	🛒	🛒
Naturally Yours Degreaser ✓	🛒	🛒	🛒	🛒	🛒	🛒	🛒
Naturally Yours Gentle Soap ✓	🛒	🛒	🛒	🛒	🛒	🛒	🛒
Pine Magic II Multi-Purpose Cleaner 71, 119	🛒	🛒	🛒	🛒	🛒	🛒	🛒
Pine-Sol Broad Spectrum Formula 71, 107	🛒	🛒	🛒	🛒	🛒	🛒	🛒

Legend: 🛒 Little to No Risk 🛒 Minimal Risk 🛒 Caution ✓ Recommended

Product	Acute Health Advisory				Chronic Health Advisory		
	Flammability	Causticity	Irritants	Allergens and Strong Sensitizers	Carcinogens	Neurotoxins	Reproductive Effects
Pine-Sol Multi-Action Spray Cleaner 23, 71	🛒	🛒	🛒	🛒	🛒	🛒	🛒
Pine-Sol Spray Cleaner 23, 71	🛒	🛒	🛒	🛒	🛒	🛒	🛒
Pledge Household Cleaner 60, 153	🛒	🛒	🛒	🛒	🛒	🛒	🛒
Prevail All Purpose Cleaner with Ammonia 14, 107, 131	🛒	🛒	🛒	🛒	🛒	🛒	🛒
Prevail Liquid Scrub Mild Abrasive Cleaner 44, 130	🛒	🛒	🛒	🛒	🛒	🛒	🛒
Radiator Specialty Company General Purpose Cleaner 7, 23, 52	🛒 (Caution)	🛒 (Caution)	🛒 (Caution)	🛒	🛒	🛒	🛒
Radiator Specialty Company Liquid Concentrated Multi-Surface Cleaner 23, 71	🛒	🛒	🛒	🛒	🛒	🛒	🛒
Simmons Pure Soaps Bar Soaps ✓	🛒	🛒	🛒	🛒	🛒	🛒	🛒
Simple Green 23	🛒	🛒	🛒	🛒	🛒	🛒	🛒
Soft Scrub 25	🛒	🛒	🛒 (Caution)	🛒	🛒	🛒	🛒
Soft Scrub Mild Abrasive Cleanser with Bleach 25, 132	🛒	🛒	🛒	🛒	🛒	🛒	🛒
S.O.S. Kitchen-Safe ✓	🛒	🛒	🛒	🛒	🛒	🛒	🛒
Spic and Span Pine Cleaner Liquid Household Cleaner 71, 107	🛒	🛒	🛒	🛒	🛒	🛒	🛒
Spic and Span Liquid ✓	🛒	🛒	🛒	🛒	🛒	🛒	🛒
Spic and Span Synthetic Detergent ✓ 135	🛒	🛒	🛒	🛒	🛒	🛒	🛒
Tackle ✓ 131, 132	🛒	🛒	🛒	🛒	🛒	🛒	🛒
Top Job Liquid Household Cleaner ✓ 14	🛒	🛒	🛒	🛒	🛒	🛒	🛒
Tropical Soap Co. Sirene Coconut-Oil Bar Soaps ✓	🛒	🛒	🛒	🛒	🛒	🛒	🛒

BATHROOM CLEANERS AND DISINFECTANTS

Product Types

Aerosol; pump; gel; liquid.

Health Advisory

Some brands with sodium hydroxide, sodium hypochlorite, and phosphoric acid can severely burn eyes, skin, or internal organs. Breathing vapors can make lungs burn. People with heart or respiratory problems should not use brands rated for caution under the categories of causticity or irritation.

Safe Use Tips

- Be sure to open all windows.
- If using products rated for caution, be sure to wear a respirator and protective gloves.
- Always wear gloves to protect against the possible presence of undisclosed carcinogenic contaminants or precursors such as artificial dyes, 1,4-dioxane (found in ethoxylated alcohols), DEA, and TEA.

Recommended Alternatives

A wide range of safe, effective bathroom cleaners is available at both supermarkets and health food stores. If you make your own homemade bathroom cleaner, then you need not worry about any undisclosed contaminants.

Here are some suggestions.

- One of the best and safest disinfectant formulas is easily made by mixing 2 teaspoons of borax, 4 tablespoons of distilled white vinegar, and 3 to 4 cups of hot water and pouring the mixture into a refillable spray bottle. For stronger cleaning power, add $1/4$ teaspoon of liquid soap.
- The TSP-based cleaner discussed on page 43 also works well for removing bathroom mildew.
- Another good homemade formula for removing tub and shower mildew is to make a paste from baking soda and water. Pour $1/2$ cup of baking soda into a large bowl, adding enough water and stirring until the mixture reaches the consistency of a paste. Use a hard-bristled brush for general mildew removal and a hard-bristled toothbrush for removing mildew in between tiles.

Bathroom Cleaners and Disinfectants

Legend:
- 🛒 Little to No Risk
- 🛒 Minimal Risk
- 🛒 Caution
- ✓ Recommended

Product	Acute Health Advisory				Chronic Health Advisory		
	Flammability	Causticity	Irritants	Allergens and Strong Sensitizers	Carcinogens	Neurotoxins	Reproductive Effects
AFM Mildew Control ✓	Little/No	Little/No	Little/No	Little/No	Little/No	Little/No	Little/No
AFM Safety Clean ✓	Little/No	Little/No	Little/No	Little/No	Little/No	Little/No	Little/No
Ajax All Purpose Liquid Cleaner Lemon Fresh ✓	Little/No	Little/No	Minimal	Little/No	Little/No	Little/No	Little/No
Allen's Multi-Purpose Spray 44, 60, 135	Little/No	Little/No	Minimal	Little/No	Minimal	Little/No	Little/No
Auro Organics Cleaning Emulsion ✓	Little/No	Little/No	Little/No	Little/No	Little/No	Little/No	Little/No
Auro Organics Plant Soap ✓	Little/No	Little/No	Little/No	Little/No	Little/No	Little/No	Little/No
Aubrey Clean Up! All-Purpose Household Cleaner ✓	Little/No	Little/No	Little/No	Little/No	Little/No	Little/No	Little/No
Aubrey Liquid Sparkle Natural Spray Cleaner ✓	Little/No	Little/No	Little/No	Little/No	Little/No	Little/No	Little/No
Bathroom Duck 51, 60, 148	Little/No	Little/No	Minimal	Little/No	Minimal	Little/No	Little/No
Biofa Household Cleaner ✓	Little/No	Little/No	Little/No	Little/No	Little/No	Little/No	Little/No
Biofa Natural Toilet Cleaner ✓	Little/No	Little/No	Little/No	Little/No	Little/No	Little/No	Little/No
Clorox Regular Bleach 132	Little/No	Caution	Caution	Little/No	Little/No	Little/No	Little/No
Descale-It Bathroom Tile and Fixture ✓	Little/No	Little/No	Minimal	Little/No	Little/No	Little/No	Little/No
Dial Corporation 20 Mule Team Borax ✓	Little/No	Little/No	Little/No	Little/No	Little/No	Little/No	Little/No
DOW Disinfectant Bathroom II Cleaner 46, 47, 148	Little/No	Little/No	Minimal	Little/No	Little/No	Little/No	Little/No
Earth Friendly Toilet Cleaner ✓	Little/No	Little/No	Little/No	Little/No	Little/No	Little/No	Little/No
EarthRite Tub & Tile Cleaner ✓	Little/No	Little/No	Little/No	Little/No	Little/No	Little/No	Little/No
Eliminate Shower Clean Tub and Tile ✓	Little/No	Little/No	Little/No	Little/No	Little/No	Little/No	Little/No
Fantastik Swipes ✓	Little/No	Little/No	Little/No	Little/No	Little/No	Little/No	Little/No
Gr-eat 'N Easy Bathroom Cleaner 23	Little/No	Little/No	Minimal	Little/No	Little/No	Minimal	Little/No

Product				Acute Health Advisory				Chronic Health Advisory		
🛒 Little to No Risk	🛒 Minimal Risk	🛒 Caution	✓ Recommended	Flammability	Causticity	Irritants	Allergens and Strong Sensitizers	Carcinogens	Neurotoxins	Reproductive Effects
Harvey's All Purpose Clean ✓ 133				🛒	🛒	🛒	🛒	🛒	🛒	🛒
K-Mart Bathroom ✓				🛒	🛒	🛒	🛒	🛒	🛒	🛒
Life Tree Bathroom Cleaner 44, 98, 153				🛒	🛒	🛒	🛒	🛒	🛒	🛒
Lime-A-Way Bathroom 106				🛒	🛒	🛒	🛒	🛒	🛒	🛒
Lysol Bathroom Touch-Ups Cleaning Wipes 46, 47				🛒	🛒	🛒	🛒	🛒	🛒	🛒
Mr. Clean ✓				🛒	🛒	🛒	🛒	🛒	🛒	🛒
Mr. Clean Liquid Synthetic Detergent ✓				🛒	🛒	🛒	🛒	🛒	🛒	🛒
Naturally Yours Basin, Tub and Tile Cleaner ✓				🛒	🛒	🛒	🛒	🛒	🛒	🛒
Naturally Yours Mold and Mildew Cleaner ✓				🛒	🛒	🛒	🛒	🛒	🛒	🛒
Neo-Life Green Personal Care Cleanser ✓				🛒	🛒	🛒	🛒	🛒	🛒	🛒
Pine Magic II Multi-Purpose Cleaner 71, 119				🛒	🛒	🛒	🛒	🛒	🛒	🛒
Pine Power All Purpose Cleaner ✓				🛒	🛒	🛒	🛒	🛒	🛒	🛒
Pine-Sol Broad Spectrum Formula 71, 107				🛒	🛒	🛒	🛒	🛒	🛒	🛒
Pine-Sol Multi-Action Spray Cleaner 23, 71				🛒	🛒	🛒	🛒	🛒	🛒	🛒
Pine-Sol Spray Cleaner 23, 71				🛒	🛒	🛒	🛒	🛒	🛒	🛒
Prevail Bathroom Cleaner Aerosol 21, 23, 112, 134				🛒	🛒	🛒	🛒	🛒	🛒	🛒
Scrub Free Bathroom Lemon Scent 106				🛒	🛒	🛒	🛒	🛒	🛒	🛒
Spic and Span Pine ✓				🛒	🛒	🛒	🛒	🛒	🛒	🛒
Tilex 131, 132				🛒	🛒	🛒	🛒	🛒	🛒	🛒
Tilex Clean Scent Formula 131, 132				🛒	🛒	🛒	🛒	🛒	🛒	🛒
Tilex Mildew Stain Remover 131, 132				🛒	🛒	🛒	🛒	🛒	🛒	🛒

Product			Recommended	Acute Health Advisory				Chronic Health Advisory		
Little to No Risk	Minimal Risk	Caution	Recommended	Flammability	Causticity	Irritants	Allergens and Strong Sensitizers	Carcinogens	Neurotoxins	Reproductive Effects
Tilex Plus Instant Mildew Stain Remover 131, 132				Little to No Risk	Caution	Minimal Risk	Minimal Risk	Little to No Risk	Little to No Risk	Little to No Risk
Tilex Soap Scum Remover & Disinfectant 60, 148, 155				Little to No Risk	Minimal Risk	Minimal Risk	Little to No Risk	Caution	Little to No Risk	Little to No Risk
Tough Act Bathroom 46, 47, 148				Little to No Risk	Minimal Risk	Minimal Risk	Little to No Risk	Little to No Risk	Little to No Risk	Little to No Risk
Tough Act Heavy Duty Bathroom Cleaner 46, 47, 148				Little to No Risk	Minimal Risk	Minimal Risk	Little to No Risk	Little to No Risk	Little to No Risk	Little to No Risk
X-14 Instant Mildew Stain Remover 132				Little to No Risk	Caution	Caution	Minimal Risk	Little to No Risk	Little to No Risk	Little to No Risk

BLEACHES AND SUBSTITUTES

Product Type

Liquid.

Health Advisory

Sodium hypochlorite, the primary ingredient in bleach, can cause sensitization. If redness develops after its use, switch to one of the safer alternatives discussed below.

Safe Use Tips

- If bleach is swallowed, it will cause vomiting; milk, egg white, starch paste, or milk of magnesia should be used as an antidote. Call a physician or poison control center immediately.
- Keep bleach away from children.
- Never mix bleach with ammonia compounds and acids. The mixture can generate toxic chloramine gas. Products that contain ammonia or quaternium compounds (derived from ammonia) include some of the all-purpose and bathroom cleaners, dishwashing detergents, and metal polishes.

Recommended Alternatives

Consumers are beginning to learn they don't need to rely on highly caustic bleaching chemicals such as sodium hypochlorite. Even major corporations, like Clorox, are giving consumers more choices than ever when it comes to buying bleaching compounds. Several recommended alternative brands are listed in the accompanying charts. You should also know about these homemade alternatives:

- Hydrogen peroxide is less caustic than typical household bleach. It can be bought as an over-the-counter antiseptic or food grade formula and used as a bleaching agent.
- Sodium perborate and sodium percarbonate (available from chemical supply companies) are slightly less toxic than typical household bleach.
- Sunshine will whiten cotton and linen fabrics.

Bleaches and Substitutes

Legend: 🛒 Little to No Risk 🛒 Minimal Risk 🛒 Caution ✓ Recommended

Product	Acute Health Advisory				Chronic Health Advisory		
	Flammability	Causticity	Irritants	Allergens and Strong Sensitizers	Carcinogens	Neurotoxins	Reproductive Effects
Bleach (Generic) 132	Little to No Risk	Caution	Caution	Little to No Risk	Little to No Risk	Little to No Risk	Little to No Risk
Clorox 132	Little to No Risk	Caution	Caution	Little to No Risk	Little to No Risk	Little to No Risk	Little to No Risk
Clorox II ✓	Little to No Risk	Little to No Risk	Little to No Risk	Little to No Risk	Little to No Risk	Little to No Risk	Little to No Risk
Country Save Chlorine Free Bleach ✓ 159	Little to No Risk	Little to No Risk	Little to No Risk	Little to No Risk	Little to No Risk	Little to No Risk	Little to No Risk
Ecover ✓	Little to No Risk	Little to No Risk	Little to No Risk	Little to No Risk	Little to No Risk	Little to No Risk	Little to No Risk
Hydrogen Peroxide (antiseptic or food grade) ✓	Little to No Risk	Little to No Risk	Minimal Risk	Little to No Risk	Little to No Risk	Little to No Risk	Little to No Risk
Naturally Yours Natural Bleach and Softener ✓	Little to No Risk	Little to No Risk	Little to No Risk	Little to No Risk	Little to No Risk	Little to No Risk	Little to No Risk
Purex 132	Little to No Risk	Caution	Caution	Little to No Risk	Little to No Risk	Little to No Risk	Little to No Risk
Sodium Perborate ✓	Little to No Risk	Little to No Risk	Little to No Risk	Little to No Risk	Little to No Risk	Little to No Risk	Little to No Risk
Sodium Percarbonate ✓	Little to No Risk	Little to No Risk	Little to No Risk	Little to No Risk	Little to No Risk	Little to No Risk	Little to No Risk
Vivid Color Safe Bleach ✓	Little to No Risk	Little to No Risk	Little to No Risk	Little to No Risk	Little to No Risk	Little to No Risk	Little to No Risk

CARPET CLEANERS AND DEODORIZERS

Product Types

Aerosol; pump; liquid; powder.

Health Advisory

Some of the most toxic ingredients in carpet cleaners include various kinds of petroleum solvents and butyl cellosolve. Both pose nervous system hazards. Products from 3M contain butyl cellosolve; we recommend against their use.

Safe Use Tip

Wear gloves when using carpet cleaners. Detergents used in these products can irritate the skin and, because the specific detergents are not always clearly disclosed, it is wise to presume some contain the carcinogen 1,4-dioxane.

Recommended Alternatives

Many safe, effective brands available in supermarkets and health food stores are listed in the charts. You also can buy various minerals, such as baking soda or borax, which also do a good job of cleaning, disinfecting, and deodorizing your carpet. You sprinkle the minerals on your rug or carpet until it is thoroughly covered. (You might need several pounds of baking soda or borax for a nine-by-twelve-foot carpet.) Then rub the powder into the nap. Wait twenty-four hours and vacuum. For particularly moldy or foul smelling carpets, several applications will be needed. You will also find many baking soda cleaners with fragrance available in supermarkets. The only difference between these and plain baking soda is the use of a masking fragrance. Buying plain baking soda is less expensive and reduces your exposure to chemicals used in producing synthetic fragrances.

Two cautions: (1) Before applying any or all of the ingredients listed below, make sure your carpet is completely dry. (2) If you are chemically sensitive or have respiratory illness, you might want to wear an inexpensive respirator or dust mask for protection.

- Baking soda deodorizes.
- Borax disinfects.
- Stained carpets or rugs require a different approach. Mix $1/4$ cup of liquid soap with 3 or more tablespoons of water in a small bowl or pot to make a foamy cleaner that can be rubbed into the stained area. Do not forget to rinse well.
- It is always best to take a preventive approach with carpet stains. If food or another staining substance is spilled, immediately rub with undiluted distilled white vinegar or lemon juice.

- Club soda is an all-purpose spot remover. It can be rubbed into the spot and cleaned off with a sponge.

Carpet Cleaners and Deodorizers

Product	Acute Health Advisory				Chronic Health Advisory		
	Flammability	Causticity	Irritants	Allergens and Strong Sensitizers	Carcinogens	Neurotoxins	Reproductive Effects
AFM Carpet Cleaner ✓	Minimal	Minimal	Minimal	Minimal	Minimal	Minimal	Minimal
AFM Carpet Guard ✓	Minimal	Minimal	Minimal	Minimal	Minimal	Minimal	Minimal
Airwick Carpet Fresh (all) ✓	Minimal	Minimal	Minimal	Minimal	Minimal	Minimal	Minimal
Ball Liquid Carpet Mop Shampoo 8	Minimal	Minimal	Little to No Risk	Minimal	Minimal	Caution	Minimal
Bissell Wall-to-Wall Rug Shampoo ✓	Minimal	Minimal	Minimal	Minimal	Minimal	Minimal	Minimal
Glade Potpourri Carpet & Room Deodorizer (all) ✓ 136	Minimal	Minimal	Little to No Risk	Little to No Risk	Minimal	Minimal	Minimal
Glamorene Apply 'n Vac ✓	Minimal	Minimal	Little to No Risk	Minimal	Minimal	Minimal	Minimal
Glamorene Spray 'n Vac ✓	Minimal	Minimal	Little to No Risk	Minimal	Minimal	Minimal	Minimal
Glory Rug Cleaner 68	Caution	Minimal	Little to No Risk	Minimal	Minimal	Minimal	Minimal
Granny's Karpet Kleen Carpet Shampoo ✓	Minimal	Minimal	Minimal	Minimal	Minimal	Minimal	Minimal
Harvey's Organic Power Carpet & Upholstery Clean 68, 112, 133	Minimal	Minimal	Caution	Minimal	Minimal	Minimal	Minimal
Lestoil Deodorizing Rug Shampoo ✓ 14, 21, 68	Minimal	Minimal	Little to No Risk	Minimal	Minimal	Minimal	Minimal
Naturally Yours Carpet and Upholstery Extraction Detergent ✓	Minimal	Minimal	Minimal	Minimal	Minimal	Minimal	Minimal
Naturally Yours Carpet and Upholstery Shampoo ✓	Minimal	Minimal	Minimal	Minimal	Minimal	Minimal	Minimal
3M Brand Carpet Spray Cleaner (aerosol) 23, 71	Caution	Minimal	Caution	Minimal	Minimal	Little to No Risk	Minimal
3M Brand Carpet Protector Concentrate 23, 71	Caution	Minimal	Little to No Risk	Minimal	Minimal	Little to No Risk	Minimal
O'Cedar Carpet Science Spot & Stain Remover ✓ 71	Minimal	Minimal	Minimal	Minimal	Minimal	Minimal	Minimal

Legend: 🛒 Little to No Risk 🛒 Minimal Risk 🛒 Caution ✓ Recommended

Product				Acute Health Advisory				Chronic Health Advisory		
Little to No Risk	Minimal Risk	Caution	Recommended	Flammability	Causticity	Irritants	Allergens and Strong Sensitizers	Carcinogens	Neurotoxins	Reproductive Effects
Prevail Carpet Cleaner (aerosol) 142				(Minimal)	(Little)	(Caution)	(Little)	(Little)	(Little)	(Little)
Prevail Rug Shampoo ✓				(Minimal)	(Little)	(Minimal)	(Little)	(Little)	(Little)	(Little)
Resolve Carpet Cleaner (pump) ✓ 71, 114				(Little)	(Little)	(Little)	(Little)	(Little)	(Little)	(Little)
Resolve Self-Cleaning Carpet Cleaner (aerosol) 68, 112				(Minimal)	(Little)	(Caution)	(Little)	(Little)	(Little)	(Little)
Woolite Deep Cleaning Rug Cleaner ✓				(Little)	(Little)	(Minimal)	(Little)	(Little)	(Little)	(Little)
Woolite Spot & Stain Rug Cleaner ✓				(Little)	(Little)	(Little)	(Little)	(Little)	(Little)	(Little)
Woolite Tough Stain Rug Cleaner ✓				(Little)	(Little)	(Little)	(Little)	(Little)	(Little)	(Little)

CLEANSERS (SCOURING POWDERS AND SOFT SCRUBS)

Product Types

Liquid; powder; pump.

Health Advisory

Acute

Chemically sensitive people may be sensitive to products containing bleach (sodium hypochlorite).

Chronic

Crystalline silica causes cancer. Safer alternatives are available.

Safe Use Tips

- Do not mix cleansers containing bleach or chlorine with products containing ammonia.
- Avoid inhalation of dust; make sure area is well ventilated.

Recommended Alternatives

Quite apart from recommended cleansers such as Bon Ami, there are many excellent homemade cleansers.

- Instead of using a commercial powdered cleanser, use plain baking soda. It will remove stains, as well as deodorize and whiten.
- Our standard formula works well. Mix 1 teaspoon of borax, 2 tablespoons of distilled white vinegar, 2 cups of hot water, and pour into a refillable spray bottle. Shake well.
- For cleaning up grease, you need more cleaning power. Nontoxic-cleaning expert Annie Berthold-Bond recommends using $1/2$ teaspoon of washing soda (also known as sodium carbonate, soda ash, or sal soda), 2 tablespoons of distilled white vinegar, $1/4$ teaspoon liquid soap, and 2 cups of hot water. Pour into a refillable spray bottle and shake. Be sure to wear gloves when working with washing soda.
- For a light and airy fragrance, add a few drops of your favorite essential oil to the above recipes. Essential oils, available at health food stores, come in many aromas, from rose to lavender to orange. They are the distilled essence of the plant or herb and safer than fragrances found in commercial products because they are based on oil from a single source. If you are allergic to one essential oil, try another. Be sure that the label specifies the oil is naturally derived, containing no synthetic fragrance ingredients.
- For bleaching, instead of using sodium hypochlorite (standard bleach), use sodium perborate, available at health food stores.
- Or try a mix of $1/2$ cup of baking soda and 3 tablespoons of sodium perborate. Pour the baking soda in a bowl with the sodium perborate. Lightly to moderately saturate a wet sponge with the mixture and rub on areas that need to be whitened, allowing the mixture to remain ten to fifteen minutes.

Cleansers (Scouring Powders and Soft Scrubs)

Product				Acute Health Advisory				Chronic Health Advisory		
Little to No Risk	Minimal Risk	Caution	Recommended ✓	Flammability	Causticity	Irritants	Allergens and Strong Sensitizers	Carcinogens	Neurotoxins	Reproductive Effects
AFM Enterprises Super Clean ✓				🛒	🛒	🛒	🛒	🛒	🛒	🛒
AFM Enterprises Safety Clean ✓				🛒	🛒	🛒	🛒	🛒	🛒	🛒

	Product			Acute Health Advisory				Chronic Health Advisory		
Little to No Risk	Minimal Risk	Caution	✓ Recommended	Flammability	Causticity	Irritants	Allergens and Strong Sensitizers	Carcinogens	Neurotoxins	Reproductive Effects
Ajax Cleanser 33, 132, 159				🛒	🛒	🛒	🛒	⬛	🛒	🛒
Auro Organics Plant Soap ✓				🛒	🛒	🛒	🛒	🛒	🛒	🛒
Auro Organics Cleansing Emulsion ✓				🛒	🛒	🛒	🛒	🛒	🛒	🛒
Bar Keepers Friend 97				🛒	🛒	🛒	🛒	🛒	🛒	🛒
Biofa Household Cleaner ✓				🛒	🛒	🛒	🛒	🛒	🛒	🛒
Bon Ami Cleaning Cake ✓ 57				🛒	🛒	🛒	🛒	🛒	🛒	🛒
Bon Ami Cleaning Powder ✓ 57				🛒	🛒	🛒	🛒	🛒	🛒	🛒
Cal Ben Soap Company Pure Soap ✓				🛒	🛒	🛒	🛒	🛒	🛒	🛒
Cal Ben Seafoam Dish Glow ✓				🛒	🛒	🛒	🛒	🛒	🛒	🛒
Comet Cleanser Regular & Lemon Fresh ✓ 25, 132, 159				🛒	🛒	🛒	🛒	🛒	🛒	🛒
Dr. Bronner's Pure Castile Soaps ✓				🛒	🛒	🛒	🛒	🛒	🛒	🛒
Dr. Bronner's Sal Suds ✓				🛒	🛒	🛒	🛒	🛒	🛒	🛒
Ecover Cream Cleaner ✓				🛒	🛒	🛒	🛒	🛒	🛒	🛒
Granny's Old Fashioned Products Aloe Care ✓				🛒	🛒	🛒	🛒	🛒	🛒	🛒
Mr. Clean Soft Cleanser ✓ 25, 142				🛒	🛒	🛒	🛒	🛒	🛒	🛒
Soft Scrub With Bleach ✓ 25, 132				🛒	🛒	🛒	🛒	🛒	🛒	🛒
Zud Heavy Duty Cleanser 33, 97				🛒	🛒	🛒	🛒	⬛	🛒	🛒

DISHWASHING LIQUIDS (HAND)

Product Types

Some dishwashing liquids are petroleum-based, containing detergents such as diethanolamine and sodium dodecylbenzenesulfonate. Others use plant-based soaps. Petroleum-based detergents have replaced more natural soaps because they are generally thought of as more effective cleaning agents than soaps—especially in hard-water areas. Most mainstream brands are petroleum-based. Many alternative brands use vegetable-based soaps.

Health Advisory

Some so-called pure and natural brands found in health food stores contain ethoxylated alcohols, which may be contaminated with the carcinogen 1,4-dioxane, or DEA, a nitrosamine precursor.

Information on which specific dyes and colors are used in dishwashing products is disclosed neither in manufacturers' MSDSs nor in product labels. Although we were not able to evaluate specific brands in this area of concern, it should be noted that many dyes are known to be carcinogenic or contaminated with carcinogenic impurities, including metals such as arsenic and lead. Dyes may penetrate the skin and residues may be deposited on dishes. We have rated for minimal caution all products containing undisclosed artificial dyes, which we were able to determine through visual inspection. In the case of dishwashing liquids, although you may wear gloves to prevent absorption of artificial dyes through the skin, dyes will leave residues on your utensils, and you really should avoid artificially colored products.

Safe Use Tips

- Wear latex gloves to prevent irritation of the skin and absorption of carcinogenic contaminants, including nitrosamines, dyes and colors, and 1,4-dioxane.
- Some products contain ammonia, which may react with chlorine and form potentially toxic chloramine gas. Do not mix brands containing ammonia with bleach or products containing it. Be sure to check your brand's label.
- Products colored amber, yellow, green, or blue are obviously dyed with artificial colors and should be avoided.

Recommended Alternatives

Supermarkets usually carry many good brands that contain neither fragrances nor dyes.

Liquid soaps are satisfactory for washing dishes. They are even more effective when used with a water softener such as borax.

Dishwashing Liquids (Hand)

Product				Acute Health Advisory				Chronic Health Advisory		
🛒 Little to No Risk	🛒 Minimal Risk	🛒 Caution	✓ Recommended	Flammability	Causticity	Irritants	Allergens and Strong Sensitizers	Carcinogens	Neurotoxins	Reproductive Effects
Ajax Dishwashing Liquid with Lemon				🛒	🛒	🛒	🛒	🛒	🛒	🛒
Allen's Naturally Dishwashing Liquid 44, 121				🛒	🛒	🛒	🛒	🛒	🛒	🛒
Aloe Care ✓				🛒	🛒	🛒	🛒	🛒	🛒	🛒
Arm & Hammer Baking Soda ✓				🛒	🛒	🛒	🛒	🛒	🛒	🛒
Arm & Hammer Super Washing Soda ✓				🛒	🛒	🛒	🛒	🛒	🛒	🛒
Biofa Natural Dishwashing Liquid ✓				🛒	🛒	🛒	🛒	🛒	🛒	🛒
Cal Ben Soap Company Pure Soap ✓				🛒	🛒	🛒	🛒	🛒	🛒	🛒
Cal Ben Soap Company Seafoam Dish Glow ✓				🛒	🛒	🛒	🛒	🛒	🛒	🛒
Chef's Soap ✓				🛒	🛒	🛒	🛒	🛒	🛒	🛒
Dawn Sureshot				🛒	🛒	🛒	🛒	🛒	🛒	🛒
Dermassage Dishwashing Liquid ✓				🛒	🛒	🛒	🛒	🛒	🛒	🛒
Dial Corporation 20 Mule Team Borax ✓				🛒	🛒	🛒	🛒	🛒	🛒	🛒
Dove Light Duty Dishwashing Liquid ✓				🛒	🛒	🛒	🛒	🛒	🛒	🛒
EarthRite Dishwashing Liquid ✓				🛒	🛒	🛒	🛒	🛒	🛒	🛒
Ecover Dishwashing Liquid ✓				🛒	🛒	🛒	🛒	🛒	🛒	🛒
Granny's E.Z. Maid/Dish and All-Purpose Cleaner 51				🛒	🛒	🛒	🛒	🛒	🛒	🛒
Heavenly Horsetail All-Purpose Cleaner 44				🛒	🛒	🛒	🛒	🛒	🛒	🛒
Ivory Dishwashing Liquid ✓				🛒	🛒	🛒	🛒	🛒	🛒	🛒
Joy				🛒	🛒	🛒	🛒	🛒	🛒	🛒
Life Tree Premium Dishwashing Liquid 44, 98, 153				🛒	🛒	🛒	🛒	🛒	🛒	🛒
Naturally Yours Gentle Soap ✓				🛒	🛒	🛒	🛒	🛒	🛒	🛒

Product				Acute Health Advisory				Chronic Health Advisory		
🛒 Little to No Risk	🛒 Minimal Risk	🛒 Caution	✓ Recommended	Flammability	Causticity	Irritants	Allergens and Strong Sensitizers	Carcinogens	Neurotoxins	Reproductive Effects
Naturally Yours Dishwashing Detergent ✓				🛒	🛒	🛒	🛒	🛒	🛒	🛒
Neo-Life Mellow Yellow ✓				🛒	🛒	🛒	🛒	🛒	🛒	🛒
Octagon Crystal White Dishwashing Liquid				🛒	🛒	🛒	🛒	🛒	🛒	🛒
Palmolive Dishwashing Liquid (no dyes) ✓				🛒	🛒	🛒	🛒	🛒	🛒	🛒
Palmolive Dishwashing Liquid with Lemon				🛒	🛒	🛒	🛒	🛒	🛒	🛒
Simmons Pure Soaps ✓				🛒	🛒	🛒	🛒	🛒	🛒	🛒
SOS Steel Wool Soap Pads ✓				🛒	🛒	🛒	🛒	🛒	🛒	🛒
Sunlight Dishwashing Liquid				🛒	🛒	🛒	🛒	🛒	🛒	🛒
Tropical Soap Company Sirena Coconut-Oil Bar Soaps ✓				🛒	🛒	🛒	🛒	🛒	🛒	🛒
Vista Lemon Scented Dish Detergent				🛒	🛒	🛒	🛒	🛒	🛒	🛒

DISHWASHING DETERGENTS (AUTOMATIC)

Product Types

Liquid; powder.

Health Advisory

Some products contain dry chlorine that is activated when it encounters water in the dishwasher. Chlorine fumes are released in the steam that leaks out of the dishwasher, and they can cause eye irritation and difficulty in breathing, especially for the hypersensitive.

Recommended Alternatives

You will need to buy a commercial product rather than making your own homemade automatic dishwashing formula. Of major brands available in supermarkets, the two that contain the lowest amounts of phosphates, according to results from tests conducted by the Washington Toxics Coalition, based in Seattle, Washington, are All Powder Automatic Dishwashing Detergent and Sunlight Powder Automatic Dishwashing Detergent. Phosphates cause rivers and lakes to become clogged with masses of algae, a process known as *eutrophication.* Phosphates also contain arsenic. Because detergents end up in treatment plants and sewage sludge is being increasingly applied as fertilizer, the heavy metal content of sludge could limit its usefulness. The use of low- or no-phosphate detergents will help keep our environment healthier.

The following brands, available in health food stores and through mail order, contain no phosphates or chlorine, according to test results from the Washington Toxics Coalition:

Bio Pac Powder
Kleer II Liquid
Kleer III Powder
Life Tree Automatic Dishwashing Detergent
Shaklee Basic D (new)
Shaklee Basic D (old)

Church & Dwight, makers of Arm & Hammer Baking Soda, reports that sprinkling baking soda over dishes can reduce by half the amount of detergent used.

Powdered brands contain fewer hazardous ingredients than liquid products. They are safer. In either case, although we did not designate which brands contain artificial colors, try to avoid products containing them when you're in the supermarket. They will leave residues on your eating utensils.

Dishwashing Detergents (Automatic)

Product				Acute Health Advisory				Chronic Health Advisory		
Little to No Risk	Minimal Risk	Caution	Recommended	Flammability	Causticity	Irritants	Allergens and Strong Sensitizers	Carcinogens	Neurotoxins	Reproductive Effects
All Automatic Dishwashing Liquid 131, 135, 159				Little to No Risk	Little to No Risk	Minimal Risk	Little to No Risk	Little to No Risk	Little to No Risk	Little to No Risk
All Automatic Dishwashing Powder ✓ 135, 159				Little to No Risk	Little to No Risk	Minimal Risk	Little to No Risk	Little to No Risk	Little to No Risk	Little to No Risk
Allen's Naturally Automatic Dishwasher Detergent 127, 133, 159				Little to No Risk	Minimal Risk	Caution	Little to No Risk	Little to No Risk	Minimal Risk	Little to No Risk
Bio Pac Powder ✓				Little to No Risk	Little to No Risk	Caution	Little to No Risk	Little to No Risk	Little to No Risk	Little to No Risk

Legend: 🛒 Little to No Risk | 🛒 Minimal Risk | 🛒 Caution | ✓ Recommended

Product	Acute Health Advisory				Chronic Health Advisory		
	Flammability	Causticity	Irritants	Allergens and Strong Sensitizers	Carcinogens	Neurotoxins	Reproductive Effects
Cascade Automatic Dishwashing Detergent 132, 135	🛒	🛒	🛒	🛒	🛒	🛒	🛒
Cascade Lemon Liquigel 132	🛒	🛒	🛒	🛒	🛒	🛒	🛒
Cal Ben Seafoam Destain for Automatic Dishwashers ✓	🛒	🛒	🛒	🛒	🛒	🛒	🛒
Cal Ben Seafoam Dishmachine Granules Concentrate ✓ 133	🛒	🛒	🛒	🛒	🛒	🛒	🛒
Electrasol Powder 135	🛒	🛒	🛒	🛒	🛒	🛒	🛒
Kleer II Liquid ✓	🛒	🛒	🛒	🛒	🛒	🛒	🛒
Kleer III Powder ✓	🛒	🛒	🛒	🛒	🛒	🛒	🛒
Life Tree Automatic Dishwashing Detergent 44, 121	🛒	🛒	🛒	🛒	🛒	🛒	🛒
Palmolive Liquid Gel Fresh Scent 131, 132	🛒	🛒	🛒	🛒	🛒	🛒	🛒
Palmolive Liquid Gel Lemon 131, 132	🛒	🛒	🛒	🛒	🛒	🛒	🛒
Shaklee Basic D (New) ✓	🛒	🛒	🛒	🛒	🛒	🛒	🛒
Shaklee Basic D (Old) ✓	🛒	🛒	🛒	🛒	🛒	🛒	🛒
Sunlight Liquid Dishwashing Detergent 131, 132, 135	🛒	🛒	🛒	🛒	🛒	🛒	🛒
Sunlight Powder Dishwashing Detergent ✓ 135, 159	🛒	🛒	🛒	🛒	🛒	🛒	🛒

DRAIN OPENERS

Product Types

Liquid; crystal; biological.

Health Advisory

Sodium hydroxide and sodium hypochlorite, found highly concentrated in many drain openers, can quickly and permanently burn eyes and skin, or burn internally if ingested. These products may be fatal if ingested.

Safe Use Tips

- Avoid eye or skin contact and inhalation of vapor or mist.
- Always provide adequate ventilation.
- Wear safety glasses and protective gloves if using conventional drain openers.
- Do not mix with ammonia-containing products, including toilet bowl and household cleaners.
- Always be sure to keep drain cleaners in a childproof area.
- If ingested, drink generous amounts of milk or water. Call poison center, emergency room, or physician immediately.
- Crystal drain cleaners are safer than liquid. If you spill crystals, they can be brushed off before much damage is done.

Recommended Alternatives

Several safe, effective drain openers have recently come on the market, including biological drain openers from Drano, Earth Friendly Drain Opener, and Biological Drain Opener (Dasun Company). They are available in supermarkets, in health food stores, and by mail order, respectively. Each contains an effective blend of stabilized enzymes and bacteria. Not only are they safer than the most popular brands, but also users have found them about as effective as the more dangerous products. You simply pour them down the drain and wait the amount of time specified on the label. As with all drain openers, they work best with lightly clogged pipes.

Prevention is the key to clear drains: Keeping drains from becoming plugged is easier and smarter than waiting for a crisis. In the long run this will save you aggravation, time, and money.

Follow these guidelines:

- Do not throw large food scraps like coffee grounds or potato peelings down the drain. Place them in the trash or make a compost pile in your garden and throw them there.
- Put a filter cover over the drain in your shower to prevent hair from clogging pipes.
- Make a habit of picking up all hair that accumulates around the shower drain after each bath or shower.
- Occasionally pouring a mixture of baking soda followed by boiling hot water down the drain can help keep pipes clear.
- Buy a plumber's snake. When drains do become clogged, a plumber's snake is often much more effective than chemical drain openers and will perform a more thorough job of reopening the pipes. It will also save you money in the long run.

Drain Openers

Product	Acute Health Advisory				Chronic Health Advisory		
	Flammability	Causticity	Irritants	Allergens and Strong Sensitizers	Carcinogens	Neurotoxins	Reproductive Effects
Dasun Biological Drain Opener ✓							
Drano Biological Drain Opener ✓							
Drano Crystal All Purpose Drain Opener 12, 131							
Drano Instant Plunger 21, 42							
Drano Liquid Drain Opener 131, 132							
Drano Liquid Professional Strength Plus 131, 132							
Earth Friendly Drain Opener ✓							
Liquid-Plumr 131, 132							
Liquid Plumr Professional Strength 131, 132							
Naturally Yours Enz-Away ✓							
Plumber's Snake (Generic) ✓							
Plunge Liquid Drain Opener 131, 132							

Risk key: Little to No Risk · Minimal Risk · Caution · Recommended ✓

FLOOR CLEANERS, WAXES, AND POLISHES

Product Types

Aerosol; liquid; paste.

Generally, products contain predominantly either (1) petroleum distillates and solvents, or (2) water-based detergents.

Health Advisory

We strongly recommend that you use water-based detergents as your first choice in a floor cleaning product. Many good products are available in both supermarkets and health food stores.

Dial 5-Minute Wax & Acrylic Remover (known in generic form as Wax Remover with Ammonia) contains tripropylene glycol monomethyl ether. Prolonged and repeated skin exposure to large doses of this chemical has resulted in narcosis and kidney injury.

Safe Use Tips

- Wear impermeable gloves.
- Use in well-ventilated areas.
- Wear a respirator.

Recommended Alternatives

You can make your own homemade formulations, as reported in *Clean & Green*:

- The simplest floor cleaner is made by adding 1 cup of vinegar to a pail of water.
- If you need a disinfecting formula, add $1/2$ cup of borax to 2 gallons of hot water. To avoid splashing and ensure that the borax is thoroughly dissolved, pour the borax into the bucket first, then pour in the hot water.
- For cutting through grease, you will need a stronger formula. Combine $1/4$ cup of washing soda with 1 tablespoon of liquid soap, $1/4$ cup of distilled white vinegar, and 2 gallons of hot water. Add the washing soda to the bucket before pouring the water to avoid splashing and ensure it is thoroughly dissolved. Warning: This formula should not be used on waxed floors. Be sure to wear protective gloves.
- For wood floors, combine $1/4$ cup of liquid soap with $1/2$ to 1 cup of distilled white vinegar or lemon juice, and 2 gallons of warm water. Use as you would any floor cleaner. For a fragrant addition to this mixture, add 1 cup of your favorite freshly brewed herb tea.
- For linoleum floors, combine 6 tablespoons of cornstarch for every cup of water. Mix these ingredients in a bucket and use as you would any floor polish.

Floor Cleaners, Waxes, and Polishes

Product				Acute Health Advisory				Chronic Health Advisory		
Little to No Risk	Minimal Risk	Caution	Recommended	Flammability	Causticity	Irritants	Allergens and Strong Sensitizers	Carcinogens	Neurotoxins	Reproductive Effects
AFM Safety Clean ✓				🛒	🛒	🛒	🛒	🛒	🛒	🛒
AFM Super Clean ✓				🛒	🛒	🛒	🛒	🛒	🛒	🛒

Product	Acute Health Advisory				Chronic Health Advisory		
Little to No Risk / *Minimal Risk* / *Caution* / *Recommended* ✓	Flammability	Causticity	Irritants	Allergens and Strong Sensitizers	Carcinogens	Neurotoxins	Reproductive Effects
Auro Organics Floor Wax-Balm Cleaner ✓							
Auro Organics Floor Wax-Balm Plant Soap ✓							
Auro Organics Cleansing Emulsion ✓							
Auro Organics Plant Thinner ✓							
Auro Organics Plant Alcohol Thinner ✓							
Auro Organics Boiled Linseed Oil ✓							
Auro Organics Boiled Herbal Linseed Oil ✓							
Bon Ami Cleaning Powder ✓ 57							
Bissell One Step Wood Floor Care 83							
Brite ✓ 60							
Bruce 1-Step with Lemon Oil 103							
Country Garden Pledge 21, 70, 112							
Dial 5-Minute Wax & Acrylic Remover 14, 44, 154							
EarthRite All Surface Floor Cleaner ✓							
Ecover Floor Soap ✓							
Future ✓							
Glo-Coat ✓ 60							
Karen's Nontoxic Products Lemon Oil ✓							
Karen's Nontoxic Products Pine Oil ✓ 107							
Livos Avi-Soap Concentrate ✓							
Livos Kiros-Alcohol Thinner ✓							

Product				Acute Health Advisory				Chronic Health Advisory		

Legend: 🛒 Little to No Risk — 🛒 Minimal Risk — 🛒 Caution — ✓ Recommended

Product	Flammability	Causticity	Irritants	Allergens and Strong Sensitizers	Carcinogens	Neurotoxins	Reproductive Effects
Livos Landis-Shellac ✓	Minimal	Minimal	Minimal	Minimal	Minimal	Minimal	Minimal
Livos Latis-Natural Concentrate ✓	Minimal	Minimal	Minimal	Minimal	Minimal	Minimal	Minimal
Livos Trebo-Shellac ✓	Minimal	Minimal	Minimal	Minimal	Minimal	Minimal	Minimal
Minwax Dura Seal Hardwood Floor Cleaner 7	Caution	Minimal	Caution	Minimal	Minimal	Caution	Minimal
Minwax Dura Top 49, 100	Caution	Minimal	Caution	Minimal	Minimal	Caution	Minimal
Minwax Paste Wax Coffee Brown 140	Caution	Minimal	Caution	Minimal	Minimal	Caution	Minimal
Minwax Paste Wax Natural 140	Caution	Minimal	Caution	Minimal	Minimal	Caution	Minimal
Minwax Renovator 140	Caution	Minimal	Caution	Minimal	Minimal	Caution	Minimal
Minwax Wax & Cleaner Coffee Brown 100, 140	Caution	Minimal	Caution	Minimal	Minimal	Caution	Minimal
Minwax Wax & Cleaner #200 Natural 100, 140	Caution	Minimal	Caution	Minimal	Minimal	Caution	Minimal
Parker's Wood Cleaner & Floor Polish ✓	Minimal	Minimal	Minimal	Minimal	Minimal	Minimal	Minimal
Paste Wax 140	Caution	Minimal	Little to No Risk	Minimal	Minimal	Little to No Risk	Minimal
Step Saver ✓	Minimal	Minimal	Little to No Risk	Minimal	Minimal	Minimal	Minimal
Wood Finishing Supply Company Beeswax ✓	Minimal	Minimal	Minimal	Minimal	Minimal	Minimal	Minimal
Wood Finishing Supply Company Carnauba Wax ✓	Minimal	Minimal	Minimal	Minimal	Minimal	Minimal	Minimal

FURNITURE POLISHES

Product Types

Liquid; spray; pump.

Health Advisory

Acute

All aerosols have been rated for caution: the microscopic particles they release can be inhaled and cause systemic damage. They should not be used.

Most furniture polishes may cause eye or skin irritation with direct contact. Many products containing various petroleum-based polishing ingredients may aggravate pre-existing skin conditions. The difference may be very slight between products posing little to no risk and those deserving minimal caution, and all products should be handled carefully to reduce skin contact.

Chronic

Old English Lemon Furniture Polish (pump) contains formaldehyde, a poisonous irritant to the skin, eyes, and mucous membranes, a carcinogen, and a neurotoxin.

Many products contain petroleum distillates with significant neurotoxic effects.

Safe Use Tips

- Always wear impermeable gloves. This is extremely important because some petroleum distillates are easily absorbed through the skin and may contain carcinogenic impurities.
- Wear a respirator if working for prolonged periods with products containing petroleum solvents.
- Before using a new furniture polish, especially in your bedroom, test it in a small area to see if its fumes cause you to suffer headaches, dizziness, or other signs of nervous system intoxication. If so, don't use. Switch to one of the many safer, recommended products listed in the charts.

Recommended Alternatives

Several safe brands are available and you should have no problem finding them in supermarkets, hardware stores, and health food stores. The following homemade polishes also work well:

- For general dusting and polishing, use 1 teaspoon of olive oil for every $1/2$ cup of distilled white vinegar. Mix together in a bowl or glass jar and apply with a soft cloth.
- For polishing, use a one-to-one mixture of olive oil with distilled white vinegar. Mix together in a bowl or glass jar and polish with a soft cloth.

The following four cleaning and polishing recipes come from an excellent Australian publication, *A-Z of Chemicals in the Home*:

- For soft woods, use a mixture of 1 part lemon juice to 2 parts olive oil. Mix together in a bowl or glass jar and apply with a soft cloth.
- For bamboo furniture, use a brush or cloth dipped in salty warm water; the salt helps to keep the original color. Mix together in a bowl or glass jar and apply with a soft cloth.

- For highly polished furniture, wipe with a chamois leather wrung out in vinegar and water and polish with a soft, dry cloth.
- For carved furniture, apply cedar oil with a cloth and then use a soft bristled brush to clean the difficult corners.

Furniture Polishes

Legend: 🛒 Little to No Risk | 🛒 Minimal Risk | 🛒 Caution | ✓ Recommended

Product	Acute Health Advisory				Chronic Health Advisory		
	Flammability	Causticity	Irritants	Allergens and Strong Sensitizers	Carcinogens	Neurotoxins	Reproductive Effects
Axiom Block Oil ✓	○	○	○	○	○	○	○
Behold Lemon Furniture Polish (aerosol) 65	●	○	●	○	○	◐	○
Behold Light Scent Furniture Polish (aerosol) 65	●	○	●	○	○	◐	○
Biofa Natural Furniture and Floor Cleaning Emulsion ✓	○	○	○	○	○	○	○
EarthRite Furniture Polish ✓	○	○	○	○	○	○	○
Endust Dusting and Cleaning Spray 65, 68	●	○	●	○	○	◐	○
Endust Lemon Dusting and Cleaning Spray 65, 68	●	○	●	○	○	◐	○
Formby's Almond Lustre 7, 68	◐	○	●	○	○	●	○
Formby's Lemon Oil Furniture Treatment 7, 160	◐	○	○	○	○	●	○
Guardsman Furniture Polish ✓	○	○	○	○	○	○	○
Herbert Stanley Beauti-Fi Cleaner 23, 85	○	○	●	○	◐	◐	○
Herbert Stanley Beauti-Fi Lemon Oil 82	○	○	○	○	○	◐	○
Herbert Stanley Burn & Stain Remover 72	◐	○	○	○	○	●	○
Herbert Stanley Candle Wax Remover 65	○	○	○	○	○	◐	○
Herbert Stanley Furniture Cream 100	○	○	○	○	○	◐	○
Herbert Stanley Furniture Cream with Lemon 100	○	○	○	○	○	○	○
Herbert Stanley Wax Remover & Cleaner 65	○	○	○	○	○	◐	○

Legend (Product risk icons): Little to No Risk · Minimal Risk · Caution · Recommended (✓)

Product	Acute Health Advisory				Chronic Health Advisory		
	Flammability	Causticity	Irritants	Allergens and Strong Sensitizers	Carcinogens	Neurotoxins	Reproductive Effects
Hope's Countertop Polish ✓	Minimal	Minimal	Minimal	Minimal	Minimal	Minimal	Minimal
Howard Feed-N-Wax 5, 94	Minimal	Minimal	Minimal	Minimal	Caution	Minimal	Minimal
Howard Orange Oil 94, 101	Minimal	Minimal	Minimal	Minimal	Caution	Minimal	Minimal
Jubilee Liquid 6	Minimal	Minimal	Minimal	Minimal	Minimal	Minimal	Minimal
Jubilee Spray 21, 68, 70, 112	Caution	Minimal	Caution	Minimal	Minimal	Minimal	Minimal
Klean 'N Shine 21, 68, 70, 112	Caution	Minimal	Caution	Minimal	Minimal	Minimal	Minimal
Meguiar's Dull Finish Preserver 100	Caution	Minimal	Minimal	Minimal	Minimal	Minimal	Minimal
Meguiar's Furniture Polish 100	Caution	Minimal	Minimal	Minimal	Minimal	Minimal	Minimal
Meguiar's Lemon Oil 100	Caution	Minimal	Minimal	Minimal	Minimal	Minimal	Minimal
Naturally Yours Furniture Cleaner and Protector ✓	Minimal	Minimal	Minimal	Minimal	Minimal	Minimal	Minimal
Old English Furniture Polishes 160	Minimal	Minimal	Minimal	Minimal	Minimal	Minimal	Minimal
Old English Lemon Furniture Polish (Cream) 101	Minimal	Minimal	Minimal	Minimal	Minimal	Minimal	Minimal
Old English Lemon Furniture Polish Aerosol 21, 101, 112	Minimal	Minimal	Caution	Minimal	Minimal	Minimal	Minimal
Old English Lemon Furniture Polish (Pump) 59	Minimal	Minimal	Caution	Caution	Caution	Minimal	Minimal
Old English Potpourri Furniture Polish (Aerosol) 21, 101, 112	Minimal	Minimal	Caution	Minimal	Minimal	Minimal	Minimal
Old English Scratch Cover for Dark Wood 100, 160	Minimal	Minimal	Minimal	Minimal	Minimal	Minimal	Minimal
Old English Scratch Cover for Light/Medium 160	Minimal	Minimal	Minimal	Minimal	Minimal	Minimal	Minimal
Old English Wood Soap ✓	Minimal	Minimal	Minimal	Minimal	Minimal	Minimal	Minimal
Parker's Perfect Polish Butcher Block ✓	Minimal	Minimal	Minimal	Minimal	Minimal	Minimal	Minimal
Parker's Perfect Polish Classic Potpourri Oil ✓	Minimal	Minimal	Minimal	Minimal	Minimal	Minimal	Minimal

Legend: 🛒 Little to No Risk 🛒 Minimal Risk 🛒 Caution ✓ Recommended

Product	Flammability	Causticity	Irritants	Allergens and Strong Sensitizers	Carcinogens	Neurotoxins	Reproductive Effects
Parker's Perfect Polish Kitchen Cabinet Clean ✓	🛒	🛒	🛒	🛒	🛒	🛒	🛒
Parker's Perfect Polish Lemon Oil ✓	🛒	🛒	🛒	🛒	🛒	🛒	🛒
Parker's Perfect Polish Wood Finish Creme ✓	🛒	🛒	🛒	🛒	🛒	🛒	🛒
Pledge Lemon 21, 70, 112	🛒	🛒	🛒	🛒	🛒	🛒	🛒
Pledge Spring Fresh Aerosol 21, 68, 70, 112	🛒	🛒	🛒	🛒	🛒	🛒	🛒
Prevail Dust and Shine (Aerosol) 21, 65, 112	🛒	🛒	🛒	🛒	🛒	🛒	🛒
Prevail Furniture Polish (Aerosol) 21, 65, 112	🛒	🛒	🛒	🛒	🛒	🛒	🛒
Prevail Furniture Polish (Non-aerosol) ✓	🛒	🛒	🛒	🛒	🛒	🛒	🛒
Scott's Liquid Gold Wood Cleaner (Aerosol) 102, 158	🛒	🛒	🛒	🛒	🛒	🛒	🛒
Scott's Liquid Gold Wood Cleaner (Pourable) 102, 158	🛒	🛒	🛒	🛒	🛒	🛒	🛒
Vernax 156	🛒	🛒	🛒	🛒	🛒	🛒	🛒
Weiman Aerosol Furniture Cream 68, 100, 112	🛒	🛒	🛒	🛒	🛒	🛒	🛒
Weiman Aerosol Furniture Cream with Lemon 68, 100, 112	🛒	🛒	🛒	🛒	🛒	🛒	🛒
Weiman Aerosol Panel Bright 68, 100, 112	🛒	🛒	🛒	🛒	🛒	🛒	🛒
Weiman Aerosol Wood Soap	🛒	🛒	🛒	🛒	🛒	🛒	🛒
Wood Plus Furniture Polish & Cleaner ✓ 53	🛒	🛒	🛒	🛒	🛒	🛒	🛒

GLASS AND WINDOW CLEANERS

Product Types

Aerosol; pump.

Health Advisory

As shown in the chart below, some popular window cleaners contain butyl cellosolve, which is neurotoxic. We recommend that consumers avoid products containing butyl cellosolve.

Recommended Alternatives

You can make your own glass and window cleaners. Two standard formulas:

- A half-and-half mixture of water and distilled white vinegar poured into a refillable spray bottle.
- One-half teaspoon of liquid soap, 3 tablespoons of distilled white vinegar, and 2 cups of water poured into a refillable spray bottle. Shake well.

Glass and Window Cleaners

Product	Acute Health Advisory				Chronic Health Advisory		
	Flammability	Causticity	Irritants	Allergens and Strong Sensitizers	Carcinogens	Neurotoxins	Reproductive Effects
Allen's Naturally Nontoxic Glass Cleaner ✓ 60	🛒	🛒	🛒	🛒	🛒	🛒	🛒
EarthRite Glass Cleaner ✓	🛒	🛒	🛒	🛒	🛒	🛒	🛒
Cinch Glass and Multi-surface Cleaner ✓	🛒	🛒	🛒	🛒	🛒	🛒	🛒
Dr. Harvey's Glass Clean ✓	🛒	🛒	🛒	🛒	🛒	🛒	🛒
409 Glass and Surface Cleaner ✓	🛒	🛒	🛒	🛒	🛒	🛒	🛒
Glass Plus 16, 23	🛒	🛒	🛒	🛒	🛒	🛒	🛒
Kmart Aerosol Window Cleaner 14, 23, 68	🛒	🛒	🛒	🛒	🛒	🛒	🛒
Kmart Liquid Window Cleaner 14, 23	🛒	🛒	🛒	🛒	🛒	🛒	🛒

Legend: 🛒 Little to No Risk — 🛒 Minimal Risk — 🛒 Caution — ✓ Recommended

Product				Acute Health Advisory				Chronic Health Advisory		
🛒 *Little to No Risk* 🛒 *Minimal Risk* 🛒 *Caution* ✓ *Recommended*				Flammability	Causticity	Irritants	Allergens and Strong Sensitizers	Carcinogens	Neurotoxins	Reproductive Effects
Mr. Clean Glass and Surface Spray Cleaner ✓				🛒	🛒	🛒	🛒	🛒	🛒	🛒
Natural Chemistry Glass Cleaner ✓				🛒	🛒	🛒	🛒	🛒	🛒	🛒
Naturally Yours Glass and Window Cleaner ✓				🛒	🛒	🛒	🛒	🛒	🛒	🛒
Radiator Specialty Company Glass Cleaner (Aerosol) 23				🛒	🛒	🛒	🛒	🛒	🛒	🛒
Radiator Specialty Company Glass Cleaner (Pump) 23				🛒	🛒	🛒	🛒	🛒	🛒	🛒
S.O.S. Ammonia Plus Glass Cleaner 23				🛒	🛒	🛒	🛒	🛒	🛒	🛒
S.O.S. Vinegar Glass Cleaner 23				🛒	🛒	🛒	🛒	🛒	🛒	🛒
Windex Glass Cleaner Aerosol 23, 68, 112				🛒	🛒	🛒	🛒	🛒	🛒	🛒
Windex Blue Glass Cleaner 23				🛒	🛒	🛒	🛒	🛒	🛒	🛒
Windex Enviro-Refill Glass Cleaner (Blue) 23				🛒	🛒	🛒	🛒	🛒	🛒	🛒
Windex Green Glass Cleaner 23				🛒	🛒	🛒	🛒	🛒	🛒	🛒
Windex Lemon Glass Cleaner (Yellow) 23				🛒	🛒	🛒	🛒	🛒	🛒	🛒
Windex Professional Strength Multisurface and Glass Cleaner 23				🛒	🛒	🛒	🛒	🛒	🛒	🛒
Windex Vinegar Glass Cleaner (Green) 23				🛒	🛒	🛒	🛒	🛒	🛒	🛒

LAUNDRY DETERGENTS AND SOAPS

Product Types

Liquid; powder. Products are either (1) petroleum-based synthetic detergents or (2) plant-based soaps.

Health Advisory

Acute

If you are chemically sensitive, seek fragrance-free laundry detergents. Allergic reactions to fragrances include asthma, flulike symptoms, and respiratory irritation. Residues remaining on clothing and bed sheets can cause severe skin rashes for chemically sensitive people. Most brands are fragranced (i.e., perfumed), unless the label specifically states they are fragrance-free.

Chronic

Ethoxylated alcohols, most often found in liquid brands, including many alleged "natural" brands, can contain 1,4-dioxane that is carcinogenic and volatile (meaning you end up inhaling it).

Safe Use Tips

- Be careful to avoid eye contact with laundry detergents. If detergent gets in eyes, flush with lukewarm, clean water for fifteen minutes. If irritation persists, seek medical attention.
- If working with detergents for long periods, especially at work, wear a dust respirator and protective goggles.
- Store in childproof area. Laundry detergent is a leading cause of poisoning among young children in America.
- If accidentally ingested, drink one or two glasses of water. If symptoms of distress persist, seek medical attention.

Recommended Alternatives

Brands gentlest to consumers and the environment use vegetable-based, replenishable, renewable resources instead of petrochemicals and eliminate fragrances or choose only scents derived from natural oils. These "alternative" brands are available in a few supermarkets, at health food stores, and by mail order.

The following brands are petroleum-free:

Bi-O-Kleen Laundry Powder
Cal Ben Seafoam Laundry Soap
Dr. Bronner's Pure Castile Soap
Dr. Bronner's Sal Suds
EarthRite Laundry Detergent
Eco Bella Laundry Powder
Eco Bella Laundry Liquid
EcoSource
Ecover Liquid Laundry Wash
Ecover Unique Washing Powder
Ecover Wool Wash Laundry Liquid
4 The Planet 4 Your Laundry
Keep America Clean

Naturally Yours Laundry
  Detergent
Seventh Generation Laundry Liquid
Seventh Generation Laundry Powder
Shaklee Basic L
Shaklee Liquid L
Simmons Pure Soaps
  Vegetarian Bar Soaps
Sodasan Soap Washing Powder
Winter White Laundry
  Detergent Powder
Winter White Liquid
  Laundry Detergent

Some major brands now come in perfume- and dye-free versions. Two examples: All and Cheerfree.

Laundry Detergents and Soaps

Icon legend: ○ = Little to No Risk · ◐ = Minimal Risk · ● = Caution · ✓ = Recommended

Product	Acute Health Advisory				Chronic Health Advisory		
	Flammability	Causticity	Irritants	Allergens and Strong Sensitizers	Carcinogens	Neurotoxins	Reproductive Effects
Ajax Laundry Detergent 39	○	○	◐	○	○	○	○
Ajax Laundry Detergent Liquid 39	○	○	◐	○	○	○	○
Ajax Ultra Concentrated Detergent 39	○	○	◐	○	○	○	○
Ajax Ultra Concentrated Detergent (Phosphate) 39	○	○	◐	○	○	○	○
All Concentrated Powdered Laundry Detergent 135, 159	○	○	◐	○	○	○	○
All Free and Clear Liquid Laundry Detergent ✓ 135	○	○	○	○	○	○	○
All Liquid Laundry Detergent 135	○	○	◐	○	○	○	○
Allen's Naturally Liquid Laundry Detergent 153	○	○	○	○	◐	○	○
Arm & Hammer Heavy Duty Detergent 51, 159	○	○	●	○	◐	○	○
Arm & Hammer Heavy Duty Liquid Detergent 91, 135	○	○	◐	○	○	○	○
Arm & Hammer Super Washing Soda 159	○	●	●	○	○	○	○
Arm & Hammer Ultra Fresh Heavy Duty Detergent 51, 159	○	●	●	○	◐	○	○
Biofa Natural Wool Washing Liquid ✓	○	○	○	○	○	○	○
Bi-O-Kleen Laundry Powder ✓	○	○	○	○	○	○	○
Bold Liquid 53	○	○	◐	○	○	○	○
Cal Ben Seafoam Laundry Soap ✓	○	○	○	○	○	○	○
Cheer Laundry Granules 39, 135, 136, 159	○	○	◐	○	○	○	○

Product	Little to No Risk	Minimal Risk	Caution	Recommended

Product	Acute Health Advisory			Chronic Health Advisory		
	Flammability	Causticity	Irritants	Allergens and Strong Sensitizers	Carcinogens	Neurotoxins	Reproductive Effects
Cheer Free Laundry Granules ✓ 39, 135, 136, 159	○	○	●	○	○	○	○
Citrus Natural Laundry Soap ✓	○	○	○	○	○	○	○
Country Safe Laundry Detergent ✓ 159	○	○	●	○	○	○	○
Dash Lemon Fresh 39, 135, 136, 159	○	○	●	○	○	○	○
Dial Heavy Duty Dry Detergent 135, 136, 159	○	○	●	○	○	○	○
Dr. Bronner's Pure Castile Soap ✓	○	○	○	○	○	○	○
Dr. Bronner's Sal Suds ✓	○	○	○	○	○	○	○
Dreft Laundry Granules 39, 135, 136, 159	○	○	●	○	○	○	○
Dreft Ultra 135, 136, 159	○	○	●	○	○	○	○
Dynamo 2 Heavy Duty Detergent 39, 53	○	○	●	○	○	○	○
EarthRite Laundry Detergent ✓	○	○	○	○	○	○	○
Ecco Bella Laundry Powder/Liquid ✓	○	○	○	○	○	○	○
Ecco Bella Suds Soap ✓	○	○	○	○	○	○	○
Ecover Liquid Laundry Wash ✓	○	○	○	○	○	○	○
Ecover Unique Washing Powder ✓	○	○	○	○	○	○	○
Ecover Wool Wash Laundry Liquid ✓	○	○	○	○	○	○	○
ERA Liquid Laundry Detergent 39	○	○	●	○	○	○	○
4 The Planet 4 Your Laundry 51	○	○	○	○	●	○	○
Fab with Fabric Softener Laundry Detergent 39	○	○	●	○	○	○	○
Fab Ultra Super Concentrated Detergent 39	○	○	●	○	○	○	○
Fresh Start (Phosphate & Nonphosphate) 39	○	○	●	○	○	○	○
Gain (Phosphate & Nonphosphate) 39, 135, 159	○	○	●	○	○	○	○

Product				Acute Health Advisory				Chronic Health Advisory		
🛒 Little to No Risk	🛒 Minimal Risk	🛒 Caution	✔ Recommended	Flammability	Causticity	Irritants	Allergens and Strong Sensitizers	Carcinogens	Neurotoxins	Reproductive Effects
Granny's Old Fashioned Products Power Plus ✔				🛒	🛒	🛒	🛒	🛒	🛒	🛒
Ivory Snow Soap Granules ✔				🛒	🛒	🛒	🛒	🛒	🛒	🛒
Life Tree Premium Laundry Liquid 51				🛒	🛒	🛒	🛒	🛒	🛒	🛒
Naturally Yours Laundry Detergent ✔				🛒	🛒	🛒	🛒	🛒	🛒	🛒
Neo-Life Super Plus ✔ 52, 133				🛒	🛒	🛒	🛒	🛒	🛒	🛒
Oxydol Laundry Granules 39, 135, 136, 159				🛒	🛒	🛒	🛒	🛒	🛒	🛒
Seventh Generation Laundry Liquid ✔				🛒	🛒	🛒	🛒	🛒	🛒	🛒
Seventh Generation Laundry Powder ✔				🛒	🛒	🛒	🛒	🛒	🛒	🛒
Shaklee Basic L 51, 136, 159				🛒	🛒	🛒	🛒	🛒	🛒	🛒
Shaklee Liquid L 51, 53				🛒	🛒	🛒	🛒	🛒	🛒	🛒
Simmons Pure Soaps Vegetarian Bar Soaps ✔				🛒	🛒	🛒	🛒	🛒	🛒	🛒
Sodasan Soap Washing Powder ✔				🛒	🛒	🛒	🛒	🛒	🛒	🛒
Sun Laundry Detergent 39				🛒	🛒	🛒	🛒	🛒	🛒	🛒
Surf Liquid Laundry Detergent 39				🛒	🛒	🛒	🛒	🛒	🛒	🛒
Surf New System Liquid Detergent 135, 159				🛒	🛒	🛒	🛒	🛒	🛒	🛒
Surf New System Powder Detergent 39, 159				🛒	🛒	🛒	🛒	🛒	🛒	🛒
Surf Ultra Zeolite Powder Laundry Detergent 135, 159				🛒	🛒	🛒	🛒	🛒	🛒	🛒
Tide Laundry Granules 39, 135, 136, 159				🛒	🛒	🛒	🛒	🛒	🛒	🛒
Tide Laundry Granules with Bleach 39, 132, 135				🛒	🛒	🛒	🛒	🛒	🛒	🛒

Product				Acute Health Advisory				Chronic Health Advisory		
Little to No Risk	Minimal Risk	Caution	Recommended	Flammability	Causticity	Irritants	Allergens and Strong Sensitizers	Carcinogens	Neurotoxins	Reproductive Effects
Tide Liquid 39, 53				🛒	🛒	🛒	🛒	🛒	🛒	🛒
White King Ultra Laundry Detergent 39				🛒	🛒	🛒	🛒	🛒	🛒	🛒
Winter White Laundry Detergent Powder ✓				🛒	🛒	🛒	🛒	🛒	🛒	🛒
Winter White Laundry Detergent Liquid ✓				🛒	🛒	🛒	🛒	🛒	🛒	🛒
Wisk Advanced Action Liquid 39				🛒	🛒	🛒	🛒	🛒	🛒	🛒
Wisk Power Scoop Powder 39, 159				🛒	🛒	🛒	🛒	🛒	🛒	🛒
Woolite Cold Water Wash ✓				🛒	🛒	🛒	🛒	🛒	🛒	🛒

LAUNDRY FABRIC SOFTENERS

Product Types

Aerosol; liquid; sheet.

Safe Use Tip

Avoid aerosol products. Laundry rooms often have poor ventilation and vapors can end up becoming concentrated. You end up inhaling the microscopic particles that damage the lungs.

Recommended Alternatives

- Add ¹/₄ cup of baking soda or borax to the wash cycle for softening clothing.
- Add ¹/₄ cup of distilled white vinegar to the wash cycle for both softening and eliminating cling.

Laundry Fabric Softeners

Product				Acute Health Advisory				Chronic Health Advisory		
Little to No Risk · Minimal Risk · Caution · Recommended ✓				Flammability	Causticity	Irritants	Allergens and Strong Sensitizers	Carcinogens	Neurotoxins	Reproductive Effects
Allen's Naturally Fabric Softener ✓ 71, 119				○	○	○	○	○	○	○
Arm & Hammer Fabric Softener Sheets ✓				○	○	◐	○	○	○	○
Bounce Scented				○	○	◐	○	○	○	○
Bounce Unscented ✓				○	○	◐	○	○	○	○
Bounce with Staingard				○	○	◐	○	○	○	○
Downy Liquid Fabric Softener				○	○	◐	○	○	○	○
Downy Sheets Fabric Softener				○	○	◐	○	○	○	○
Dryer Fresh ✓				○	○	○	○	○	○	○
Ecover Fabric Conditioner ✓				○	○	○	○	○	○	○
Faultless Aerosol Fabric Finish 21, 68, 112				○	○	●	○	○	○	○
Final Touch Liquid Fabric Softener				○	○	◐	○	○	○	○
Naturally Yours Natural Bleach and Softener ✓				○	○	○	○	○	○	○
Shaklee Softer Than Soft Fabric Conditioner ✓ 71				○	○	○	○	○	○	○
Snuggle Fabric Softener Dry Sheet				○	○	◐	○	○	○	○
Snuggle Liquid Fabric Softener Blue				○	○	○	○	○	○	○
Snuggle Liquid Fabric Softener Yellow				○	○	◐	○	○	○	○

LAUNDRY SOIL AND STAIN REMOVERS

Product Types

Aerosol; liquid; pump.

Health Advisory

Avoid use of products containing petroleum distillates such as Shout Aerosol and Spray 'n Wash Tough Stain Remover (aerosol).

Safe Use Tips

- Wear impermeable gloves.
- Use in a well-ventilated area.

Recommended Alternatives

You will find safer, equally effective brands recommended in the charts.

These homemade alternatives also work well at spot and stain removal:

- For an all-purpose stain remover, mix $1/4$ cup of borax with 2 cups of cold water. Use this mixture as a soak for clothing and fabrics or apply with a sponge and allow to dry. It is reported to work for blood, chocolate, coffee, mildew, mud, and urine.
- You can also try adding baking soda, pumice, or washing soda to this mixture for additional stain-removing power and for removing odors, mold, and grease. By decreasing the amount of water in the mixture, you can increase the power of the formula. Additional rinsing will be required. **Caution**: Do not use baking soda on wool fabrics. Wear gloves when using washing soda.

Laundry Soil and Stain Removers

Product				Acute Health Advisory				Chronic Health Advisory		
Little to No Risk	Minimal Risk	Caution	Recommended	Flammability	Causticity	Irritants	Allergens and Strong Sensitizers	Carcinogens	Neurotoxins	Reproductive Effects
Bi-O-Kleen ✓				🛒	🛒	🛒	🛒	🛒	🛒	🛒
Earth Wise ✓				🛒	🛒	🛒	🛒	🛒	🛒	🛒
Easy Wash Concentrated Soil & Stain Remover 49, 157				🛒	🛒	🛒	🛒	🛒	🛒	🛒

Product				Acute Health Advisory				Chronic Health Advisory		
Little to No Risk	Minimal Risk	Caution	✓ Recommended	Flammability	Causticity	Irritants	Allergens and Strong Sensitizers	Carcinogens	Neurotoxins	Reproductive Effects
Easy Wash Laundry Soil & Stain Remover 49, 157				🛒	🛒	🛒	🛒	🛒	🛒	🛒
Naturally Yours All-Purpose Spotter ✓				🛒	🛒	🛒	🛒	🛒	🛒	🛒
Naturally Yours Enviro-Bright ✓				🛒	🛒	🛒	🛒	🛒	🛒	🛒
Naturally Yours Natural Solvent Spotter ✓				🛒	🛒	🛒	🛒	🛒	🛒	🛒
Shaklee Nature Bright ✓ 9, 116, 159				🛒	🛒	🛒	🛒	🛒	🛒	🛒
Shout Aerosol 21, 68, 83, 112				🛒	🛒	🛒	🛒	🛒	🛒	🛒
Shout Liquid ✓				🛒	🛒	🛒	🛒	🛒	🛒	🛒
Shout Stick Laundry Prespotter 51, 90, 130				🛒	🛒	🛒	🛒	🛒	🛒	🛒
Spray 'n Wash Stain Stick ✓				🛒	🛒	🛒	🛒	🛒	🛒	🛒
Spray 'n Wash Tough Stain Remover (aerosol) 9, 60, 103, 116				🛒	🛒	🛒	🛒	🛒	🛒	🛒
Spray 'n Wash Tough Stain Remover (liquid) 51				🛒	🛒	🛒	🛒	🛒	🛒	🛒

LAUNDRY STARCHES

Product Type

Aerosol.

Health Advisory

Although we recommend against the use of aerosols because their tiny particles are easily inhaled and can cause lung damage, we could not find any nonaerosol brands to recommend.

Recommended Alternatives

Two homemade recipes from *Clean & Green* work well and are far less hazardous.

To starch light-colored clothing, dissolve 2 or 3 teaspoons of cornstarch in 1 cup of water, pour into a spray bottle, and shake well.

To starch dark-colored clothing, add about $1/2$ cup of black tea, brewed and cooled, to the starch formula described above. This will prevent the starch from showing through darker clothing.

Laundry Starches

Legend: Little to No Risk · Minimal Risk · Caution · ✓ Recommended

Product	Acute Health Advisory				Chronic Health Advisory		
	Flammability	Causticity	Irritants	Allergens and Strong Sensitizers	Carcinogens	Neurotoxins	Reproductive Effects
Faultless Spray Starch 21, 68, 112, 139	Little to No Risk	Little to No Risk	Caution	Minimal Risk	Little to No Risk	Little to No Risk	Little to No Risk
Niagara Spray Professional Finish Heavy 68, 112, 139	Little to No Risk	Little to No Risk	Caution	Minimal Risk	Little to No Risk	Little to No Risk	Little to No Risk
Niagara Spray Professional Finish Original 68, 139	Little to No Risk	Little to No Risk	Caution	Minimal Risk	Little to No Risk	Little to No Risk	Little to No Risk
Niagara Sizing 68	Little to No Risk	Little to No Risk	Caution	Little to No Risk	Little to No Risk	Little to No Risk	Little to No Risk

LIME REMOVERS

Product Types

Liquid; pump.

These products are used to remove mineral buildup from bathroom fixtures, shower doors, curtains, and other areas and appliances of the home such as humidifiers.

Health Advisory

Sodium hypochlorite can strongly irritate the lungs if inhaled. Individuals with respiratory illnesses such as asthma or heart disease may be most severely affected and should avoid use of products containing highly concentrated sodium hypochlorite. Such products include Easy-Off, Tile Plus, Tilex, and X-14.

Phosphoric acid can also be extremely irritating to the lungs. It is found in Lime-A-Way. We recommend against its use unless each of the safe use tips outlined below is followed.

Safe Use Tips

- Use in a well-ventilated area.
- Wear nonpermeable gloves.
- If you use any products for which caution is recommended, wear a respirator.
- If you become dizzy or have trouble breathing, leave the area immediately and get fresh air.

Recommended Alternatives

- A baking soda paste applied with a hard-bristled brush works well to clean up lime. Pour $1/2$ cup of baking soda into a bowl, adding enough water to make a paste. Use a hard-bristled brush or toothbrush on areas between tiles.
- For hardened mineral deposits, mix 1 teaspoon alum with $1/4$ cup of distilled white vinegar or lemon juice in a bowl. Saturate a rag and scrub the mineral buildup until clean. Alum can be found in the herb and spice section of supermarkets.
- Shower curtains can be cleaned with a sponge saturated with vinegar. The vinegar is a mild disinfectant and eliminates mold and mildew.

Lime Removers

Product				Acute Health Advisory				Chronic Health Advisory		
Little to No Risk	Minimal Risk	Caution	Recommended	Flammability	Causticity	Irritants	Allergens and Strong Sensitizers	Carcinogens	Neurotoxins	Reproductive Effects
Descale-It Bathroom Tile and Fixture ✔				Little to No Risk	Little to No Risk	Little to No Risk	Little to No Risk	Little to No Risk	Little to No Risk	Little to No Risk
EarthRite Tub & Tile Cleaner ✔				Little to No Risk	Little to No Risk	Little to No Risk	Little to No Risk	Little to No Risk	Little to No Risk	Little to No Risk
Easy-Off 132				Little to No Risk	Minimal Risk	Caution	Recommended	Little to No Risk	Little to No Risk	Little to No Risk
Lime-A-Way 106				Little to No Risk	Minimal Risk	Caution	Little to No Risk	Little to No Risk	Little to No Risk	Little to No Risk
Tile Plus 132				Little to No Risk	Minimal Risk	Caution	Recommended	Little to No Risk	Little to No Risk	Little to No Risk
Tilex 132				Little to No Risk	Minimal Risk	Caution	Recommended	Little to No Risk	Little to No Risk	Little to No Risk
X-14 132				Little to No Risk	Minimal Risk	Caution	Recommended	Little to No Risk	Little to No Risk	Little to No Risk

MARBLE CLEANERS AND POLISHES

Product Type

Liquid.

Health Advisory

Some products contain ethylene glycol, which is neurotoxic and causes reproductive effects.

Safe Use Tips

- Use nonpermeable gloves and avoid all skin contact.
- Pregnant women should not use brands containing ethylene glycol.

Marble Cleaners and Polishes

Product				Acute Health Advisory				Chronic Health Advisory		
🛒 Little to No Risk	🛒 Minimal Risk	🛒 Caution	✓ Recommended	Flammability	Causticity	Irritants	Allergens and Strong Sensitizers	Carcinogens	Neurotoxins	Reproductive Effects
Marble Cleaner 23				🛒	🛒	🛒	🛒	🛒	🛒	🛒
Marble Shine 55				🛒	🛒	🛒	🛒	🛒	🛒	🛒
Weiman Marble Polish ✓				🛒	🛒	🛒	🛒	🛒	🛒	🛒

METAL POLISHES

Product Types

Aerosol; liquid.

Health Advisory

Although the MSDSs for some of the products from Hagerty & Sons did not list specific hazardous ingredients, they noted that these products can cause skin irritation with prolonged exposure. Such products include: Chanda Cleaner Chandelier Cleaner; Coppersmith's Polish; Dry Silver Polish; Heavy-Duty Copper, Brass, Metal Polish; Jewel Clean; Silversmith's Polish.

Safe Use Tips

- Wash-off brands are more irritating to the eyes and skin than wipe-off brands.
- Wear nonpermeable gloves.
- Use wash-off products in well-ventilated areas, as inhaling fumes can cause headaches.

Recommended Alternatives

Recommended safe and effective metal polishes are available at hardware stores and supermarkets. One standard formula, described in *The Nontoxic Home & Office,* works well for silverware and relies on the principle of magnetism. The combination of aluminum and a salt such as table salt or baking soda acts as a magnet to "lure" tarnish away from the silverware.

Cover the bottom of a pan with aluminum foil, adding two to three inches of water, 1 teaspoon salt, and 1 teaspoon baking soda. Place on stove and bring to a boil, adding silverware. Make sure that the water covers all the silverware. After boiling for two to three minutes, remove the silverware, and dry.

This procedure can be used for large silver pieces as well. Instead of boiling the water on the stove, simply add hot water from the tap.

Metal Polishes

Product				Acute Health Advisory				Chronic Health Advisory		
Little to No Risk	Minimal Risk	Caution	Recommended	Flammability	Causticity	Irritants	Allergens and Strong Sensitizers	Carcinogens	Neurotoxins	Reproductive Effects
Hagerty & Sons Chanda Cleaner Chandelier Cleaner ✓ 71				🛒	🛒	🛒	🛒	🛒	🛒	🛒
Hagerty & Sons Coppersmith's Polish ✓ 71				🛒	🛒	🛒	🛒	🛒	🛒	🛒
Hagerty & Sons Dry Silver Polish 83				🛒	🛒	🛒	🛒	🛒	🛒	🛒
Hagerty & Sons Heavy-Duty Copper, Brass, Metal Polish 5				🛒	🛒	🛒	🛒	🛒	🛒	🛒
Hagerty & Sons Jewel Clean ✓				🛒	🛒	🛒	🛒	🛒	🛒	🛒
Hagerty & Sons Silversmith's Polish ✓ 71				🛒	🛒	🛒	🛒	🛒	🛒	🛒
Hagerty & Sons Silversmith Spray Polish 68, 71, 112, 151				🛒	🛒	🛒	🛒	🛒	🛒	🛒

Product	Acute Health Advisory				Chronic Health Advisory		
	Flammability	Causticity	Irritants	Allergens and Strong Sensitizers	Carcinogens	Neurotoxins	Reproductive Effects
Hope's Brass Polish ✓	Little to No Risk	Little to No Risk	Little to No Risk	Little to No Risk	Little to No Risk	Little to No Risk	Little to No Risk
Hope's Copper Polish 106	Little to No Risk	Caution	Caution	Little to No Risk	Little to No Risk	Little to No Risk	Little to No Risk
Hope's Silver Polish ✓	Little to No Risk	Little to No Risk	Little to No Risk	Little to No Risk	Little to No Risk	Little to No Risk	Little to No Risk
Hope's Stainless Steel Cleaner 106	Little to No Risk	Caution	Caution	Little to No Risk	Little to No Risk	Little to No Risk	Little to No Risk
Kleen King Aluminum Brightener 33	Little to No Risk	Little to No Risk	Minimal Risk	Little to No Risk	Caution	Little to No Risk	Little to No Risk
Kleen King Copper & Stainless Steel Cleaner 33	Little to No Risk	Little to No Risk	Minimal Risk	Little to No Risk	Caution	Little to No Risk	Little to No Risk
Kleen King Copper & Stainless Steel Cleaner Liquid ✓	Little to No Risk	Little to No Risk	Little to No Risk	Little to No Risk	Little to No Risk	Little to No Risk	Little to No Risk
Parker's Perfect Polish Aluminum Stainless Steel ✓	Little to No Risk	Little to No Risk	Little to No Risk	Little to No Risk	Little to No Risk	Little to No Risk	Little to No Risk
Twinkle Silver Polish ✓	Little to No Risk	Little to No Risk	Little to No Risk	Little to No Risk	Little to No Risk	Little to No Risk	Little to No Risk
Weiman Royal Sterling Silver Polish ✓	Little to No Risk	Little to No Risk	Little to No Risk	Little to No Risk	Little to No Risk	Little to No Risk	Little to No Risk

Legend: Little to No Risk · Minimal Risk · Caution · ✓ Recommended

OVEN CLEANERS

Product Types

Aerosol; vapor cleaner.

Health Advisory

When sodium hydroxide is highly concentrated as it is in oven cleaners, it can burn eyes, skin, and internal organs. Take care not to inhale the fumes, ingest the foam, liquid, or powder, or allow products to contact the skin.

Safe Use Tips

Your best strategy is to buy a self-cleaning oven. If you choose to use products rated for extreme caution, observe the following precautions:

- Wear a respirator.
- Use nonpermeable gloves and goggles.

- Open windows and be sure that others, especially children, are out of the room.
- Leave the area until fumes have subsided.
- If the fumes begin to affect you, close the oven door, leave the room, and get fresh air immediately.

Recommended Alternatives

Several new "fume-free" products, which have come on the market, are much safer, but require longer to work.

The following homemade recipes work well:

- Use baking soda, water, and a small amount of liquid plant-based soap. Cover the bottom of the oven with water; be sure not to flood it. Next, sprinkle baking soda over the water; then add another light layer of water. Let it sit for about twelve hours or overnight. Then use a cloth to remove the grease. Follow with a soapy sponge to wash the inside of the oven and rinse.
- Microwave oven interiors can be cleaned by making a paste from 3 or 4 tablespoons of baking soda mixed with water. Use a sponge lightly saturated with the mixture, then rinse.

Oven Cleaners

Legend: ○ = Little to No Risk · ◐ = Minimal Risk · ● = Caution · ✓ = Recommended

Product	Acute Health Advisory				Chronic Health Advisory		
	Flammability	Causticity	Irritants	Allergens and Strong Sensitizers	Carcinogens	Neurotoxins	Reproductive Effects
Ball Oven Cleaner Aerosol 131	○	●	●	○	○	○	○
Bon Ami Cleaning Powder 57	○	○	◐	○	○	○	○
Easy-Off Fume Free Oven Cleaner (Pump) ✓	○	○	○	○	○	○	○
Easy-Off Non-Caustic Oven Cleaner Aerosol 68	○	○	●	○	○	○	○
Easy-Off Oven Cleaner Original Heavy Duty Aerosol 21, 131	○	●	●	○	○	○	○
Ecover Cream Cleaner ✓	○	○	○	○	○	○	○
Mr. Muscle Oven Cleaner Aerosol 21, 68, 131	◐	●	●	○	○	○	○
Prevail Oven Cleaner Aerosol 21, 68, 131	◐	●	●	○	○	○	○

SPOT REMOVERS

Product Types

Aerosol; liquid; pump.

Health Advisory

Spot removers often rely on highly toxic petrochemical solvents such as petroleum distillates, xylene, and toluene. These can cause a wide range of acute and chronic effects, including eye and skin irritation, cancer, central nervous system damage, and reproductive effects. Seek recommended brands first.

Safe Use Tips

- Use adequate ventilation.
- Wear a respirator for products with neurotoxic effects.
- Wear safety glasses or goggles.
- Wear impermeable gloves.

Recommended Alternatives

Safe, effective alternative brands are available at supermarkets and health food stores.

A standard formula for a general spot remover calls for $1/4$ cup borax dissolved in 2 cups cold water. Make sure that the borax is completely mixed without residues falling to the bottom of the bowl. The formula can be sponged on fabrics or rubbed on more durable carpets.

Quick action is essential for removing stains. One tablespoon of baking soda mixed with 1 cup of liquid soap in a bowl and then applied to the stained area with a saturated cloth will help remove many stains and deodorize.

Spot Removers

Product				Acute Health Advisory				Chronic Health Advisory		
Little to No Risk	Minimal Risk	Caution	Recommended	Flammability	Causticity	Irritants	Allergens and Strong Sensitizers	Carcinogens	Neurotoxins	Reproductive Effects
AFM Safety Clean ✓				●	●	●	●	●	●	●
AFM Super Clean ✓				●	●	●	●	●	●	●
Arm & Hammer Baking Soda ✓				●	●	●	●	●	●	●

Product				Acute Health Advisory				Chronic Health Advisory		
🛒 *Little to No Risk*	🛒 *Minimal Risk*	🛒 *Caution*	✓ *Recommended*	Flammability	Causticity	Irritants	Allergens and Strong Sensitizers	Carcinogens	Neurotoxins	Reproductive Effects
Arm & Hammer Super Washing Soda 159				🛒	🛒	🛒	🛒	🛒	🛒	🛒
Auro Organics Cleansing Emulsion ✓				🛒	🛒	🛒	🛒	🛒	🛒	🛒
Auro Organics Plant Thinner ✓				🛒	🛒	🛒	🛒	🛒	🛒	🛒
Bi-O-Kleen ✓				🛒	🛒	🛒	🛒	🛒	🛒	🛒
Citra-Solv 75, 92, 94				🛒	🛒	🛒	🛒	🛒	🛒	🛒
Dial Corporation 20 Mule Team Borax ✓				🛒	🛒	🛒	🛒	🛒	🛒	🛒
Didi 7 74, 129, 153				🛒	🛒	🛒	🛒	🛒	🛒	🛒
Earth Wise ✓				🛒	🛒	🛒	🛒	🛒	🛒	🛒
Energine Cleaning Fluid 151				🛒	🛒	🛒	🛒	🛒	🛒	🛒
Energine Spot Remover 150				🛒	🛒	🛒	🛒	🛒	🛒	🛒
Granny's Old Fashioned Products Soil Away ✓				🛒	🛒	🛒	🛒	🛒	🛒	🛒
Greenspan Healthy Cleaner ✓				🛒	🛒	🛒	🛒	🛒	🛒	🛒
Kleenol 1 103				🛒	🛒	🛒	🛒	🛒	🛒	🛒
Kleenol 2 (All Purpose) ✓ 60, 71				🛒	🛒	🛒	🛒	🛒	🛒	🛒
K2r Spot-Lifter 151				🛒	🛒	🛒	🛒	🛒	🛒	🛒
3M Brand Carpet Spot Remover & Upholstery Cleaner (Aerosol) 23				🛒	🛒	🛒	🛒	🛒	🛒	🛒
NaturCare ✓				🛒	🛒	🛒	🛒	🛒	🛒	🛒
Naturally Yours Natural Solvent Spotter ✓				🛒	🛒	🛒	🛒	🛒	🛒	🛒
O'Cedar Carpet Science Spot & Stain Remover ✓				🛒	🛒	🛒	🛒	🛒	🛒	🛒
Shoe Goo 144				🛒	🛒	🛒	🛒	🛒	🛒	🛒
Spray 'n Wash Stain Stick ✓				🛒	🛒	🛒	🛒	🛒	🛒	🛒

TOILET BOWL CLEANERS AND DEODORIZERS

Product Types

Crystal; liquid; solid.

Health Advisory

Many products are highly caustic, so be sure to follow *Safe Use Tips.*

People with asthma should know that the sulfate-based compounds in toilet bowl cleaners may cause asthmatic attacks. An increased risk for such attacks has been reported in the general population to be correlated with elevated levels of sulfate particles in the air.

Safe Use Tips

- Wear impermeable gloves.
- Always ensure adequate ventilation when using foaming products.
- Do not mix with chlorine-based products such as cleansers and all-purpose cleaners.

Recommended Alternatives

- The standard formula for cleaning toilet bowls requires pouring 1 cup of borax and $1/4$ cup of distilled white vinegar or lemon juice into the bowl. Allow the mixture to remain there for a few hours or as long as overnight, then scrub with toilet bowl brush. Flush.
- A few drops of pine oil added to the above formula will disinfect. (Remember that pine oil is a weak allergen; its use may not be appropriate for some people.)

Toilet Bowl Cleaners and Deodorizers

Product				Acute Health Advisory				Chronic Health Advisory		
Little to No Risk	Minimal Risk	Caution	Recommended	Flammability	Causticity	Irritants	Allergens and Strong Sensitizers	Carcinogens	Neurotoxins	Reproductive Effects
AFM Safety Clean ✓				◻	◻	◻	◻	◻	◻	◻
Arm & Hammer Baking Soda ✓				◻	◻	◻	◻	◻	◻	◻
Depend-O Blue Automatic Toilet Cleaner 3				◻	◻	◻	◻	●	◻	◻

Product				Acute Health Advisory				Chronic Health Advisory		

Legend:
🛒 Little to No Risk 🛒 Minimal Risk 🛒 Caution ✓ Recommended

Product	Flammability	Causticity	Irritants	Allergens and Strong Sensitizers	Carcinogens	Neurotoxins	Reproductive Effects
Dial Corporation 20 Mule Team Borax ✓	Little/No	Little/No	Little/No	Little/No	Little/No	Little/No	Little/No
Earth Friendly Toilet Cleaner ✓	Little/No	Little/No	Little/No	Little/No	Little/No	Little/No	Little/No
EarthRite Toilet Bowl Cleaner ✓	Little/No	Little/No	Little/No	Little/No	Little/No	Little/No	Little/No
Ecover Toilet Cleaner ✓	Little/No	Little/No	Little/No	Little/No	Little/No	Little/No	Little/No
Lysol Cling Thick Liquid Toilet Bowl Cleaner (Fresh & Pine) 15	Little/No	Caution	Caution	Little/No	Little/No	Little/No	Little/No
Lysol Liquid Disinfectant Toilet Bowl Cleaner 66	Little/No	Caution	Caution	Little/No	Little/No	Little/No	Little/No
Sani-Flush Automatic Toilet Cleaner (Solid) ✓	Little/No	Little/No	Minimal	Little/No	Little/No	Little/No	Little/No
Sani-Flush Toilet Bowl Cleaner 136, 159	Little/No	Little/No	Caution	Caution	Little/No	Little/No	Little/No
Sno Bol Toilet Bowl Cleaner 66	Little/No	Caution	Caution	Little/No	Little/No	Little/No	Little/No
Sno Drops Toilet Bowl Cleaner 136	Minimal	Caution	Caution	Caution	Little/No	Little/No	Little/No
Ty-D-Bol Automatic Toilet Cleaner 67	Little/No	Little/No	Caution	Little/No	Little/No	Little/No	Little/No
Ty-D-Bol Bleach Tabs 127	Little/No	Caution	Little/No	Little/No	Little/No	Little/No	Little/No
Ty-D-Bol Power Tabs 67	Little/No	Little/No	Caution	Little/No	Little/No	Little/No	Little/No
VANISH Blue Automatic Toilet Cleaner 39	Little/No	Little/No	Minimal	Little/No	Little/No	Little/No	Little/No
VANISH Bowl Freshener ✓	Little/No	Little/No	Little/No	Little/No	Little/No	Little/No	Little/No
VANISH Clear Drop-Ins-Tank Automatic Bowl Cleaner 66	Little/No	Caution	Caution	Little/No	Little/No	Little/No	Little/No
VANISH Crystal Toilet Bowl Cleaner 136	Little/No	Little/No	Caution	Caution	Little/No	Little/No	Little/No
VANISH DROP-INS Solid Automatic Toilet Bowl ✓	Little/No	Little/No	Little/No	Little/No	Little/No	Little/No	Little/No
VANISH Extra Strength Fragrance Bowl Freshener ✓	Little/No	Little/No	Little/No	Little/No	Little/No	Little/No	Little/No

Product				Acute Health Advisory				Chronic Health Advisory		
Little to No Risk	Minimal Risk	Caution	Recommended	Flammability	Causticity	Irritants	Allergens and Strong Sensitizers	Carcinogens	Neurotoxins	Reproductive Effects
VANISH Foamin' Toilet Bowl Cleaner (aerosol) 21, 112				◧	◻	◼	◻	◻	◻	◻
VANISH Fresh Scent Thick Liquid Toilet Bowl Cleaner 66				◻	◼	◧	◻	◻	◻	◻
VANISH Green Automatic Toilet Cleaner 39*				◻	◻	◻	◻	◻	◻	◻
VANISH Solid Automatic Toilet Bowl Cleaner ✓				◻	◻	◧	◻	◻	◻	◻
VANISH Thick Liquid Toilet Bowl Cleaner 66				◻	◼	◧	◻	◻	◻	◻

UPHOLSTERY CLEANERS AND PROTECTORS

Product Types

Aerosol; liquid; pump.

Health Advisory

Because the microscopic particulates from aerosol upholstery cleaners and protectors can be inhaled, causing systemic effects, we recommend against their use.

Recommended Alternatives

Several easily obtainable brands have been recommended, but you can also use the following homemade recipe for cleaning upholstery.

- A basic upholstery cleaner can be made by mixing $1/4$ cup of liquid soap with 3 tablespoons of water. Ingredients should be blended in a bowl and the foam rubbed into the upholstery with a cotton cloth, then rinsed with a clean sponge.

This product contains an uncharacterized artificial color.

Upholstery Cleaners and Protectors

Legend: 🛒 Little to No Risk · 🛒 Minimal Risk · 🛒 Caution · ✓ Recommended

Product	Acute Health Advisory				Chronic Health Advisory		
	Flammability	Causticity	Irritants	Allergens and Strong Sensitizers	Carcinogens	Neurotoxins	Reproductive Effects
AFM Safety Clean ✓	Little	Little	Little	Little	Little	Little	Little
AFM Super Clean ✓	Little	Little	Little	Little	Little	Little	Little
Auro Organics Cleansing Emulsion ✓	Little	Little	Little	Little	Little	Little	Little
Auro Organics Plant Thinner ✓	Little	Little	Little	Little	Little	Little	Little
Arm & Hammer Baking Soda ✓	Little	Little	Little	Little	Little	Little	Little
Bissell Upholstery Shampoo (aerosol)	Minimal	Little	Caution	Little	Little	Little	Little
Dial Corporation 20 Mule Team Borax ✓	Little	Little	Little	Little	Little	Little	Little
Dr. Harvey's Organic Power Carpet & Upholstery Clean 68, 112, 133	Little	Little	Caution	Little	Little	Little	Little
Glamorene Spray 'n Brush (aerosol) 68	Minimal	Little	Caution	Little	Little	Little	Little
Granny's Old Fashioned Products Soil Away ✓	Little	Little	Little	Little	Little	Little	Little
Greenspan Friendly Cleaner ✓	Little	Little	Little	Little	Little	Little	Little
Kmart Aerosol Upholstery Shampoo	Minimal	Little	Caution	Little	Little	Little	Little
3M Brand Aerosol Carpet Spot Remover & Upholstery Clean 23	Minimal	Little	Caution	Little	Little	Minimal	Little
Naturally Yours ✓	Little	Little	Little	Little	Little	Little	Little
Woolite Upholstery Cleaner 68	Minimal	Little	Caution	Little	Little	Little	Little

CHAPTER 2

Paint and Related Products

PAINTS

Product Types

Oil-based; water-based (latex); plant-based; spray.

Health Advisory

Acute

Oil-based and latex paints can cause mucous membrane and/or skin irritation. Painters may also suffer from nonallergic contact dermatitis, chronic bronchitis, and asthma.

Oil-based and latex paints often cause allergic sensitization. Painters may also suffer from allergic contact dermatitis.

Chronic

The reports most relevant for assessing cancer risk associated with occupational exposures in painting are three large epidemiological studies of painters that showed a consistent excess of a wide range of cancers, including cancers of the esophagus, stomach, and bladder, at about 20 percent above the national average, and a consistent excess of lung cancers, at about 40 percent above the national average. Children of painters are also at risk for cancer. Studies have shown an excess of childhood cancer when their mothers or fathers are exposed to the chemicals in paint. Additional studies have shown an excess risk for brain tumors in the children of male painters.

Sanding or removing paint generates crystalline silica (also known as quartz or cristobalite) dust, which is then inhaled. Crystalline silica is carcinogenic. It is hazardous in the dry, not liquid, state, and it is important to note that the hazard from crystalline silica occurs only during paint removal.

Neurotoxins: Although it is commonly believed that new latex paints are lead-free, in fact they may contain up to 0.06 percent lead, according to Ken Giles of the Consumer Product Safety Commission. Lead is neurotoxic. The greatest risk for exposure to lead in paint is in inhalation of dusts, fumes, mists, or vapors and by ingestion of lead compounds introduced into the mouth on food, fingers, or other objects. Typically, such exposures occur during renovation of old homes when old paint is removed without adequate protection, contaminating areas of the home. In some cases children swallow paint chips from flaking walls, window frames, and doorjambs. Extreme caution is recommended whenever paint-removal and paint-sanding projects are undertaken. Wear respirators and consult a professional.

Both oil-based and latex paints are neurotoxic because of the solvents they contain. Oil-based paints pose the greater risk. Use them with caution.

Latex paints containing mercury-based fungicides were to have been taken off the market because of neurotoxic effects. However, product MSDSs from the Kelly-Moore company report some products contain mercury-based fungicides.

Reproductive Toxins: Ethylene glycol and ethylene glycol ethylether are readily absorbed by the lungs and skin, and they are teratogenic.

Paints manufactured before 1990 may contain mercury-based fungicides; some may still be sold to consumers. One such mercury-based fungicide still found in paints, acetoxyphenylmercury, is teratogenic.

Sanding or scraping paints may result in exposure to lead, which causes reproductive effects.

Safe Use Tips

- Always provide adequate ventilation.
- Wear a respirator for all painting.
- Extinguish pilot lights when painting indoors. Most solvents are highly flammable. Vapors from a solvent-based product can build up in seconds.
- Do not leave paint containers opened. Airborne organic solvent fumes from open paint containers are unhealthy and a fire hazard.
- *Never use aerosols* because of the microscopic particles that are present in them. These particles can be inhaled and cause systemic effects.
- Keep paint products in their original containers. The risk of child poisoning is increased when toxics are transferred into empty food containers.

Furthermore, in the event of poisoning the product label is essential for determining the ingredients.

- If pregnant, avoid exposure to toxic chemicals. The chemicals in even household paint products can cause birth defects. Nursing mothers, infants, and youngsters should also avoid exposure to all toxic products. Pregnant women should never paint!
- To prevent lung damage or cancer, wear appropriate respirators when sanding or scraping paint.
- To prevent paint fumes that might be emitted for days to months after paint is applied, use a sealing product such as Pace Chem Industries' Crystal Aire Acrylic Clear Finish.
- Never sand and scrape paint without thoroughly investigating its lead content. If there is lead, such work should be done by professionally trained experts.
- Wait at least forty-eight hours before reinhabiting freshly painted rooms.
- All new paints should be tested before you paint entire living areas with them. To determine their safety from acute effects, paint an unneeded piece of wood or other material with the brand you are considering using. Leave this freshly painted wood in your bedroom while you sleep. If the freshly applied paint does not bother you overnight, it is probably safe to use.
- Some alternative brands may cause problems for chemically sensitive people. Natural oil-based paint used indoors has been known to cause severe respiratory irritation. This points up the fact that oil-based paints, whether mainstream or "alternative," should *never* be used indoors. Also, always sample new paints, including recommended brands, in smaller areas; use the safety test discussed *above* before investing substantial sums of money (or living space) in them.

Paints

Product				Acute Health Advisory				Chronic Health Advisory		
Little to No Risk	Minimal Risk	Caution	✓ Recommended	Flammability	Causticity	Irritants	Allergens and Strong Sensitizers	Carcinogens	Neurotoxins	Reproductive Effects
Allsafe Paints (entire line) ✓				🛒	🛒	🛒	🛒	🛒	🛒	🛒
Auro Organics Coloured Top Coat Gloss ✓ *149*				🛒	🛒	🛒	🛒	🛒	🛒	🛒
Auro Organics Metal Primer and Undercoat ✓ *149*				🛒	🛒	🛒	🛒	🛒	🛒	🛒

Product				Acute Health Advisory				Chronic Health Advisory		
🛒 Little to No Risk	🛒 Minimal Risk	🛒 Caution	✓ Recommended	Flammability	Causticity	Irritants	Allergens and Strong Sensitizers	Carcinogens	Neurotoxins	Reproductive Effects
Auro Organics White Top Coat Eggshell ✓ 149				🛒	🛒	🛒	🛒	🛒	🛒	🛒
Auro Organics White Top Coat Gloss ✓ 149				🛒	🛒	🛒	🛒	🛒	🛒	🛒
Auro Organics White Undercoat ✓ 149				🛒	🛒	🛒	🛒	🛒	🛒	🛒
Biofa Black Natural Enamel Paint (1190) ✓				🛒	🛒	🛒	🛒	🛒	🛒	🛒
Biofa Blue Natural Enamel Paint (1150) ✓				🛒	🛒	🛒	🛒	🛒	🛒	🛒
Biofa Dark Brown Natural Enamel Paint (1180) ✓				🛒	🛒	🛒	🛒	🛒	🛒	🛒
Biofa Glossy White Natural Enamel Paint (1110) ✓ 149				🛒	🛒	🛒	🛒	🛒	🛒	🛒
Biofa Green Natural Enamel Paint (1160) ✓				🛒	🛒	🛒	🛒	🛒	🛒	🛒
Biofa Light Brown Natural Enamel Paint (1170) ✓				🛒	🛒	🛒	🛒	🛒	🛒	🛒
Biofa Ochre Natural Enamel Paint (1130) ✓				🛒	🛒	🛒	🛒	🛒	🛒	🛒
Biofa Red Brown Natural Enamel Paint (1140) ✓				🛒	🛒	🛒	🛒	🛒	🛒	🛒
Biofa Yellow Natural Enamel Paint (1120) ✓				🛒	🛒	🛒	🛒	🛒	🛒	🛒
Biofa Wall Paints (all) ✓ 13, 149				🛒	🛒	🛒	🛒	🛒	🛒	🛒
Biofa White Priming Paint (1210) ✓ 149				🛒	🛒	🛒	🛒	🛒	🛒	🛒
Crystal Shield Latex Paint (all colors) ✓				🛒	🛒	🛒	🛒	🛒	🛒	🛒
Dutch Boy Architectural Alkyd Semi-Gloss Enamel 55, 83, 149				🛒	🛒	🛒	🛒	🛒	🛒	🛒(Caution)
Dutch Boy Architectural Exterior Latex Flat Paint 33, 55, 149				🛒	🛒	🛒	🛒	🛒(Caution)	🛒	🛒(Caution)

Product				Acute Health Advisory				Chronic Health Advisory		
🛒 Little to No Risk	🛒 Minimal Risk	🛒 Caution	✓ Recommended	Flammability	Causticity	Irritants	Allergens and Strong Sensitizers	Carcinogens	Neurotoxins	Reproductive Effects
Dutch Boy Architectural Latex Flat Wall Paint 33, 55, 149				🛒	🛒	🛒	🛒	🛒	🛒	🛒
Dutch Boy Architectural Latex Semi-Gloss Enamel 23, 55, 149				🛒	🛒	🛒	🛒	🛒	🛒	🛒
Dutch Boy Confident Exterior Latex Flat Finishes; and Primer 33, 55, 149				🛒	🛒	🛒	🛒	🛒	🛒	🛒
Dutch Boy Confident Exterior Latex Gloss Finish 23, 55, 149				🛒	🛒	🛒	🛒	🛒	🛒	🛒
Dutch Boy Dirt Fighter Exterior Latex Satin Finish 23, 33, 55, 149				🛒	🛒	🛒	🛒	🛒	🛒	🛒
Dutch Boy Dirt Fighter Exterior Oil/Alkyd Gloss Finish 23, 55, 83, 149				🛒	🛒	🛒	🛒	🛒	🛒	🛒
Dutch Boy Dirt Fighter Interior Latex All Prep 33, 55				🛒	🛒	🛒	🛒	🛒	🛒	🛒
Dutch Boy Dirt Fighter Interior Latex Flat Finish 33, 55, 149				🛒	🛒	🛒	🛒	🛒	🛒	🛒
Dutch Boy Dirt Fighter Interior Latex Satin Finish (all colors) 23, 33, 55, 149				🛒	🛒	🛒	🛒	🛒	🛒	🛒
Dutch Boy Dirt Fighter Interior Latex Semi-Gloss 23, 55, 149				🛒	🛒	🛒	🛒	🛒	🛒	🛒
Dutch Boy Dirt Fighter Latex Wall & Wood Primer 33, 55, 149				🛒	🛒	🛒	🛒	🛒	🛒	🛒
Dutch Boy Dirt Fighter Interior Oil/Alkyd Satin Finish; Semi-Gloss 55, 83, 149				🛒	🛒	🛒	🛒	🛒	🛒	🛒
Dutch Boy Rust Beater Oil/Alkyd Gloss Enamel 55, 83, 149				🛒	🛒	🛒	🛒	🛒	🛒	🛒
Dutch Boy Super Exterior Latex Flat Finish 33, 55, 149				🛒	🛒	🛒	🛒	🛒	🛒	🛒
Dutch Boy Super Exterior Latex Gloss Finish 23, 55, 149				🛒	🛒	🛒	🛒	🛒	🛒	🛒
Dutch Boy Super Exterior Latex Satin Finish (all colors) 23, 33, 55, 149				🛒	🛒	🛒	🛒	🛒	🛒	🛒

Product				Acute Health Advisory				Chronic Health Advisory		
🛒 Little to No Risk	🛒 Minimal Risk	🛒 Caution	✓ Recommended	Flammability	Causticity	Irritants	Allergens and Strong Sensitizers	Carcinogens	Neurotoxins	Reproductive Effects
Dutch Boy Super Interior Latex Satin Finish (all colors) 33, 55, 149				🛒	🛒	🛒	🛒	🛒	🛒	🛒
Dutch Boy Super Interior Latex Semi-Gloss Finish (all colors) 23, 55, 149				🛒	🛒	🛒	🛒	🛒	🛒	🛒
Glidden Spred 2000 Flat Wall Paint ✓ 149				🛒	🛒	🛒	🛒	🛒	🛒	🛒
Kelly-Moore Acrylic Primer-Sealer 2, 33, 55, 149				🛒	🛒	🛒	🛒	🛒	🛒	🛒
Kelly-Moore Acry-Plex Flat Wall Enamel 33, 149				🛒	🛒	🛒	🛒	🛒	🛒	🛒
Kelly-Moore All Purpose Q.D. Undercoat 33, 83, 161,				🛒	🛒	🛒	🛒	🛒	🛒	🛒
Kelly Moore Exterior Primer 18, 33, 83				🛒	🛒	🛒	🛒	🛒	🛒	🛒
Kelly-Moore Kel-Bond Primer/Surface Conditioner 33, 83				🛒	🛒	🛒	🛒	🛒	🛒	🛒
Kelly-Moore Kel-Cote Alkyd Semi-Gloss Enamel 33, 83				🛒	🛒	🛒	🛒	🛒	🛒	🛒
Kelly-Moore Kel Guard Epoxy Enamel 33, 56, 149				🛒	🛒	🛒	🛒	🛒	🛒	🛒
Kelly-Moore Latex Flat Wall Paint (all colors in 505 series) 33, 149				🛒	🛒	🛒	🛒	🛒	🛒	🛒
Kelly-Moore Latex Flat Wall Paint (all colors in 510 series) 55, 149				🛒	🛒	🛒	🛒	🛒	🛒	🛒
Kelly-Moore Latex Flat Wall Paint (all colors in 515 series) 55, 149				🛒	🛒	🛒	🛒	🛒	🛒	🛒
Kelly-Moore Latex Flat Wall Paint (all colors in 575 series) 55, 149				🛒	🛒	🛒	🛒	🛒	🛒	🛒
Kelly-Moore Latex Flat Wall Paint (all colors in 581 series) 55, 149				🛒	🛒	🛒	🛒	🛒	🛒	🛒
Kelly-Moore Latex Flat Wall Paint (all colors in 585 series) 55, 149				🛒	🛒	🛒	🛒	🛒	🛒	🛒
Kelly-Moore Painter's Alkyd Gloss Enamel 83, 149				🛒	🛒	🛒	🛒	🛒	🛒	🛒

Product				Acute Health Advisory				Chronic Health Advisory		
Little to No Risk	Minimal Risk	Caution	Recommended ✓	Flammability	Causticity	Irritants	Allergens and Strong Sensitizers	Carcinogens	Neurotoxins	Reproductive Effects
Kelly-Moore Stain-Resistant Acrylic Primer 33, 55, 149								●		
Kelly-Moore Super Latex Flat Wall Paint 33, 55, 149								●		●
Livos Vindo-Enamel Paint 45, 70										
Miller Paint Co. Acri-Lite ✓										
Miller Paint Co. Acri-Lite Semigloss Trim ✓										
Miller Paint Co. Acro Latex Enamel Interior Semigloss ✓										
Miller Paint Co. Pro-Jex Satin Interior Latex ✓										
Miller Paint Co. PVA Primer for Wallboards & Plaster ✓										
Miller Paint Co. Rubber Lustre Velvet Latex ✓										
The Old Fashioned Milk Paint Co. Milk Paint 13, 33								●		

PAINT REMOVERS AND STRIPPERS

Product Types

Chemical stripper (aerosol, liquid); heat gun; mechanical (sander).

Health Advisory

Many paint removers and strippers contain methanol, which can cause permanent blindness. Exposure can occur through inhalation, skin absorption, and ingestion.

A review of MSDSs for all paint strippers indicates that the majority can cause eye and skin irritation, as well as mucous membrane and upper respiratory irritation.

Be aware that although methylene chloride has been removed from many other consumer products, many brands of paint stripper contain this chemical.

Quite apart from carcinogenicity and neurotoxicity, methylene chloride can cause irregular heartbeat, even heart attack, when inhaled.

Others contain 1,1,1-trichloroethane, which can cause an irregular heartbeat.

Safe Use Tips

- Wear impermeable gloves.
- Wear respirator and goggles.
- Always keep a wet rag and bucket of water nearby when using heat guns in case of fire.
- Never touch the metal nozzle of a heat gun or allow yourself to be blasted by its heat.
- Keep heat guns away from areas frequented by children or pets.
- For removal of lead-based paint, a professional who specializes in lead paint removal is recommended; however, if you remove lead-based paint yourself, always use one of the safer brands of chemical strippers to avoid dust generated through mechanical stripping or the use of heat guns.
- We recommend against heat guns because they volatilize chemicals. Heat guns spew air hotter than 800°F, making the paint blister and bubble, ready to be scraped. They can easily burn skin and start fires. If your home has lead-based paint, you should never use a heat gun. *Consumer Reports* notes, "If you're stripping lead paint, [heat guns] can increase your exposure to lead by whipping paint dust into the air, where you can inhale it. When the dust settles, it can still be hazardous to young children."
- Note that the safest paint strippers take longer to work. They may require more than one application, and may take overnight to soften several coats.

Paint Removers and Strippers

Product				Acute Health Advisory				Chronic Health Advisory		
Little to No Risk	Minimal Risk	Caution	Recommended	Flammability	Causticity	Irritants	Allergens and Strong Sensitizers	Carcinogens	Neurotoxins	Reproductive Effects
Auro Paint Remover Paste No. 461 ✓				⊕	⊕	⊕	⊕	⊕	⊕	⊕
Custom Building Products Finish Stripper 23, 84				⊕	⊕	🛒	⊕	⊕	⊕	⊕
Easy-Off Paint Stripper ✓				⊕	⊕	⊕	⊕	⊕	⊕	⊕
Formby's Aerosol Paint Remover 78, 81				🛒	⊕	🛒	🛒	🛒	🛒	⊕

Product				Acute Health Advisory				Chronic Health Advisory		
🛒 Little to No Risk	🛒 Minimal Risk	🛒 Caution	✓ Recommended	Flammability	Causticity	Irritants	Allergens and Strong Sensitizers	Carcinogens	Neurotoxins	Reproductive Effects
Formby's Paint Remover (non-methylene chloride) 78, 150				🛒	🛒	🛒	🛒	🛒	🛒	🛒
Formby's Paint Remover Wash 78, 150				🛒	🛒	🛒	🛒	🛒	🛒	🛒
Jasco Adhesive Remover 78, 81, 150				🛒	🛒	🛒	🛒	🛒	🛒	🛒
Jasco Premium Remover Aerosol 78, 81				🛒	🛒	🛒	🛒	🛒	🛒	🛒
Livos Paint Remover ✓				🛒	🛒	🛒	🛒	🛒	🛒	🛒
3M Safest Stripper ✓				🛒	🛒	🛒	🛒	🛒	🛒	🛒
Parks Furniture Refinisher 78, 150				🛒	🛒	🛒	🛒	🛒	🛒	🛒
Parks Liquid Strip 78, 81, 150				🛒	🛒	🛒	🛒	🛒	🛒	🛒
Parks No Drip Strip 78, 150				🛒	🛒	🛒	🛒	🛒	🛒	🛒
Parks Pro Stripper 78, 81				🛒	🛒	🛒	🛒	🛒	🛒	🛒
Parks Pro Stripper Spray 78, 81				🛒	🛒	🛒	🛒	🛒	🛒	🛒
Parks Quit-N Time 78, 81, 150				🛒	🛒	🛒	🛒	🛒	🛒	🛒
Parks Rough 'N Ready 150				🛒	🛒	🛒	🛒	🛒	🛒	🛒
Peel Away 6 ✓				🛒	🛒	🛒	🛒	🛒	🛒	🛒
Rock Miracle Paint and Varnish Remover 103				🛒	🛒	🛒	🛒	🛒	🛒	🛒
Savogran FinishOff 103				🛒	🛒	🛒	🛒	🛒	🛒	🛒
Savogran StrypSafer ✓				🛒	🛒	🛒	🛒	🛒	🛒	🛒
Sunnyside Gloss Remover and Pre-Paint Cleaner 151, 161				🛒	🛒	🛒	🛒	🛒	🛒	🛒
Sunnyside HB Paint and Varnish Remover 1, 150				🛒	🛒	🛒	🛒	🛒	🛒	🛒
Sunnyside Liquid Paint and Varnish Remover 78, 81, 161				🛒	🛒	🛒	🛒	🛒	🛒	🛒
Sunnyside Premium Paint and Varnish Remover 78, 81, 161				🛒	🛒	🛒	🛒	🛒	🛒	🛒
Sunnyside Tile Adhesive Remover 78, 81, 161				🛒	🛒	🛒	🛒	🛒	🛒	🛒

STAINS

Product Types

Aerosol; liquid.

Health Advisory

Many brands contain formaldehyde, which is a sensitizer and a poisonous irritant to skin, eyes, and mucous membranes. It is also carcinogenic and neurotoxic.

Many brands contain carcinogenic crystalline silica. Dust generated through sanding or scraping is thus dangerous.

Safe Use Tips

- Wear a respirator for extended periods of exposure whether you are working indoors or outdoors.
- Wear impermeable gloves.
- Avoid all skin contact.

Stains

Product				Acute Health Advisory				Chronic Health Advisory		
Little to No Risk	Minimal Risk	Caution	Recommended ✓	Flammability	Causticity	Irritants	Allergens and Strong Sensitizers	Carcinogens	Neurotoxins	Reproductive Effects
Auro Natural Resin Floor Oil No. 126 ✓				Little/No	Little/No	Little/No	Little/No	Little/No	Little/No	Little/No
Auro Natural Resin-Oil Lasur No. 131 ✓				Little/No	Little/No	Little/No	Little/No	Little/No	Little/No	Little/No
Endurance Oil Stain Solid Color Series 33, 55, 59				Caution	Little/No	Caution	Little/No	Caution	Caution	Caution
Kel-Lac Lacquer Stain 23, 80, 158				Caution	Little/No	Caution	Little/No	Little/No	Caution	Caution
Kel-Tone Semi-Transparent Stain 83, 149				Caution	Little/No	Caution	Little/No	Minimal	Caution	Little/No
Livos Kalet Resin and Oil 45, 70				Little/No	Little/No	Minimal	Minimal	Minimal	Minimal	Minimal
Lucas Latex Solid Color Wood Stain (all colors) 33, 55, 149				Little/No	Little/No	Caution	Little/No	Caution	Caution	Caution
Lucas Oil Base Solid Color Stain 55, 83, 149				Caution	Little/No	Minimal	Little/No	Minimal	Caution	Caution
Lucas Semi-transparent Oil Stain & Wood Preservative 55, 83, 149				Caution	Little/No	Minimal	Little/No	Minimal	Caution	Caution

THINNERS

Product Type

Liquid.

Health Advisory

Virtually all brands can cause central nervous depression, including permanent brain cell damage from prolonged inhalation. Use with caution.

Many brands contain methyl ethyl ketone or toluene. Both cause reproductive effects.

Safe Use Tips

- Wear protective clothing, including a respirator when using thinners for an extended time.
- Avoid all skin contact.

Thinners

Legend: 🛒 Little to No Risk 🛒 Minimal Risk 🛒 Caution ✓ Recommended

Product	Acute Health Advisory				Chronic Health Advisory		
	Flammability	Causticity	Irritants	Allergens and Strong Sensitizers	Carcinogens	Neurotoxins	Reproductive Effects
Auro Plant Alcohol Thinner ✓							
Biofa Thinner ✓							
Jasco Lacquer Thinner 1, 23, 71, 150							
Jasco Paint Thinner 7							
Kelly-Moore Lacquer Thinner 80, 161							
Kelly-Moore Mineral Spirits Paint Thinner 83							
Kelly-Moore Synthetic Thinner 80, 150, 161							
Livos Natural Citrus Thinner 45							
Parks Lacquer Thinner 78, 80, 150							
Sunnyside Lacquer Thinner 1, 23, 71, 150							
Sunnyside Paint Thinner 83, 140							

VARNISHES

Product Types

Aerosol; liquid.

Safe Use Tips

- Use in a well-ventilated area. Open all windows if indoors.
- Avoid use of aerosol products.
- Wear a respirator.
- Wear impermeable gloves.
- Avoid all skin contact.

Recommended Alternative

Although some of the recommended varnishes may contain crystalline silica or titanium dioxide, these substances present hazards only when dry and scraped, and the products are clearly the safest available. Alternatively, use pure shellac.

Varnishes

Product		Acute Health Advisory				Chronic Health Advisory		
Little to No Risk / Minimal Risk / Caution / Recommended		Flammability	Causticity	Irritants	Allergens and Strong Sensitizers	Carcinogens	Neurotoxins	Reproductive Effects
Auro Clear Varnish 5, 45		🛒	🛒	🛒	🛒	🛒	🛒	🛒
Biofa Wood Varnish Clear ✓ 33		🛒	🛒	🛒	🛒	🛒	🛒	🛒
Biofa Wood Varnish Colors ✓ 33, 149		🛒	🛒	🛒	🛒	🛒	🛒	🛒
Biofa Hard Varnish ✓		🛒	🛒	🛒	🛒	🛒	🛒	🛒
Dutch Boy Crystaloid Oil/Alkyd Varnish 33, 55, 83, 149		🛒	🛒	🛒	🛒	🛒	🛒	🛒
Dutch Boy Interior/Exterior Gloss Varnish 83		🛒	🛒	🛒	🛒	🛒	🛒	🛒
Dutch Boy Oil/Alkyd Spar Varnish 83		🛒	🛒	🛒	🛒	🛒	🛒	🛒
Dutch Boy Oil/Alkyd Sanding Sealer Semi-Gloss 83, 158		🛒	🛒	🛒	🛒	🛒	🛒	🛒
Dutch Boy Polyurethane Clear Varnish Aerosol 1, 23, 80, 149, 150, 161		🛒	🛒	🛒	🛒	🛒	🛒	🛒

Product				Acute Health Advisory				Chronic Health Advisory		
Little to No Risk	Minimal Risk	Caution	Recommended	Flammability	Causticity	Irritants	Allergens and Strong Sensitizers	Carcinogens	Neurotoxins	Reproductive Effects
Dutch Boy Urethane Sealer 83				🛒	🛒	🛒	🛒	🛒	🛒	🛒
Kel-Thane Clear Polyurethane Gloss Varnish 83				🛒	🛒	🛒	🛒	🛒	🛒	🛒
Kel-Thane Clear Polyurethane Satin Varnish 83				🛒	🛒	🛒	🛒	🛒	🛒	🛒
Kelly-Moore Rhino Spar Varnish (clear) 83				🛒	🛒	🛒	🛒	🛒	🛒	🛒
Parks Varnish Sanding Sealer 83, 158				🛒	🛒	🛒	🛒	🛒	🛒	🛒

Pesticides

HOME AND GARDEN PESTICIDES

This chapter reports on pesticides used in lawn care and pest treatment. For information on pesticides applied to food crops, see part III, "Foods and Beverages."

There are two sources of exposure for consumers: from personal use of products and from professional applicators who will come into your home and apply pesticides for pest treatments ranging from ants and fleas to termites. This section will deal primarily with products available in stores, and only in a limited fashion with professional applicators.

Product Types

Aerosol; bait; fogger; powder; pump. Professional applicators who apply pesticides.

Health Advisory

Acute

Irritants: The following pesticides are often used in products for home or garden. All can cause severe eye, skin, and respiratory irritation as a result of both direct skin contact and inhalation. Use with caution.

acephate	benomyl
atrazine	betasan
balan	carbaryl
bendiocarb	chlorothalonil

chlorpyrifos
2,4-D
Dichlorvos (DDVP)
DSMA
dacthal
diazinon
diphenamid
dicamba
glyphosate
MCPA
MCPP
MSMS
malathion

maneb
methoxychlor
methyl bromide
oftanol
PCNB
pronamide
siduron
sulfur
sulfuryl fluoride (Vikane)
trichlorfon
Triumph
ziram

Allergens and strong sensitizers: The following pesticides, often used for home and gardens, can cause allergic reactions and sensitization. Use products containing these ingredients with caution.

acephate
atrazine
balan
bendiocarb
benomyl
betasan
carbaryl
chlorothalonil
chlorpyrifos
2,4-D
DDVP
DSMA
dacthal
diazinon
diphenamid

dicamba
glyphosate
MCPA
MCPP
MSMS
malathion
maneb
oftanol
PCNB
pronamide
siduron
sulfur
trichlorfon
Triumph
ziram

Chronic

Carcinogens: Beware of home and garden pesticides. There is growing evidence that they are hazardous to your health and to the health of your children.

A highly increased risk for leukemia was found for children whose parents used pesticides in their home or garden before giving birth. Home pesticide use resulted in a risk some four times higher than normal for childhood leukemia. The risk was some six to seven times higher for children of parents who used garden pesticides. The risk was greater with more frequent use.

Childhood brain cancer is associated with use of pesticides to control nuisance pests in the home, no-pest strips in the home, pesticides to control termites, shampoos containing the pesticide lindane, flea collars on pets, diazinon in the garden or orchard, and herbicides to control weeds in the yards, pesticide bombs in the home, and carbaryl (Sevin) in the garden or orchard.

Yet another study has found a significant relationship between insecticides and weed killers and leukemia.

Commercially available no-pest strips, which are hung from ceilings, are associated with cancer. The active ingredient used in many is dichlorvos (DDVP), which is carcinogenic. Pest strips emit continous vapors of DDVP. According to the EPA, people who use the strips as directed and are exposed to them over a lifetime have an increased chance of getting cancer: the risk is as much as one in one hundred. This is ten thousand times higher than the risk considered to be of significant concern. The EPA estimates that members of a household using the pest strips face a cancer risk ten times greater than pest-control workers who apply DDVP thousands of times a year without wearing protective clothing.

The cancer danger of the use of some pesticides extends to pets who are in very close contact with contaminated soils, lawns, and plants. Flea collars with DDVP put pets at a similarly increased cancer risk.

The following pesticides are carcinogenic and should never be used:

acephate	dacthal (DCPA)
atrazine	isoxaben
benomyl	maneb
chlorothalonil	permethrin
2,4-D	pronamide
DDVP	

Neurotoxins: Many of the pesticides used for home and garden are neurotoxic. The following pesticides, which are often used for home and garden pest control, are neurotoxic. Use products containing these pesticides with caution.

acephate	MCPA
atrazine	MCPP
bendiocarb	MSMA
benomyl	malathion
betasan	maneb
carbaryl	methyl bromide
chlorpyrifos	oftanol
2,4-D	sulfuryl fluoride (Vikane)
DDVP	trichlorfon
DSMA	Triumph
diazinon	ziram

Reproductive toxins: These generic pesticides are frequently used in home and garden pest control and are capable of causing reproductive effects. Use with caution:

benomyl	dicamba
carbaryl	MCPA
chlorpyrifos	MCPP
2,4-D	

Safe Use Tips

- The use of pesticides poses extreme hazards—except for some of the botanically derived pesticides such as pyrethrum and pyrethrin and some of the inorganic materials such as diatomaceous earth or fatty acid soaps. We strongly recommend against the use of any pesticides in the home and garden other than natural pyrethrum or pyrethrin extracts, fatty acid soaps, and other natural biological and physicial pesticides. If you insist on using pesticides, follow these precautions:
- Protect the label. Store substances in their original container. If the item is not in its original container, clearly label the current container with the product name and date. Write **DANGER** on the container. Also keep in mind that the label precautions are generally grossly misleading and grossly misstate harmful effects.

- If possible, store pesticides in a locked cabinet. Do not store pesticides near food. Do not store metal cans containing pesticides in wet areas where metal can rust. Freezing can ruin the effectiveness of some pesticides—check with your county agricultural extension service if you plan to store a pesticide outside.

- Never store pesticides in glass jars or other breakable containers. Use plastic containers. Surround the container in turn with a nonflammable absorbent, such as clay-based cat litter, to help contain any small leaks that may occur; using flammable materials, such as nonclay cat litter or newspaper, may lead to spontaneous combustion. Clearly label the outside container with the contents and date. Write **DANGER** on the outside container.

- If the pesticide is flammable be certain that it is stored away from all sources of heat, sparks, and flames. Remember that light switches, electrical appliances, and garage door openers can all be sources of sparks.

- Store out of the reach of children and pets.

- Always follow label precautions carefully when using pesticides. Follow all label directions for preparation and application. When using sprays, a pesticide-approved respirator should be worn. In most instances heavy rubber gloves, clothing that covers exposed skin, boots, and eye protection (wraparound goggles) should be worn. Wash exposed clothing separately from other laundry in a full load setting with hot water and detergent to remove pesticide residues. Put the washer, emptied of all clothing, through two to three more cycles to help remove any residue that may be contaminating its fixtures. Dry clothing that has made contact with pesticides on a line outside to avoid contaminating other clothing or the dryer.

- When through with a pesticide, unless it is banned or restricted, use it up as directed or give it to someone who can completely use it up. Empty containers of pesticides should be filled with water three times, and the rinse water used as the pesticide in accordance with label direction. After triple rinsing, the containers of some pesticides can be placed in the trash. Unopened pesticides should be taken back to the place of purchase. If a pesticide is banned or restricted, or if you cannot use it, then it must be taken to a licensed hazardous waste handler or secured and held for a hazardous waste collection.

- Pesticides should never be burned, buried, put in the trash, poured on the ground, or poured down the drain. Such improper disposal can pollute ground, surface, and drinking water supplies.

- Do not water pesticide-treated areas right after application unless directed to do so by label directions. The pesticide could run off with the excess water into a storm drain or nearby stream. It is probably preferable to water the lawn or garden before application rather than after application, unless otherwise directed.

- Do not fall victim to misleading safety assurances from professional applicators. Misleading advertising is common. Claims range from "completely safe for humans and environment," to "materials have passed scientific tests for safety," and "approved by the EPA [or state government]." In fact, most pesticides pose a wide range of human and environmental hazards, and EPA does not "approve" pesticides, but simply registers them under a risk-benefit standard.

Recommended Alternatives

To Foil Ants and Cockroaches

- Take away their food. Keep food covered or in the refrigerator.
- Put garbage in sealed metal containers with tight covers and keep cans outside.
- Wash your cabinets, counters, tables, and dishes immediately following use.
- Use sealed containers with tight-fitting lids to store your flour, sugar, cereal, and crackers.
- Clean storage, shelves, and drawers. Carefully dust corners and undersides of shelves, drawers, and other spaces.
- Paint shelves with enamel. Do not use paper.
- Take away the pests' water. Fix all leaks. Keep areas under sinks and basins clean and dry.
- Take away their hiding places. Clean out junk and clutter. Throw out old newspapers, empty bottles, carboard boxes, and other clutter. Get rid of unused furniture, appliances, food, and clothing.
- If these remedies fail, then call a professional pest exterminator and have him or her apply boric acid to infested areas inside and outside of the house. Boric acid is one of the least toxic pesticides that exterminators use regularly. Don't let them talk you into using far more toxic pesticides like chlorpyrifos (Dursban).

To Foil Garden Pests

- *Aphids, earwigs, grasshoppers, mites, whiteflies:* Use plenty of yellow sticky traps, available from most garden shops. Release lacewing larvae; they are available through nurseries, garden shops, and mail-order catalogs. Pyrethrins with piperonyl butoxide (for synergy) work extremely well. So will fatty acid soaps (bought from garden shops) sprayed on infested plants.
- *Corn earworms, mealybugs:* Release lacewings and ladybugs. Pyrethrins and fatty acid soaps also work well when sprayed on infested plants.

- *Fungi:* Use sulfur dusts. Also spray fatty acid soaps on infested plants.
- *Red spider mites, scale:* Use oil sprays without copper additives. Also try fatty acid soaps sprayed on infested areas.
- *Snails:* Use diatomaceous earth or predator snails known as *Rumina decollata,* available at nurseries, garden shops, and through mail-order catalogs. They will kill the pest snails and then disappear underground, providing continuous protection.

For Lawn Care

- Dandelions can be eliminated easily by digging them with a fishtail weeder. Young dandelion leaves make excellent, nutrient-rich additions to your salad.
- Release natural predators such as praying mantises and beneficial species of nematodes. They can be bought from your local nursery.
- Clover should not be considered a weed; its root nodules contain bacteria that have the ability to convert nitrogen to a form available to plants.
- Fungus often grows in wet, thatchy, over-fertilized lawns. Drain, dry out, de-thatch, re-add soil bacteria (from compost or manure). Then reseed.
- Aerate twice a year. Compacted soil promotes weeds. Add soil loosener (compost, gypsum) and reseed.
- To control Japanese beetles, in the fall spread milky spore over your entire lawn. Milky spore is a disease that specifically attacks the Japanese beetle grubs. It takes a couple of years after application for milky spore to be fully effective, because it takes time for it to spread densely throughout the lawn. But one application lasts for years inasmuch as the spore continues to multiply in the soil. It's harmless to humans, animals, and friendly insects. You can also use Japanese beetle traps, which are widely available in hardware and garden supply stores.
- Nematodes are also helpful. *Neoplectana* and *Heterorhabditis,* two beneficial nematodes, are capable of repressing over two hundred pests, including cutworms, chinch bugs, flea larvae, sod webworms, and Japanese beetles. The Ortho Chemical Company has recently come out with a new product containing beneficial nematodes. It is available at garden shops.
- Finally, remember to mow often; mow high. Do not rake; leave clippings on the lawn to act as a natural fertilizer and mulch.

To Foil Termites

Avoid the use of Dursban (chlorpyrifos), Vikane, and methyl bromide. Alternatives include: heat, cold, electricity, microwaving, nematodes, and preventive barriers.

- *Subterranean termites:* Many companies now use nematodes, a nontoxic biological approach that has been known to work but has also been criticized. Some experts maintain that the nematodes will not necessarily destroy all of the termites' nests. Another alternative is to use a product called Timbor, made by U.S. Borax, which is mixed with soap and applied into voids with a foaming machine.

- *Drywood termites:* Replacing the wood is often sufficient. Cold treatment using nontoxic liquid nitrogen is an excellent strategy. Heat treatment using tenting and applying heat is another effective method. The use of electricity is also gaining acceptance. In the hands of a trained operator, electrical currents at extremely high voltage but low wattages are sent into the wood, killing insects within the wood without leaving toxic residues or harming the operator or house. For more information on the use of electricity and suppliers of this service in your area, write to ETEX, Ltd., 916 S. Casino Center, Las Vegas, NV 89101 or call (702) 382-3966.

- *Prevention:* Barrier sand is a new preventive subterranean termite method. It can be applied before new construction or around an existing structure. For further information on barrier sand, as well as desiccating dusts that can be injected into the walls during construction or after termite treatment to prevent further infestations, write the Bio-Integral Resource Center (BIRC), PO Box 7414, Berkeley, CA 94707 or call (510) 524-2567. BIRC offers a booklet, *Least Toxic Pest Management for Termites.* BIRC is an excellent resource for information about dealing with other pest problems using least toxic methods.

Home and Garden Pesticides

Product				Acute Health Advisory				Chronic Health Advisory		
🛒 Little to No Risk	🛒 Minimal Risk	🛒 Caution	✓ Recommended	Flammability	Causticity	Irritants	Allergens and Strong Sensitizers	Carcinogens	Neurotoxins	Reproductive Effects
Antrol Ant Control System 29				🛒	🛒	🛒	🛒	🛒	🛒	🛒
Bag-A-Bug Gypsy Mother Lure 43				*	*	🛒	🛒	🛒	🛒	🛒
Black Flag Ant & Roach Killer 113				*	*	🛒	🛒	🛒	🛒	🛒
Black Flag Ant & Roach Killer New Pine Scent 113				*	*	🛒	🛒	🛒	🛒	🛒
Black Flag Flea & Roach Fogger 43				*	*	🛒	🛒	🛒	🛒	🛒

Information not available.

Legend:
- 🛒 (open cart) = Little to No Risk
- 🛒 (shaded cart) = Minimal Risk
- 🛒 (dark cart) = Caution
- ✓ = Recommended

Product	Acute Health Advisory				Chronic Health Advisory		
	Flammability	Causticity	Irritants	Allergens and Strong Sensitizers	Carcinogens	Neurotoxins	Reproductive Effects
Black Flag Professional Ant & Roach Killer 43	*	*	🛒	🛒	●	●	●
Black Flag Roach Ender Roach Control System ✓	🛒	🛒	🛒	🛒	🛒	🛒	🛒
Black Flag Special City Formula Roach Killer 43	*	*	🛒	🛒	●	●	●
Combat Ant Control System 64	🛒	🛒	🛒	🛒	●	🛒	🛒
Combat Flying Insect Killer 68, 100, 105, 112, 147	◐	🛒	●	●	🛒	🛒	🛒
Combat Roach Control System 64	🛒	🛒	🛒	🛒	●	🛒	🛒
Combat Room Fogger 68, 99, 100, 112, 147	◐	🛒	●	🛒	🛒	🛒	🛒
Enforcer Ant & Roach Home Pest Control II 99	🛒	🛒	●	●	●	🛒	🛒
Enforcer Ant & Roach Killer III 88, 99, 118	🛒	🛒	🛒	🛒	●	🛒	🛒
Enforcer Ant Trap 20	🛒	🛒	●	🛒	●	🛒	🛒
Enforcer Fire Ant Killer Granules 40	🛒	●	●	🛒	●	🛒	🛒
Enforcer Flying Insect Killer III 105, 147	◐	🛒	●	🛒	●	🛒	🛒
Enforcer Four Hour Fogger 58, 100, 147, 151	●	🛒	●	🛒	◐	🛒	🛒
Enforcer Overnight Roach Spray II 105	◐	🛒	●	🛒	🛒	🛒	🛒
Enforcer Roach Rid ✓	🛒	🛒	◐	🛒	🛒	🛒	🛒
Enforcer Wasp & Hornet Killer 100, 122, 151	●	🛒	●	🛒	◐	🛒	🛒
Enforcer Wasp & Yellow Jacket Foam V 105, 147	🛒	🛒	●	🛒	🛒	🛒	🛒
Off Insect Repellant 21, 38, 53, 68, 112	●	🛒	🛒	🛒	🛒	🛒	🛒
Ortho Weed-B-Gon Lawn Weed Killer 128	🛒	🛒	●	🛒	🛒	🛒	●
Perma Proof Diacide ✓ 118, 143	🛒	🛒	🛒	◐	◐	🛒	🛒
Perma Proof Diatomaceous Earth ✓	🛒	🛒	🛒	🛒	🛒	🛒	🛒

*Information not available.

Legend (Product icons):
🛒 Little to No Risk | 🛒 Minimal Risk | 🛒 Caution | ✓ Recommended

Product	Acute Health Advisory				Chronic Health Advisory		
	Flammability	Causticity	Irritants	Allergens and Strong Sensitizers	Carcinogens	Neurotoxins	Reproductive Effects
Perma Proof Drax Ant Gel ✓	🛒	🛒	🛒	🛒	🛒	🛒	🛒
Perma Proof Drax PF ✓	🛒	🛒	🛒	🛒	🛒	🛒	🛒
Perma Proof It Works Discs ✓	🛒	🛒	🛒	🛒	🛒	🛒	🛒
Perma Proof Roach Killer ✓	🛒	🛒	🛒	🛒	🛒	🛒	🛒
Raid Ant and Roach Killer 103, 113	🛒	🛒	🛒	🛒	🛒	🛒	🛒
Raid Ant Baits 29	🛒	🛒	🛒	🛒	🛒	🛒	🛒
Raid Flea Killer Plus II 21, 68, 88, 112	🛒	🛒	🛒	🛒	🛒	🛒	🛒
Raid Flying Insect Killer Formula 12 21, 37, 68, 105, 147	🛒	🛒	🛒	🛒	🛒	🛒	🛒
Raid Fumigator 27, 99	🛒	🛒	🛒	🛒	🛒	🛒	🛒
Raid Indoor Fogger 68, 70, 88, 112, 151	🛒	🛒	🛒	🛒	🛒	🛒	🛒
Raid Indoor Fogger II 68, 88, 105, 147, 151	🛒	🛒	🛒	🛒	🛒	🛒	🛒
Raid Max Fogger 36, 68, 70, 88, 112, 151	🛒	🛒	🛒	🛒	🛒	🛒	🛒
Raid Professional Strength Home Insect Killer 29, 142	🛒	🛒	🛒	🛒	🛒	🛒	🛒
Raid Roach and Ant Killer 29, 68, 103, 112, 147	🛒	🛒	🛒	🛒	🛒	🛒	🛒
Raid Roach Controller and Large Roach Bait 29	🛒	🛒	🛒	🛒	🛒	🛒	🛒
Raid Wasp & Hornet Killer 103, 113, 147, 151	🛒	🛒	🛒	🛒	🛒	🛒	🛒
Raid Weed Killer 128	*	*	🛒	🛒	🛒	🛒	🛒
Safer African Violet Insect Attack ✓	🛒	🛒	🛒	🛒	🛒	🛒	🛒
Safer Beetle Trap Attack Floral Lure ✓	🛒	🛒	🛒	🛒	🛒	🛒	🛒

*Information not available.

Legend:
- ◒ *Little to No Risk*
- ◓ *Minimal Risk*
- ● *Caution*
- ✓ *Recommended*

In the table below, "Minimal" = Minimal Risk icon and "Caution" = Caution (shaded) icon.

Product	Flammability	Causticity	Irritants	Allergens and Strong Sensitizers	Carcinogens	Neurotoxins	Reproductive Effects
Safer Beetle Trap Attack Sex Lure ✓	Minimal	Minimal	Minimal	Minimal	Minimal	Minimal	Minimal
Safer B.t. Caterpillar Attack ✓	Minimal	Minimal	Minimal	Minimal	Minimal	Minimal	Minimal
Safer B.t. Leaf Beetle Attack M-One ✓	Minimal	Minimal	Minimal	Minimal	Minimal	Minimal	Minimal
Safer Crawling Insect Attack 118	Minimal	Minimal	Minimal	Caution	Minimal	Caution	Minimal
Safer Fruit/Vegetable Insect Attack/Soap ✓	Minimal	Minimal	Minimal	Minimal	Minimal	Minimal	Minimal
Safer Garden Fungicide ✓ 141	Minimal	Minimal	Caution	Caution	Minimal	Minimal	Minimal
Safer Garden Fungicide Concentrate ✓ 141	Minimal	Minimal	Caution	Caution	Minimal	Minimal	Minimal
Safer Insecticidal Soap Concentrate ✓	Minimal	Minimal	Minimal	Minimal	Minimal	Minimal	Minimal
Safer Insecticidal Soap for Houseplants ✓	Minimal	Minimal	Minimal	Minimal	Minimal	Minimal	Minimal
Safer Leaf Clean & Lustre RTU ✓	Minimal	Minimal	Minimal	Minimal	Minimal	Minimal	Minimal
Safer Moss & Algae Attack ✓	Minimal	Minimal	Minimal	Minimal	Minimal	Minimal	Minimal
Safer Moss Attack for Lawns Concentrate ✓	Minimal	Minimal	Minimal	Minimal	Minimal	Minimal	Minimal
Safer Rose/Flower Insect Attack ✓	Minimal	Minimal	Minimal	Minimal	Minimal	Minimal	Minimal
Safer Sharpshooter Weed & Grass Killer ✓	Minimal	Minimal	Minimal	Minimal	Minimal	Minimal	Minimal
Safer Tree & Shrub Insect Attack/Soap ✓	Minimal	Minimal	Minimal	Minimal	Minimal	Minimal	Minimal
Safer Vegetable Insect Attack Squeeze Duster ✓	Minimal	Minimal	Minimal	Minimal	Minimal	Minimal	Minimal
Safer Yard & Garden Insect Attack ✓ 118	Minimal	Minimal	Minimal	Caution	Minimal	Caution	Minimal

Pesticide Chemicals

Product				Acute Health Advisory				Chronic Health Advisory		
🛒 *Little to No Risk*	🛒 *Minimal Risk*	🛒 *Caution*	✓ *Recommended*	Flammability	Causticity	Irritants	Allergens and Strong Sensitizers	Carcinogens	Neurotoxins	Reproductive Effects
Acephate				*	*	🛒	🛒	🛒	🛒	🛒
Atrazine				*	*	🛒	🛒	🛒	🛒	🛒
Balan				*	*	🛒	🛒	🛒	🛒	🛒
Bayleton				*	*	🛒	🛒	🛒	🛒	🛒
Bendiocarb				*	*	🛒	🛒	🛒	🛒	🛒
Benomyl				*	*	🛒	🛒	🛒	🛒	🛒
Betasan				*	*	🛒	🛒	🛒	🛒	🛒
Carbaryl				*	*	🛒	🛒	🛒	🛒	🛒
Chlorothalonil				*	*	🛒	🛒	🛒	🛒	🛒
Chlorpyrifos				*	*	🛒	🛒	🛒	🛒	🛒
2,4-D				*	*	🛒	🛒	🛒	🛒	🛒
DDVP				*	*	🛒	🛒	🛒	🛒	🛒
DSMA				*	*	🛒	🛒	🛒	🛒	🛒
Dacthal				*	*	🛒	🛒	🛒	🛒	🛒
Diazinon				*	*	🛒	🛒	🛒	🛒	🛒
Dicamba				*	*	🛒	🛒	🛒	🛒	🛒
Diphenamid ✓				🛒	🛒	🛒	🛒	🛒	🛒	🛒
Endothall				🛒	🛒	🛒	🛒	🛒	🛒	🛒
Glyphosate				*	*	🛒	🛒	🛒	🛒	🛒
Isoxaben				*	*	🛒	🛒	🛒	🛒	🛒
MCPA				*	*	🛒	🛒	🛒	🛒	🛒
MCPP				*	*	🛒	🛒	🛒	🛒	🛒
MSMA				*	*	🛒	🛒	🛒	🛒	🛒

Information not available.

Product				Acute Health Advisory				Chronic Health Advisory		
Little to No Risk	Minimal Risk	Caution	Recommended	Flammability	Causticity	Irritants	Allergens and Strong Sensitizers	Carcinogens	Neurotoxins	Reproductive Effects
Malathion				*	*					
Maneb				*	*					
Methoxychlor				*	*					
Oftanol				*	*					
PCNB				*	*					
Pronamide				*	*					
Siduron				*	*					
Sulfur				*	*					
Trichlorfon				*	*					
Triumph				*	*					
Ziram				*	*					

* Information not available.

CHAPTER 4

Pet Supplies

CAT LITTER

Product Types

Gravel; compressed pellets.

Health Advisory

Crystalline silica, found in many cat litter products, is irritating to the lungs. It is also carcinogenic. This hazard is particularly relevant for workers in occupational settings. But while the presence of this carcinogen isn't a major hazard for most cat owners, you may want to use brands that do not contain crystalline silica, or that are dust-free, to avoid even minimal unnecessary pollution to your indoor air.

Cat feces can transmit a disease called toxoplasmosis. Pregnant women are most susceptible and should follow *Safe Use Tips*.

Safe Use Tips

- If your occupation requires you to work around cat litter, a particle mask or respirator is recommended to avoid inhalation of crystalline silica.
- Avoid rubbing eyes after handling cat litter.
- Always wash hands thoroughly after handling used cat litter.
- Pregnant women should not handle cat litter.

Cat Litter

Product				Acute Health Advisory				Chronic Health Advisory		
🛒 Little to No Risk	🛒 Minimal Risk	🛒 Caution	✓ Recommended	Flammability	Causticity	Irritants	Allergens and Strong Sensitizers	Carcinogens	Neurotoxins	Reproductive Effects
Control Cat Litter 33, 107				🛒	🛒	🛒	🛒	●	🛒	🛒
Fresh Step 33				🛒	🛒	🛒	🛒	🛒	🛒	🛒
Jonny Cat 33				🛒	🛒	🛒	🛒	●	🛒	🛒
Jonny Cat Scoop Formula 33				🛒	🛒	🛒	🛒	🛒	🛒	🛒
Kitty Litter Maxx Superior Cat Box Filler ✓				🛒	🛒	🛒	🛒	🛒	🛒	🛒
Litter Green ✓				🛒	🛒	🛒	🛒	🛒	🛒	🛒
Oil-Dri Corp. Cat Litter Natural 33				🛒	🛒	🛒	🛒	●	🛒	🛒
Oil-Dri Corp. Cat Litter Scented 33				🛒	🛒	🛒	🛒	●	🛒	🛒
Scamp Cat Box Filler 33				🛒	🛒	🛒	🛒	🛒	🛒	🛒
Scoop Away Cat Litter 33				🛒	🛒	🛒	🛒	🛒	🛒	🛒
Tidy Cat 3 Cat Box Filler 33				🛒	🛒	🛒	🛒	●	🛒	🛒
Tidy Cat MC Cat Box Filler ✓				🛒	🛒	🛒	🛒	🛒	🛒	🛒
Tidy Scoop Clean-Scooping Cat Filler 33				🛒	🛒	🛒	🛒	●	🛒	🛒

FLEA COLLARS

Product Types

Cotton; plastic.

Health Advisory

We advise owners *not* to use standard flea collars. Collars continuously expose pets to compounds that are toxic to mammals as well as insects. If the pet suffers from a chronic infestation, try improving your pet's diet and skin condition; also, see our flea-control tips on page 125.

Safe Use Tip

Avoid use of standard flea collars on puppies, kittens, and pregnant pets.

Recommended Alternatives

- Herbal-based flea collars (available at health food stores) work well. They do not necessarily kill fleas but they do ward off infestations.
- Apply pyrethrum and pyrethrins to your pet; these are among the most effective, safest pesticides.
- Hire professional exterminators, such as Flea Busters, that use nontoxic flea eradication methods.
- For further flea eradication tips, see *Flea and Tick Products* on page 124.

Flea Collars

Product	Acute Health Advisory				Chronic Health Advisory		
	Flammability	Causticity	Irritants	Allergens and Strong Sensitizers	Carcinogens	Neurotoxins	Reproductive Effects
Bansect Flea and Tick Collar for Dogs 86	🛒	🛒	🛒	🛒	🛒	🛒	🛒
Hartz 2-in-1 Flea & Tick Collars for Puppies, Dogs 145	🛒	🛒	🛒	🛒	🛒	🛒	🛒
Longlife Flea Killing Collar for Cats 43	🛒	🛒	🛒	🛒	🛒	🛒	🛒
Longlife Flea Killing Collar for Dogs 43	🛒	🛒	🛒	🛒	🛒	🛒	🛒
Natural Pet Company Flea Collars ✓	🛒	🛒	🛒	🛒	🛒	🛒	🛒
Pet Agree 5-Month Flea & Tick Collar for Cats 40	🛒	🛒	🛒	🛒	🛒	🛒	🛒
Pet Agree 11-Month Flea & Tick Collar for Dogs 29	🛒	🛒	🛒	🛒	🛒	🛒	🛒
Scratchex Flea & Tick Collar for Cats 29	🛒	🛒	🛒	🛒	🛒	🛒	🛒
Scratchex Flea & Tick Collar for Dogs 29	🛒	🛒	🛒	🛒	🛒	🛒	🛒
Sergeant's Dual Action Flea & Tick Collar 86	🛒	🛒	🛒	🛒	🛒	🛒	🛒
Sergeant's Dual Action Flea & Tick Collar for Cats 86	🛒	🛒	🛒	🛒	🛒	🛒	🛒

Legend: Little to No Risk · Minimal Risk · Caution · Recommended ✓

Product				Acute Health Advisory				Chronic Health Advisory		
🛒 Little to No Risk	🛒 Minimal Risk	🛒 Caution	✓ Recommended	Flammability	Causticity	Irritants	Allergens and Strong Sensitizers	Carcinogens	Neurotoxins	Reproductive Effects
Trader Joe's Herbal Flea Collar for Cats or Dogs ✓				🛒	🛒	🛒	🛒	🛒	🛒	🛒
Wow-Bow Rechargeable Herbal Flea Collar ✓				🛒	🛒	🛒	🛒	🛒	🛒	🛒
Zodiac Clear Flea Collar for Cats 113				🛒	🛒	🛒⬤	🛒⬤	🛒⬤	🛒⬤	🛒
Zodiac Clear Flea Collar for Dogs 113				🛒	🛒	🛒⬤	🛒⬤	🛒⬤	🛒⬤	🛒

FLEA AND TICK PRODUCTS

Product Types

Aerosol; liquid; powder; pump; vapor release.

Health Advisory

Flea and tick dip, spray, and dust pose hazards not only to owners, but also to their pets. The EPA reports that Hartz Mountain Blockade cat, flea, and tick repellent, which contains two powerful pesticides, DEET and fenvalerate, was responsible for over two hundred known dog and cat poisonings, including twenty-six pet deaths during 1987. (The label for Blockade now warns that your pet may experience salivation, tremors, or vomiting on application.) *Consumer Reports* asserts that carbaryl, a common pet flea killer, may cause birth defects among canines. Remember, fleas are persistent and even the most heavy-duty poisons are only temporary measures.

D-Limonene Warning for Cat Owners

Cat owners should be wary of using flea sprays that contain d-limonene. This chemical can cause vomiting, nausea, salivation, muscle tremors, staggering, imbalance, and other symptoms of nervous system poisoning. It is especially hazardous when used on cats.

Chronic

Carcinogens: Bladder cancer in dogs is associated with lifetime exposure to tick and flea dips. Each time a pet is treated with tick and flea dip, substantial human exposure is likely to occur, primarily by absorption through the skin while handling the pet.

Neurotoxins: Dipping pets is likely to cause muscle weakness and tingling of the extremities. Dusting is associated with increased frequency of nausea and headaches. Sponging is associated with increased frequency of convulsions and mental confusion. Caution is recommended.

- Foggers and bombs, particularly those that contain more potent insecticides, unnecessarily expose everyone and everything in the house to the chemical residues. Some contain flammable propellants or solvents, making their use around appliances with pilot lights dangerous. Never use!

Safe Use Tips

- Shampooing *is not* associated with acute symptoms of irritation or neurotoxicity.
- Workers who use protective clothing and equipment and follow protective work practices are not at increased risk for acute and chronic health hazard.
- Always wear a respirator, nonpermeable gloves, and apron.
- After dipping, dusting, or spraying, wash your hands thoroughly, shower immediately, and change your clothing.
- Store products in childproof, vapor-tight areas.
- Always choose the least toxic brands.

Recommended Alternatives

Several excellent brands of flea products are available at supermarkets, health food stores, and pet shops. Seek these out. But also use the following strategies to enhance their effectiveness.

Fleas

- Controlling fleas requires treating the pet and the pet's environment to kill eggs and larvae. We recommend a two-step approach: (1) Remove fleas from pet without poison by using a flea comb. (2) Treat the indoor environment.
- Least toxic soaps, powders, and dips contain diatomaceous earth, silica gel or insecticidal soaps, or pyrethrum/pyrethrins.
- To get rid of larvae and adult fleas around the pet—in bedding, furniture, carpets, and anything else likely to be flea-ridden—vacuum the areas thoroughly and wash the pet's bedding.
- Any substances used safely on pets can be used safely in the surrounding environment. Other useful, relatively nontoxic weapons for ridding

areas of flea larvae include insect growth regulators such as methoprene (Precor) and hydroprene. They work by preventing larvae from turning into adults. The best time to use insect growth regulators is before flea season, sometime in the spring. Diatomaceous earth, made from pre-historic shells, is an abrasive crystal that cuts insects. It is another safe alternative. Dust areas of your house and garden where fleas are likely to hide—carpets, floors, cracks, bookcases, and under kitchen appliances. Pyrethrum/pyrethrins with piperonyl butoxide are highly effective; these should not be confused with the synthetic pyrethroids, such as allethrin, cyfluthrin, fenvalerate, permethrin, phenothrin, resmethrin, and tetramethrin, all of which are far more neurotoxic.

- One of your first strategies for eliminating fleas in the home should be frequent vacuuming using a vacuum with strong suction and easily removable inner container. After vacuuming, immediately remove and seal the bag. Dispose of it or wrap it in a plastic bag and place it in the sun. The extreme heat will kill all the fleas. If this doesn't work, call in a service that uses nontoxic dusts to kill fleas, such as Flea Busters, which has franchises nationwide. Also place a nontoxic herbal flea collar on your pet to repel fleas. They end up jumping on the carpet or floor where they are eventually killed by the nontoxic sodium polyborate powder used by Flea Busters. Call Flea Busters at (800) 765-FLEA (3532).

- Regularly groom your pet with a flea comb, a fine-toothed metal device available at pet stores. Put petroleum or plant-based jelly on the base of the comb's teeth to make the fleas stick and flick any you find into alcohol or soapy water, or dip the whole comb.

- Fleas are attracted to dry, chapped skin. Maintain optimal skin condition by using Dr. Bronner's Almond Oil Castile Soap, which reportedly acts as a repellent, to shampoo your pet. Lemon skin tonic also reportedly works well. The recipe includes thinly slicing 1 whole lemon and adding it to 1 pint of near-boiling water. Steep overnight. Sponge the solution the next day on the pet's skin and let it dry, repeating daily for severe skin problems. Other skin therapies include rubbing in pure aloe vera gel a few times a day until the irritation is gone. Supplements containing primrose oil work well to cure canine dermatitis.

- Herbal repellents used in shampoos, dips, sprays, and flea collars rely on plant oils such as pennyroyal, mint, eucalyptus, citronella, and rosemary. They can be used on animals, carpets, furniture, and yards. They are somewhat effective, but you should not expect them to work against a serious infestation.

- One of the best nontoxic shampoos is known as insecticidal pet soap. Its active ingredients include fatty acid salts and potassium oleate that are completely nontoxic to humans and work on fleas through suffocation. If you leave some soap residue in your pet's coat, it should be effective several days following the initial shampoo. You can also use insecticidal soaps on pet bedding, baseboards, and outdoor areas. The concentrate should be diluted to 1 part soap and 10 parts water.

Ticks

- A flea comb can remove unattached large ticks. The sticky portion of a lint roller can remove small ticks. Remove attached ticks by carefully pulling them out with tweezers or small forceps. If the tick pops or tears, you expose yourself to any disease-carrying organisms in its blood. *Consumer Reports* advises that to prevent tearing the tick, you grasp it as close to its mouth parts as possible, then pull it upward steadily, without jerking. After removing the tick, disinfect the bite with rubbing alcohol or povidone iodine. Don't handle the tick—dispose of it in alcohol or flush it down the drain.
- Ingredients that are effective against fleas—diatomaceous earth, silica gel, insecticidal soap, citrus oils, and pyrethrum/pyrethrins—can be used to repel and kill ticks.
- "The best tick medicine is prevention," says *Consumer Reports*. "Try to avoid tick habitats, especially in peak tick season. If your pet suffers repeatedly from ticks, try to keep it indoors. Clean up brush, wood piles, and other places that harbor rodents, the major source of meals for larval and nymphal ticks."
- While Lyme disease has been reported in all but four states, the disease is concentrated in just eight states—Connecticut, New York, New Jersey, Rhode Island, Delaware, Wisconsin, Maryland, and Pennsylvania.

Ear Mites

- If your pet is shaking its head frequently, or scratching and pawing its ears, it may be suffering from an ear mite infestation. The best antidote for light or moderate infestations is mineral oil, which suffocates the mites. Use an eyedropper and massage the outside of the ear to work it down into the canal. Repeat at four- to five-day intervals for two weeks to eliminate new generations that may have hatched.

Flea and Tick Products

Legend:
🛒 Little to No Risk 🛒 Minimal Risk 🛒 Caution ✓ Recommended

Product	Flammability	Causticity	Irritants	Allergens and Strong Sensitizers	Carcinogens	Neurotoxins	Reproductive Effects
Ace Hardware Pet & Home Flea & Tick Killer 11, 100, 105	🛒	🛒	🛒	🛒	🛒	●	🛒
Beecham Mycodex Pet Shampoo ✓	🛒	🛒	🛒	🛒	🛒	🛒	🛒
Cardinal Flea & Tick Shampoo 118	🛒	🛒	🛒	🛒	🛒	🛒	🛒
Cardinal Shampoo for Cats and Kittens 100, 105	🛒	🛒	🛒	🛒	🛒	●	🛒
Daltek Timed-Release for Cats and Kittens 100, 105	🛒	🛒	🛒	🛒	🛒	●	🛒
Daltek Organic Flea Spray for Cats 45	🛒	🛒	🛒	🛒	🛒	🛒	🛒
Daltek Organic Flea Spray for Dogs 45	🛒	🛒	🛒	🛒	🛒	🛒	🛒
Diatom Dust ✓	🛒	🛒	🛒	🛒	🛒	🛒	🛒
Dr. Bronner's Almond Oil Castile Soap ✓	🛒	🛒	🛒	🛒	🛒	🛒	🛒
EarthSafe Organics Diatomaceous Earth ✓	🛒	🛒	🛒	🛒	🛒	🛒	🛒
Eco Safe Labs Diatom Dust ✓	🛒	🛒	🛒	🛒	🛒	🛒	🛒
Enforcer Flea & Tick Powder for Pets 33, 88, 118	🛒	🛒	🛒	🛒	●	🛒	🛒
Enforcer Flea & Tick Shampoo for Pets 88, 118	🛒	🛒	🛒	🛒	🛒	🛒	🛒
Enforcer Flea & Tick Spray for Dogs 99, 118	🛒	🛒	🛒	🛒	●	●	🛒
Flea Stop Concentrated Shampoo ✓	🛒	🛒	🛒	🛒	🛒	🛒	🛒
Flea Stop Pet Spray 45	🛒	🛒	🛒	🛒	🛒	🛒	🛒
Four Paws Flea and Tick Shampoo for Dogs 100, 118	🛒	🛒	🛒	🛒	🛒	🛒	🛒
Four Paws Flea Foam Dry Bath for Cats 100, 118	🛒	🛒	🛒	🛒	🛒	🛒	🛒

Legend:
- 🛒 *Little to No Risk*
- 🛒 *Minimal Risk*
- 🛒 *Caution*
- ✓ *Recommended*

Product	Acute Health Advisory				Chronic Health Advisory		
	Flammability	Causticity	Irritants	Allergens and Strong Sensitizers	Carcinogens	Neurotoxins	Reproductive Effects
Four Paws Flea Foam Dry Bath for Dogs 100, 118	○	○	◐	○	○	◐	○
Hartz Blockade 38	○	○	●	●	○	●	○
Hartz Cat Flea Powder 123	○	○	●	○	●	○	●
Hartz 2-in-1 Dog Flea Soap 88, 118	○	○	◐	◐	○	○	○
Hartz 2-in-1 Flea & Tick Killer (pump) 88, 118	○	○	○	○	○	○	○
Hartz 2-in-1 Flea & Tick Spray for Dogs (aerosol) 145	○	○	●	○	●	○	○
Hartz 2-in-1 Rid Flea Shampoo 88, 118	○	○	◐	◐	○	○	○
Nala Berry Pet Organics Shampoo and Yard Guard ✓	○	○	○	○	○	○	○
Natra Aloepet Shampoo for Dogs & Cats ✓ 118	○	○	○	◐	○	◐	○
Nature's Gate My Pet Herbal Shampoo ✓	○	○	○	○	○	○	○
Natural Pet Company Citrus Oil Coat Enhancer ✓	○	○	○	○	○	○	○
Natural Pet Company Flea Shampoo & Spray ✓	○	○	○	○	○	○	○
Natural Pet Company Herbal Pet Powder ✓	○	○	○	○	○	○	○
Natural Pet Company Pyrethrum Powder ✓ 118	○	○	○	◐	○	○	○
Natural Pet Company Shoo Repellent Fluid ✓	○	○	○	○	○	○	○
Ortho Pet Flea & Tick Spray Formula III ✓ 118	○	○	○	◐	○	◐	○
Perma-guard Fossil Shell Flour ✓	○	○	○	○	○	○	○
Perma-guard Pet & Animal Insecticide ✓ 118	○	○	○	◐	○	◐	○

Legend (Product risk icons):
🛒 Little to No Risk · 🛒 Minimal Risk · 🛒 Caution · ✓ Recommended

Product	Flammability	Causticity	Irritants	Allergens and Strong Sensitizers	Carcinogens	Neurotoxins	Reproductive Effects
	Acute Health Advisory				Chronic Health Advisory		
Pet Gold Pennyroyal Conditioning Shampoo ✓	Little to No Risk	Caution	Little to No Risk	Caution	Little to No Risk	Caution	Little to No Risk
Pet Gold PFT Plus Flea Spray ✓	Little to No Risk	Caution	Little to No Risk	Caution	Little to No Risk	Caution	Little to No Risk
Petland Flea/Tick Shampoo 100, 118	Little to No Risk	Little to No Risk	Minimal Risk	Caution	Little to No Risk	Minimal Risk	Little to No Risk
Raid Flea Killer 118, 147	Little to No Risk	Little to No Risk	Minimal Risk	Caution	Little to No Risk	Caution	Little to No Risk
Real-Kill Pet & Home Flea Killer 11, 100, 105	Caution	Little to No Risk	Minimal Risk	Caution	Little to No Risk	Little to No Risk	Little to No Risk
Rid-a-Flea Flea & Tick Killer for Dogs & Cats 122	Little to No Risk	Little to No Risk	Little to No Risk	Caution	Little to No Risk	Caution	Little to No Risk
Ringer Flea & Tick Attack ✓ 118	Little to No Risk	Little to No Risk	Little to No Risk	Minimal Risk	Little to No Risk	Little to No Risk	Little to No Risk
Safe Entire Flea & Tick Spray ✓ 118	Little to No Risk	Little to No Risk	Little to No Risk	Minimal Risk	Little to No Risk	Little to No Risk	Little to No Risk
Safe Flea Shampoo ✓	Little to No Risk	Little to No Risk	Little to No Risk	Little to No Risk	Little to No Risk	Little to No Risk	Little to No Risk
Safer Insecticidal Soap ✓	Little to No Risk	Little to No Risk	Little to No Risk	Little to No Risk	Little to No Risk	Little to No Risk	Little to No Risk
Scratchex Powerguard 99	Little to No Risk	Little to No Risk	Minimal Risk	Caution	Little to No Risk	Caution	Little to No Risk
Sergeant's Dog Flea & Tick Spray Pump 28	Little to No Risk	Little to No Risk	Minimal Risk	Caution	Minimal Risk	Caution	Little to No Risk
Sergeant's Flea & Tick Dip 99	Little to No Risk	Little to No Risk	Minimal Risk	Caution	Caution	Caution	Little to No Risk
Sergeant's Flea & Tick Powder for Cats 33, 79, 118	Little to No Risk	Little to No Risk	Caution	Minimal Risk	Caution	Little to No Risk	Caution
Sergeant's Flea & Tick Spray with Coat Conditioner for Cats 113	Little to No Risk	Little to No Risk	Little to No Risk	Little to No Risk	Caution	Caution	Little to No Risk
Sergeant's Skip Flea Shampoo for Dogs 11	Little to No Risk	Little to No Risk	Minimal Risk	Little to No Risk	Little to No Risk	Caution	Little to No Risk
Sudbury Flea & Tick Dip Concentrate for Dogs 99	Minimal Risk	Little to No Risk	Minimal Risk	Caution	Caution	Caution	Little to No Risk
Sulfodene Scratchex Power Dip ✓ 118	Little to No Risk	Little to No Risk	Little to No Risk	Minimal Risk	Little to No Risk	Minimal Risk	Little to No Risk
Victory Veterinary Formula Spray for Dogs 99, 118	Minimal Risk	Little to No Risk	Minimal Risk	Caution	Caution	Caution	Little to No Risk
Zenox Flea & Tick Shampoo for Dogs 118	Minimal Risk	Little to No Risk	Little to No Risk	Minimal Risk	Little to No Risk	Minimal Risk	Little to No Risk

Product				Acute Health Advisory				Chronic Health Advisory		
🛒 Little to No Risk	🛒 Minimal Risk	🛒 Caution	✓ Recommended	Flammability	Causticity	Irritants	Allergens and Strong Sensitizers	Carcinogens	Neurotoxins	Reproductive Effects
Zodiac Flea & Tick Shampoo for Dogs 100, 118				🛒	🛒	🛒	🛒	🛒	🛒	🛒
Zodiac Flea & Tick Shampoo for Dogs & Cats 100, 118				🛒	🛒	🛒	🛒	🛒	🛒	🛒
Zodiac Fleatrol Spray for Cats ✓ 118				🛒	🛒	🛒	🛒	🛒	🛒	🛒
Zodiac Fleatrol Spray for Dogs & Puppies ✓ 118				🛒	🛒	🛒	🛒	🛒	🛒	🛒
Zodiac Pyrethrin Dip for Cats ✓ 118				🛒	🛒	🛒	🛒	🛒	🛒	🛒
Zodiac Pyrethrin Dip for Dogs & Puppies ✓ 118				🛒	🛒	🛒	🛒	🛒	🛒	🛒

Flea and Tick Products for Use Around Pets

Product				Acute Health Advisory				Chronic Health Advisory		
🛒 Little to No Risk	🛒 Minimal Risk	🛒 Caution	✓ Recommended	Flammability	Causticity	Irritants	Allergens and Strong Sensitizers	Carcinogens	Neurotoxins	Reproductive Effects
Black Flag Flea & Tick Killer Rug & Room Spray 105, 147				🛒	🛒	🛒	🛒	🛒	🛒	🛒
Black Flag Flea Ender 99				🛒	🛒	🛒	🛒	🛒	🛒	🛒
Black Flag Flea Killer II 105, 147				🛒	🛒	🛒	🛒	🛒	🛒	🛒
d-Con Flea & Tick Killer II 11, 105				🛒	🛒	🛒	🛒	🛒	🛒	🛒
Diacide Pet Powder ✓ 118				🛒	🛒	🛒	🛒	🛒	🛒	🛒
Enforcer Flea Spray for Carpets & Furniture V 68, 99, 112				🛒	🛒	🛒	🛒	🛒	🛒	🛒
Enforcer Flea Killer for Carpets V 105				🛒	🛒	🛒	🛒	🛒	🛒	🛒
Enforcer Precor Concentrate for Fleas ✓				🛒	🛒	🛒	🛒	🛒	🛒	🛒
Enforcer 7-Month Flea Spray for Homes 99				🛒	🛒	🛒	🛒	🛒	🛒	🛒

Legend:
- 🛒 Little to No Risk
- 🛒 Minimal Risk
- 🛒 Caution
- ✓ Recommended

Product	Flammability	Causticity	Irritants	Allergens and Strong Sensitizers	Carcinogens	Neurotoxins	Reproductive Effects
Gro-Well No Mix Flea & Tick Spray ✓ 118	Little/No	Little/No	Little/No	Minimal	Little/No	Minimal	Little/No
Hartz 2-in-1 Household Flea & Tick Killer 88, 122	Little/No	Little/No	Minimal	Caution	Little/No	Caution	Little/No
Hartz 2-in-1 Time Release Flea & Tick Killer 118	Little/No	Little/No	Little/No	Minimal	Little/No	Minimal	Little/No
Natural Pet Care Company Diatomaceous Earth ✓	Little/No	Little/No	Little/No	Little/No	Little/No	Little/No	Little/No
Natural Pet Care Company Flea Household Spray ✓	Little/No	Little/No	Little/No	Little/No	Little/No	Little/No	Little/No
Natural Pet Care Company Precor ✓	Little/No	Little/No	Little/No	Little/No	Little/No	Little/No	Little/No
Natural Pet Care Company Ultra Carpet Powder ✓ 118	Little/No	Little/No	Little/No	Minimal	Little/No	Minimal	Little/No
Ortho Flea-B-Gone Flea Killer Formula II 105, 147	Little/No	Little/No	Minimal	Caution	Little/No	Minimal	Little/No
Ortho Insecticidal Soap ✓	Little/No	Little/No	Little/No	Little/No	Little/No	Little/No	Little/No
Perma-guard Household Insecticide 118	Little/No	Little/No	Little/No	Minimal	Little/No	Little/No	Little/No
Raid Flea Killer Plus 99, 118, 147	Little/No	Little/No	Minimal	Caution	Caution	Caution	Little/No
Raid House & Garden Formula 8 11, 100, 122	Little/No	Little/No	Minimal	Caution	Little/No	Caution	Little/No
Raid Multi-Bug Killer Formula D39 11, 122	Little/No	Little/No	Minimal	Caution	Little/No	Minimal	Little/No
Revenge Home Exterminator Kit 100, 118	Little/No	Little/No	Minimal	Little/No	Little/No	Little/No	Little/No
Safer Flea & Tick Attac Premuse Spray 118	Little/No	Little/No	Little/No	Minimal	Little/No	Little/No	Little/No
Safer Indoor Flea Guard RTU ✓	Little/No	Little/No	Little/No	Little/No	Little/No	Little/No	Little/No
Sergeant's Rug Patrol 11, 105	Little/No	Little/No	Minimal	Caution	Little/No	Caution	Little/No
Zodiac Fleatrol Indoor Concentrate ✓	Little/No	Little/No	Little/No	Minimal	Little/No	Little/No	Little/No
Zodiac Fleatrol Carpet Spray 100, 118	Little/No	Little/No	Minimal	Minimal	Little/No	Minimal	Little/No
Zodiac Fleatrol Indoor Spray 99, 100	Little/No	Little/No	Minimal	Minimal	Caution	Caution	Little/No

Foggers

Product				Acute Health Advisory				Chronic Health Advisory		
🛒 Little to No Risk	🛒 Minimal Risk	🛒 Caution	✓ Recommended	Flammability	Causticity	Irritants	Allergens and Strong Sensitizers	Carcinogens	Neurotoxins	Reproductive Effects
Black Flag Adult Flea Killer Indoor Step 2 100, 105, 147				🛒	🛒	🛒	🛒	🛒	🛒	🛒
Black Flag Automatic Room 100, 118				🛒	🛒	🛒	🛒	🛒	🛒	🛒
Black Flag Flea Killer System 100, 105, 147				🛒	🛒	🛒	🛒	🛒	🛒	🛒
Black Flag Large Area Automatic Room 100, 105, 147				🛒	🛒	🛒	🛒	🛒	🛒	🛒
Black Flag Pre-Adult Flea Killer ✓				🛒	🛒	🛒	🛒	🛒	🛒	🛒
Black Flag Roach 100, 118				🛒	🛒	🛒	🛒	🛒	🛒	🛒
Enforcer Adult & Pre-adult Flea Fogger 100, 105, 147				🛒	🛒	🛒	🛒	🛒	🛒	🛒
Enforcer Flea Fogger with Precor 112, 151				🛒	🛒	🛒	🛒	🛒	🛒	🛒
Four Paws Fast Killing Indoor 100, 147				🛒	🛒	🛒	🛒	🛒	🛒	🛒
Holiday Household Insect 58				🛒	🛒	🛒	🛒	🛒	🛒	🛒
Holiday Household Insect New Pine Scent 105, 147				🛒	🛒	🛒	🛒	🛒	🛒	🛒
Ortho Hi-Power Indoor Insect Formula IV 58, 118				🛒	🛒	🛒	🛒	🛒	🛒	🛒
Raid 100, 118				🛒	🛒	🛒	🛒	🛒	🛒	🛒
Raid Max Fogger 36, 68, 70, 88, 112, 151				🛒	🛒	🛒	🛒	🛒	🛒	🛒
Raid Fumigator 27, 99				🛒	🛒	🛒	🛒	🛒	🛒	🛒
Rid-A-Bug Flea and Roach Fogger 43				🛒	🛒	🛒	🛒	🛒	🛒	🛒
Sergeant's Indoor Fogger 11, 58, 100, 151				🛒	🛒	🛒	🛒	🛒	🛒	🛒
Spectracide Professional Flea Control ✓				🛒	🛒	🛒	🛒	🛒	🛒	🛒
Zodiac House & Kennel 99				🛒	🛒	🛒	🛒	🛒	🛒	🛒
Zodiac Fleatrol 99				🛒	🛒	🛒	🛒	🛒	🛒	🛒
Zoecon Improved Strike Flea Ender Fogger 43				🛒	🛒	🛒	🛒	🛒	🛒	🛒

CHAPTER 5

Auto Products

ANTIFREEZE AND COOLANTS

Product Type

Liquid.

Safe Use Tips

- Only trained mechanics should add antifreeze.
- If you choose to add antifreeze to your own car, be sure to wear impermeable gloves, goggles, and impermeable clothing.
- If antifreeze is swallowed, induce vomiting; immediately take victim to the hospital.
- Keep antifreeze and coolants locked away from children and pets. The sweet taste of ethylene glycol makes it a poisoning threat especially to children and pets, who may be tempted to taste it. In addition, the Humane Society estimates that tens of thousands of companion animals and wildlife die each year from ethylene glycol poisoning. Half of all poisoning deaths of dogs and cats are associated with ethylene glycol ingestion.

Recommended Alternatives

You can make an important switch in your choice of antifreeze that could save pets' lives and help the environment. Rather than using ethylene glycol–based antifreeze, which poses neurotoxic and reproductive risks, many manufacturers now produce antifreeze with propylene glycol, a milder ingredient that has been proven safe enough for many cosmetic formulations. Not only is propylene glycol far less toxic if accidentally ingested, but it also appears to last two to three times longer in automotive use than ethylene glycol. Look on the charts for these safer brands.

Antifreeze and Coolants

Product				Acute Health Advisory				Chronic Health Advisory		
🛒 Little to No Risk	🛒 Minimal Risk	🛒 Caution	✓ Recommended	Flammability	Causticity	Irritants	Allergens and Strong Sensitizers	Carcinogens	Neurotoxins	Reproductive Effects
Antifreeze (Generic) 55				Little to No Risk	Minimal Risk	Caution	Minimal Risk	Minimal Risk	Caution	Caution
Prestone Advanced Formula Anti-freeze & Coolant 55				Little to No Risk	Minimal Risk	Caution	Minimal Risk	Minimal Risk	Caution	Caution
Radiator Specialty Company Anti-freeze/ Coolant Booster 55				Minimal Risk	Minimal Risk	Caution	Minimal Risk	Minimal Risk	Minimal Risk	Caution
Radiator Specialty Company Liquid Kool Engine Coolant 55				Minimal Risk	Minimal Risk	Caution	Minimal Risk	Minimal Risk	Minimal Risk	Caution
Sierra ✓				Minimal Risk	Minimal Risk	Minimal Risk	Minimal Risk	Minimal Risk	Minimal Risk	Minimal Risk
Sta-Clean Antifreeze ✓				Minimal Risk	Minimal Risk	Minimal Risk	Minimal Risk	Minimal Risk	Minimal Risk	Minimal Risk
Trak Anti-freeze & Coolant 55				Little to No Risk	Minimal Risk	Caution	Minimal Risk	Minimal Risk	Caution	Caution

BUG, INSECT, AND TAR REMOVERS

Product Types

Aerosol; liquid.

Safe Use Tips

- Wear impermeable gloves.
- Use in well-ventilated area, never in a garage.
- Wear a respirator if your job requires you to frequently use bug, insect, and tar removers.

Recommended Alternatives

- Saturate a rag with food-grade raw linseed oil; rub until the tar has been removed. Or use Auro Organics' boiled linseed oil, which will dry faster than typical food grades.
- Saturate a rag with a plant-based thinner and rub until tar is removed. See *Thinners* on page 103 for our recommendations.

Bug, Insect, and Tar Removers

Product	Acute Health Advisory				Chronic Health Advisory		
	Flammability	Causticity	Irritants	Allergens and Strong Sensitizers	Carcinogens	Neurotoxins	Reproductive Effects
Armor All No. "7" Tar & Bug Remover 77,161	●	●	●	●	●	●	●
Kit Bug Out ✓	●	●	●	●	●	●	●
Radiator Specialty Company Tar & Bug Remover (aerosol) 7, 52	●	●	●	●	●	●	●
Radiator Specialty Company Tar & Bug Remover (liquid) 7, 52	●	●	●	●	●	●	●

Legend: Little to No Risk · Minimal Risk · Caution · Recommended (✓)

CAR CHROME POLISHES

Product Types

Liquid; paste.

Safe Use Tips

- Polish outdoors or with garage door open.
- Wear nonpermeable gloves.
- Store in childproof area.

Recommended Alternatives

From your nontoxic cleaning supplies, you can find plenty of ways to shine chrome without resorting to commercial products.

- One of the best and simplest ways to shine the chrome of your car is to combine ¹/₄ cup of baking soda with enough water to make a paste. Use a sponge saturated with the paste and rub the chrome. The abrasiveness of the baking soda will shine your chrome without scratching. Rinse with warm water and polish.

- Polish chrome by rubbing with a cotton cloth saturated with lemon juice.
- Distilled white vinegar also will work. Saturate your sponge with ¹/₄ cup of vinegar and rub the chrome until it is clean.

Car Chrome Polishes

Product				Acute Health Advisory				Chronic Health Advisory		
🛒 Little to No Risk	🛒 Minimal Risk	🛒 Caution	✓ Recommended	Flammability	Causticity	Irritants	Allergens and Strong Sensitizers	Carcinogens	Neurotoxins	Reproductive Effects
Armor All No. "7" Chrome Polish & Cleaner 77, 124				🛒	🛒	🛒	🛒	🛒	🛒	🛒
Kit Chrome Polish ✓ 14, 140				🛒	🛒	🛒	🛒	🛒	🛒	🛒
Turtle Wax Chrome Polish 100, 156				🛒	🛒	🛒	🛒	🛒	🛒	🛒

DRIVEWAY AND GARAGE FLOOR CLEANERS

Product Type

Liquid.

Safe Use Tip

Always wear gloves and a respirator; even the safest products contain undesirable ingredients capable of causing damage to internal organs with prolonged and repeated exposure.

Driveway and Garage Floor Cleaners

Product				Acute Health Advisory				Chronic Health Advisory		
🛒 Little to No Risk	🛒 Minimal Risk	🛒 Caution	✓ Recommended	Flammability	Causticity	Irritants	Allergens and Strong Sensitizers	Carcinogens	Neurotoxins	Reproductive Effects
Naturally Yours Degreaser ✓				🛒	🛒	🛒	🛒	🛒	🛒	🛒
Parks Driveway Cleaner 114, 133				🛒	🛒	🛒	🛒	🛒	🛒	🛒

Product				Acute Health Advisory				Chronic Health Advisory		
Little to No Risk	Minimal Risk	Caution	Recommended ✓	Flammability	Causticity	Irritants	Allergens and Strong Sensitizers	Carcinogens	Neurotoxins	Reproductive Effects
Radiator Specialty Company General Purpose Cleaner 7, 23, 52				🛒	🛒	🛒	🛒	🛒	🛒	🛒
Radiator Specialty Co. Liquid Concentrated Multi-Surface Cleaner 23, 71				🛒	🛒	🛒	🛒	🛒	🛒	🛒
Simple Green 23				🛒	🛒	🛒	🛒	🛒	🛒	🛒
Swab Concrete Cleaner 52, 133				🛒	🛒	🛒	🛒	🛒	🛒	🛒
Swab Concrete Spot Cleaner 23, 52, 100				🛒	🛒	🛒	🛒	🛒	🛒	🛒

INTERIOR AND EXTERIOR CLEANERS AND PROTECTANTS

Product Types

Aerosol; pump.

Health Advisory

Beware of products containing formaldehyde. Once you use it, you will be breathing this chemical every time you get in the car.

Safe Use Tips

- Open all windows.
- Allow the car to air out before driving.
- Wear nonpermeable gloves.

Recommended Alternatives

You do not need to buy commercial products for making your car shine. You can use basic cleaning supplies such as washing soda for cleaning the interior of your car.

- The basic formula for interior car cleaning is to dissolve 1 to 2 teaspoons of washing soda with 1 cup of boiling water. Use a sponge dipped in this cleaning solution and wipe off vinyl upholstery.
- Some chemically sensitive people may find the fumes of new vinyl irritating. AFM Vinyl Block helps prevent emission of these fumes.

Interior and Exterior Cleaners and Protectants

Legend for ratings: ○ = Little to No Risk · ◐ = Minimal Risk · ● = Caution · ✓ = Recommended

Product	Flammability	Causticity	Irritants	Allergens and Strong Sensitizers	Carcinogens	Neurotoxins	Reproductive Effects
	Acute Health Advisory				Chronic Health Advisory		
Armor All Leather Care ✓ 125	○	○	○	○	○	○	○
Formula 1 Premium Leather Conditioner 59	○	○	●	●	●	●	○
Kit Carpet Clean Trigger Spray ✓ 49, 114	○	○	◐	○	○	○	○
Kit Lustre Rich Creme Protectant Pump 59	○	○	●	●	●	●	○
Kit Velour Plus Trigger Spray ✓ 49	○	○	◐	○	○	○	○
K&W Products Leather/Vinyl Spray 23, 59, 71, 83	○	○	○	●	●	●	○
K&W Products Tannery Wash/Wax 51, 120	○	●	●	◐	◐	◐	○
Meguiar's Intensive Protectant ✓	○	○	○	○	○	○	○
Radiator Specialty Company Carpet Shampoo (aerosol) 68, 114	◐	○	●	○	○	○	○
Radiator Specialty Company Life for Vinyl, Leather and Rubber ✓	○	○	◐	○	○	○	○
Radiator Specialty Company Silicone Tire Shine Aerosol 23, 151	○	○	●	○	◐	●	○
Radiator Specialty Company Tire White Whitewall Tire Cleaner (aerosol) 7, 31, 68, 100, 112	○	○	●	○	○	◐	○
Radiator Specialty Company Tire White Whitewall Tire Cleaner (liquid) 23, 131, 135	●	●	●	○	○	◐	○
Simoniz Tuff Stuff Trigger Pump 23, 133, 142	○	○	◐	○	○	◐	○
STP Son of a Gun Concentrated Protectant ✓ 125	○	○	◐	○	○	○	○
Turtle Wax Carpet Cleaner & Protector (foam aerosol) ✓ 68, 114	◐	○	◐	○	○	○	○
Turtle Wax Foaming Carpet & Upholstery Cleaner (foam aerosol) 23	◐	○	◐	○	○	◐	○

Product				Acute Health Advisory				Chronic Health Advisory		
🛒 Little to No Risk	🛒 Minimal Risk	🛒 Caution	✓ Recommended	Flammability	Causticity	Irritants	Allergens and Strong Sensitizers	Carcinogens	Neurotoxins	Reproductive Effects
Turtle Wax Velour Upholstery Cleaner (foam aerosol) ✓ *68, 112, 114*				🛒	🛒	🛒	🛒	🛒	🛒	🛒
Turtle Wax Vinyl-Fabric Upholstery Cleaner (foam aerosol) ✓ *68, 100, 112*				🛒	🛒	🛒	🛒	🛒	🛒	🛒

WASHES

Product Types

Gel; liquid; powder.

Safe Use Tip

Wear impermeable gloves, as some products contain detergents that may be contaminated with carcinogens such as 1,4-dioxane, or they may contain artificial colors, some of which are also carcinogenic.

Recommended Alternative

Instead of buying commercial formulas, you can make your own car wash with basic cleaning materials on hand in your home. All you need is one of our recommended liquid soaps or dishwashing detergents and a bucket of warm water. Mix $1/4$ to $1/2$ cup of a liquid soap or dishwashing detergent into a bucket of warm water. Swirl to make suds. Use as you would a commercial car wash.

Washes

Product				Acute Health Advisory				Chronic Health Advisory		
🛒 Little to No Risk	🛒 Minimal Risk	🛒 Caution	✓ Recommended	Flammability	Causticity	Irritants	Allergens and Strong Sensitizers	Carcinogens	Neurotoxins	Reproductive Effects
Armor All Car Wash Concentrate *44*				🛒	🛒	🛒	🛒	🛒	🛒	🛒
Kit Super Wash Car Wash ✓				🛒	🛒	🛒	🛒	🛒	🛒	🛒
Meguiar's Deep Crystal Soft Wash Gel ✓				🛒	🛒	🛒	🛒	🛒	🛒	🛒

Product				Acute Health Advisory				Chronic Health Advisory		
🛒 Little to No Risk	🛒 Minimal Risk	🛒 Caution	✓ Recommended	Flammability	Causticity	Irritants	Allergens and Strong Sensitizers	Carcinogens	Neurotoxins	Reproductive Effects
Radiator Specialty Company Liquid Car Wash ✓				🛒	🛒	🛒	🛒	🛒	🛒	🛒
Radiator Specialty Company Powdered Car Wash ✓				🛒	🛒	🛒	🛒	🛒	🛒	🛒
Rain Dance Car Wash Concentrate				🛒	🛒	🛒	🛒	🛒	🛒	🛒
Rain Dance Wash & Wax Cleaning Compound 51, 119				🛒	🛒	🛒	🛒	🛒	🛒	🛒
Simoniz Super Blue Car Wash 23, 71, 153				🛒	🛒	🛒	🛒	🛒	🛒	🛒
Turtle Wax Liquid Crystal Ultimate Car Wash ✓				🛒	🛒	🛒	🛒	🛒	🛒	🛒
Westley's Concentrate Car Wash ✓				🛒	🛒	🛒	🛒	🛒	🛒	🛒

CAR WAXES

Product Types

Gel; liquid; paste.

Safe Use Tips

- Work in well-ventilated area, preferably outdoors.
- Wear nonpermeable neoprene or nitrile gloves, especially if you frequently wax your car.

Car Waxes

Product				Acute Health Advisory				Chronic Health Advisory		
🛒 Little to No Risk	🛒 Minimal Risk	🛒 Caution	✓ Recommended	Flammability	Causticity	Irritants	Allergens and Strong Sensitizers	Carcinogens	Neurotoxins	Reproductive Effects
Armor All Liquid Car Wax 72				🛒	🛒	🛒	🛒	🛒	🛒	🛒
Auri Polish 95, 140, 161				🛒	🛒	🛒	🛒	🛒	🛒	🛒

Legend:
- 🛒 Little to No Risk
- 🛒 Minimal Risk
- 🛒 Caution
- ✓ Recommended

Product	Acute Health Advisory				Chronic Health Advisory		
	Flammability	Causticity	Irritants	Allergens and Strong Sensitizers	Carcinogens	Neurotoxins	Reproductive Effects
Formula 1 Premium Creme Wax 59, 85, 140	Little	Minimal	Caution	Caution	Caution	Caution	Little
Formula I Premium Paste Wax 59, 85, 140	Little	Minimal	Caution	Caution	Caution	Caution	Little
Formula 1 Show Car Glaze ✓ 70	Little	Minimal	Little	Minimal	Little	Minimal	Little
Kit Creme Car Wax 85, 140	Little	Minimal	Caution	Minimal	Little	Minimal	Little
Kit Scratch Out ✓	Little	Minimal	Little	Minimal	Little	Little	Little
Kit Speed Shine ✓ 70, 71	Little	Minimal	Minimal	Minimal	Little	Little	Little
Liquid Lustre ✓ 7	Little	Minimal	Little	Minimal	Little	Little	Little
Meguiar's Car Cleaner Wax-Liquid 5, 101	Little	Minimal	Little	Minimal	Little	Little	Little
Meguiar's Deep Crystal Carnauba Paste Wax 5	Little	Minimal	Little	Minimal	Little	Little	Little
Meguiar's Mirror Glaze Professional High-Tech Cleaner 5, 87	Little	Minimal	Little	Minimal	Little	Little	Caution
Meguiar's Mirror Glaze Professional Hi-Tech Yellow Wax 5, 103	Little	Minimal	Little	Minimal	Little	Caution	Little
Meguiar's Professional Sealer & Resealer Glaze 5, 159	Little	Minimal	Little	Minimal	Little	Little	Little
Quad 14, 23, 85, 140	Caution	Minimal	Caution	Minimal	Little	Little	Little
Rain Dance Liquid Car Wax 8, 72, 85	Caution	Minimal	Caution	Minimal	Little	Little	Little
Rain Dance Paste Car Wax 8, 72, 85	Caution	Minimal	Caution	Minimal	Little	Little	Little
Simoniz Ultimate Liquid Gloss Car Wax 7, 12, 72, 76	Little	Minimal	Little	Minimal	Little	Little	Little
Simoniz Ultimate Paste Gloss Car Wax 7, 12, 72, 76	Little	Minimal	Little	Minimal	Little	Little	Little
Turtle Wax Clear Guard ✓ 100	Little	Minimal	Little	Minimal	Little	Little	Little
Turtle Wax Heavy Duty Rubbing Compound ✓ 100	Little	Minimal	Little	Minimal	Little	Little	Little
Turtle Wax Liquid Crystal 55, 100	Little	Minimal	Little	Minimal	Little	Caution	Caution
Turtle Wax Liquid Crystal Creme 14, 55, 100	Little	Minimal	Little	Minimal	Little	Caution	Caution

Product				Acute Health Advisory				Chronic Health Advisory		
Little to No Risk	Minimal Risk	Caution	Recommended	Flammability	Causticity	Irritants	Allergens and Strong Sensitizers	Carcinogens	Neurotoxins	Reproductive Effects
Turtle Wax Plus Liquid ✓ 100				🛒	🛒	🛒	🛒	🛒	🛒	🛒
Turtle Wax Plus Paste Wax ✓ 14, 100				🛒	🛒	🛒	🛒	🛒	🛒	🛒
Turtle Wax Super Hard Shell Liquid ✓ 100				🛒	🛒	🛒	🛒	🛒	🛒	🛒
Turtle Wax Super Hard Shell Paste ✓ 100				🛒	🛒	🛒	🛒	🛒	🛒	🛒
Turtle Wax White Polishing Compound ✓ 100, 131				🛒	🛒	🛒	🛒	🛒	🛒	🛒

CHAPTER 6

Art and Craft Supplies

Product Types

Liquid; gel; aerosol.

Health Advisory

Art and craft materials are often inadequately labeled. Manufacturers of art and craft materials that contain toxic chemicals are required to provide consumers with warnings of health dangers. However, a 1991 study found that only 36 percent of 150 art products surveyed included a statement on the label disclosing hazardous ingredients, making it impossible for consumers to determine whether the product has been checked for toxic chemicals.

Federal law requires art and craft products containing substances that can cause chronic illnesses to have warning labels. As of November 1990, art and craft supplies that pose long-term health risks must have labels that include a warning statement of the hazard, such as CANCER AGENT EXPOSURE MAY PRODUCE CANCER; identification of the hazardous ingredients; guidelines for safe use, such as AVOID INHALATION/INGESTION/SKIN CONTACT or USE NIOSH-CERTIFIED MASK FOR DUSTS/MISTS/FUMES; and the name, address, and telephone number of the manufacturer or importer.

For very thorough, updated lists of the names of safe as well as hazardous art products, write the Art and Craft Materials Institute, 100 Boylston Street, Suite 1050, Boston, MA 02116; or call (617) 426-6400.

Acute

Ceramics: produce dusts such as silica (from clay), talc, and asbestos (from white clay) that can irritate the respiratory tract and cause long-term lung damage such as mesothelioma, silicosis, and asbestosis. Kiln exhaust containing carbon monoxide also poses an acute poisoning hazard that can be fatal.

Metal working: often involves work with cadmium-containing silvery solders, which are used especially with jewelry making, metal sculptures, silver brazing, soldering, and welding. Inhalation or ingestion can result in severe chronic lung and kidney damage, and acute, severe respiratory tract irritation, lung damage, and even death.

Painting solvents: Contained in turpentine and permanent markers and used in oil painting and silk screening, painting solvents have been associated with skin disease. Prolonged or repeated exposure can cause dermatitis.

Plastics: generate dusts such as fiberglass dust and asbestos, which can cause long-term lung damage. Use such products with caution.

Silk screen solvents: have been associated with skin disease. Use such products with caution.

Solvents: Used in a wide range of art supplies, solvents not only can dry skin; many artists using oil paints, turpentine, and other solvents in poorly ventilated areas find themselves with chronic colds. Their physician may misdiagnose them as having "chronic bronchitis" when in fact they are exhibiting symptoms of overexposure to solvents. The cause of their illness remains undetected. Thus, their "cold" can progress to greater difficulty breathing.

Chronic

Carcinogens: In a death certificate study of nearly sixteen hundred professional artists, researchers found significantly elevated risks of leukemia and cancer of the bladder, colon, rectum, kidney, and brain among white male artists. Among female artists studied, excess numbers of deaths because of cancer of the rectum, lung, and breast were noted. Results from a case-control interview study by researchers of bladder cancer patients found further support for an association between bladder cancer and employment as an artistic painter. Not surprisingly, some of the nation's leading brands of oil paints contain carcinogenic ingredients such as PCBs and hexachlorobenzene. We strongly recommend avoiding these products.

Ceramics: This work involves the use of heavy metals such as arsenic, cadmium, and lead, which are used in glazes. They are carcinogenic. Use products containing these materials with caution.

Painting: can expose the artist to crystalline silica. Silica, safe in paints when wet, is carcinogenic and dangerous when the artist inhales it as in scraping and sanding. Lead and cadmium, also found in paints, are carcinogenic. Methylene chloride, used in spray paints as well as in removers and strippers, is carcinogenic. Use products containing these materials with caution.

Plastics: expose artists to polymers such as polyvinyl chloride (PVC), which contains vinyl chloride. Vinyl chloride is carcinogenic. Other plastic products may expose the artist to di(2-ethylhexyl)phthalate, which is carcinogenic.

Silk screen: artists may be exposed to heavy metals, including chromium and lead, which are carcinogenic.

Neurotoxins

Ceramics: Kiln exhaust contains carbon monoxide, which can cause acute neurotoxic effects leading to death, as well as chronic neurotoxicity.

Metal working and welding: exposes people to gases such as carbon monoxide and unburned acetylene phosgene, which can cause acute and fatal nervous system poisoning leading to death, as well as chronic neurotoxicity.

Paint solvents: can cause long-term organic brain damage. Older and even some newer paints may contain mercury antifungal agents that can cause nervous system damage. Solvents contained in turpentine and kerosene and used in permanent markers and oil paints have been associated with nervous system damage.

Silk screen: chemicals contained in inks, lacquer thinners, and screen washes include solvents such as methyl ethyl ketone and toluene, which are neurotoxic.

Reproductive Toxins

Ceramics: exposes people to glazes containing lead, which is teratogenic.

Paints: expose people to ethylene glycol, which is a reproductive toxin. Pigments in paints including lead are teratogenic. Older paints contain mercury antifungal agents, which are also teratogenic.

Safe Use Tips

- Know the hazards of the materials you are working with. Read the labels, request Material Safety Data Sheets on all products from the product manufacturer, and know what precautions, safety gear, and cleanup procedures are advised.
- Use the safest materials and procedures possible. Stay current on the new developments in your art or craft; safer, less toxic alternatives are being devised for many activities.
- Use good ventilation at all times. Local exhaust is the best, such as a hood or spray booth that vents to the outside. Next best is to use exhaust fans that pull the contaminated air away from you and exhaust it outside. An air-conditioning system is not adequate, because it recirculates most of the

air. An open window does not usually supply adequate ventilation; toxic materials may be blown back on your face.

- Wear a respirator. Artists should become used to wearing a respirator, which dramatically purifies the air.
- Use good hygiene and housekeeping. Separate work and living areas; avoid eating, drinking, or smoking in the work area. Do not store materials in food containers. Wash and change clothes after working. Wet mop or vacuum to clean up dust.
- For more information on safety in the arts also write:

Center for Safety in the Arts
5 Beekman Street, Suite 1030
New York, NY 10038

Arts, Crafts, and Theater Safety
181 Thompson Street, #23
New York, NY 10012

ART MATERIALS RECOMMENDED ESPECIALLY FOR CHILDREN

Do Not Use	Substitute
Dusts and Powders	
1. Clay in dry form. Powder clay, which is easily inhaled, contains free silica and possible asbestos. Do not sand dry clay pieces or do other dust-producing activities.	1. Order talc-free, premixed clay. Wet mop or sponge surfaces thoroughly after using clay.
2. Ceramic glazes or copper enamels.	2. Use water-based paints instead of glazes. Teachers may waterproof pieces with shellac or varnish.
3. Cold water, fiber-reactive dyes, or other commercial dyes.	3. Use vegetable and plant dyes (e.g., onionskins, tea, flowers) and food dyes.
4. Instant papier mâchés create inhalable dusts and some tempera colors contain toxic pigments and preservatives.	4. Make papier mâché from black and white newspaper and library or white paste.

ART MATERIALS RECOMMENDED ESPECIALLY FOR CHILDREN
(continued)

Do Not Use	Substitute
5. Powdered tempera colors create inhalable dusts and some tempera colors contain toxic pigments and preservatives.	5. Use liquid paints or paints the teacher premixes.
6. Pastels or chalks that create dusts.	6. Use crayons, oil pastels, or dustless chalks.

Solvents

Do Not Use	Substitute
1. Solvents (e.g., turpentine, toluene, rubber cement, thinner) and solvent-containing materials such as inks, alkyd paints, rubber cement.	1. Use water-based products only.
2. Solvent-based silk screen and other printing inks.	2. Use water-based silk screen inks, block printing, or stencil inks containing safe pigments.
3. Aerosol sprays.	3. Use water-based paints with brushes or spatter techniques.
4. Epoxy, instant glue, airplane glue, or other solvent-based adhesives	4. Use white glue or school paste.
5. Permanent felt tip markers that may contain toluene or other toxic solvents.	5. Use only watercolor markers.

Toxic Metals

Do Not Use	Substitute
1. Stained-glass projects using lead, solder, flux.	1. Use colored cellophane and black paper to simulate lead.
2. Arsenic, cadmium, chrome, mercury, lead, manganese, or other toxic metals that may occur in pigments, metal filings, metal enamels, metal casting.	2. Get ingredient information from Material Safety Data Sheets on products that are uncertified to be certain they are free of toxic metals.

Recommended Alternatives

- *Ceramics:* Instead of glazes containing heavy metals such as lead, chromium, and cadmium, use lead-free and talc-free glazes. Be sure to work "wet," use premixed glazes, wear a dust mask, and vent the kiln to the outside.
- *Jewelry:* Eliminate the use of cadmium-based solders. Use higher-melting silver solders or the new lower-melting cadmium-free silver solders. Do not buy concentrated pickling solutions that must then be diluted with water. To avoid concentrated acids, buy pickling solutions in dilute form or use Sparex. The pickling bath should be vented to the outside.
- *Paints:* Instead of using solvent-based paints, use water-based paints. Use a respirator. Avoid spray paints containing methylene chloride. Be sure to wear a respirator when using any spray paints whatsoever.

Art and Craft Supplies

Product ratings legend: 🛒 *Little to No Risk*, 🛒 *Minimal Risk*, 🛒 *Caution*, ✔ *Recommended*

Product	Flammability	Causticity	Irritants	Allergens and Strong Sensitizers	Carcinogens	Neurotoxins	Reproductive Effects
Alexander Oil Colors (all) ✔	🛒	🛒	🛒	🛒	🛒	🛒	🛒
Bond 527 Multi-Purpose Cement 1	*	*	🛒	🛒	🛒	⬤	🛒
Columbia Artists Rubber Cement 63	*	*	🛒	🛒	🛒	⬤	🛒
Copper Topper Antiquing Solution 14, 23	*	*	🛒	🛒	🛒	🛒	🛒
Decocolor Opaque Paint Marker 161	*	*	🛒	🛒	🛒	🛒	⬤
Denatured Alcohol Solvent 4, 78	⬤	*	🛒	🛒	🛒	🛒	🛒
Design Art Marker 161	*	*	🛒	🛒	🛒	⬤	⬤
Duco Cement 1	*	*	🛒	🛒	🛒	🛒	🛒
E-6000 Adhesive Sealant 150, 158	*	*	🛒	🛒	🛒	⬤	🛒
Envirospray Acrylic Water-Based Spray Paint 23	*	*	🛒	🛒	🛒	🛒	🛒
Folk Art Mud 33, 54, 100	*	*	🛒	🛒	⬤	⬤	⬤
Glitter Magic 150	*	*	🛒	🛒	🛒	⬤	⬤
Gum Spirits of Turpentine 156	*	*	🛒	⬤	🛒	🛒	🛒

* Information not available.

Product				Flammability	Causticity	Irritants	Allergens and Strong Sensitizers	Carcinogens	Neurotoxins	Reproductive Effects
Little to No Risk	Minimal Risk	Caution	Recommended							
Grumbacher Artist's Oil Colors (all) 24, 30, 62				⊞	⊞	⊞	⊞	⊞	⊞	⊞
Grumbacher Gainsborough Oil Paints (all) 19, 108				⊞	⊞	⊞	⊞	⊞	⊞	⊞
Grumbacher Pretested Artists' Oil Colors (all) 24, 30, 73				⊞	⊞	⊞	⊞	⊞	⊞	⊞
Liquitex Artists Rectified Turpentine 156				*	*	⊞	⊞	⊞	⊞	⊞
Mostenbocker Lift-Off Aerosol Cleaner 151, 161				*	*	⊞	⊞	⊞	⊞	⊞
Nankee Gum Turpentine 156				*	*	⊞	⊞	⊞	⊞	⊞
Odorless Turpenoid 100				*	*	⊞	⊞	⊞	⊞	⊞
PENTEL Correction Pen (red) 151				*	*	⊞	⊞	⊞	⊞	⊞
Sunnyside Pure Gum Spirits of Turpentine 156				*	*	⊞	⊞	⊞	⊞	⊞
Tru Bond Rubber Adhesive 100, 150				*	*	⊞	⊞	⊞	⊞	⊞
Val-Oil 100				*	*	⊞	⊞	⊞	⊞	⊞
Z-Pro Water-Based Spray Paint 23				*	*	⊞	⊞	⊞	⊞	⊞

* Information not available.

CHAPTER 7

Miscellany

AIR FILTERS

Apart from the air pollution from the outside, the obvious way to avoid indoor air pollution is to avoid introducing hazardous products into your home or office. The air quality of indoor spaces can be improved through the use of home air filters. Air contaminants include particulates and dust, microorganisms, and volatile organic chemicals. Particulates and dust often carry microorganisms; therefore, a filter that will remove particulates will also remove microorganisms.

HEPA Filters

One of the best kinds of home air filters to buy combines a high-efficiency particle air (HEPA) filter with a carbon filter made from granular coconut shell. The HEPA filter is able to remove from 95 percent to 99 percent of particulates from the air down to the .3 micron size. The carbon filter will remove volatile organic chemicals (VOCs) including chemicals, gases, and odors.

Models come in tabletop or console. Such filters cost $200 to $400 but can be as expensive as $1,000.

By the way, air filters can be bought for use in cars. Ironically, they are powered from your auto's cigarette lighter. One such brand is the Auto Aire II from AllerMed, which retails for about $200. See Appendix A for the manufacturer's address.

Plants

Plants can also help to provide a natural solution for indoor air pollution. A two-year study by the National Aeronautics and Space Administration (NASA) and the Associated Landscape Contractors of America shows that common household plants can remove harmful toxins, including formaldehyde and trichloroethylene from the air. Some plants were able to remove as much as 90 percent of the chemicals in a room in only twenty-four hours.

This information is helpful for almost any home. For example, in homes that use natural gas for cooking and heating, small amounts of benzene may be released into the air. Having house plants may play a role in reducing the concentration of this carcinogenic contaminant.

The bottom line is that "By having plants in your home, you can reduce the chemicals in the air," says NASA principal investigator Bill C. Wolverton, who recommends one ten- to twelve-inch potted plant per every one hundred square feet.

Carbon Monoxide Removal

Spider plants (*Chlorophytum elatum*) and golden pothos (*Epipremnum aureum*) are recommended.

Benzene Removal

Try Chinese evergreen, English ivy (*Hedera helix*), peace lily (*Spathiphyllum*, "Mauna Loa"), or Marginata (*Dracaena marginata*).

Formaldehyde Removal

Keep a spider plant (*Chlorophytum elatum*), mass cane/corn cane (*Dracaena massangeana*), or golden pothos (*Epipremnum aureum*).

Trichloroethylene Removal

The best plants are potted mum (*Chrysanthemum morifolium*), peace lily (*Spathiphyllum*, "Mauna Loa"), and Warneckii (*Dracaena deremeusis*, "Warneckii").

CARPETS AND CARPET BACKING

Health Advisory

There is evidence of a link between adverse health effects and the levels of VOCs emitted by new carpet, especially a substance called 4-phenylcyclohexane (4-PC). Some people report allergy or flulike symptoms caused by newly installed carpet.

When a new carpet is installed, it may produce an odor, but some people are more sensitive to odors than others. If you can smell an odor, then that will often mean VOCs are being emitted from the carpeting or the adhesives. Finally, manufacturers of carpets and related products have begun to acknowledge publicly that floor coverings and adhesives have the potential to irritate respiratory systems and eyes and to cause allergic reactions when installed. See *Safe Use Tips*.

Some of the allergic reactions that people attribute to new carpets actually may be associated with dust and other particles that become airborne when old carpeting is removed.

Chemical emissions from new carpeting, cushions, and adhesives are also a cause of allergic reactions and sensitization. The samples of carpets that have caused problems in experimental studies cut across all different types of carpet fibers and brands, both natural fiber treated with various chemicals during production, and synthetic fibers. See *Safe Use Tips* for advice on finding carpets made without the use of these and related synthetic chemicals.

Safe Use Tips

- In 1992, after many complaints from the public of eye and throat irritation, the carpet industry reached an agreement with the EPA to submit products for examination to ensure that emissions of certain VOCs fall below industry standards. Carpets whose emissions fall below industry standards will carry a label that certifies they have been tested and have passed. Be sure to request such emission information. But do not allow a certification label to lull you into a false sense of security—especially if you are chemically sensitive. The "green" label program has come under fire from some congressional representatives, Consumers Union, and attorneys general from several states. There is concern that the "green tag" labeling program may have the unintended effect of leading consumers to believe their carpet is "safe," and that any adverse health effects they might experience are not caused by carpeting. For chemically sensitive people especially, carpets with even very low VOC emissions can have what one researcher calls just absolutely "terrifying" health effects. Furthermore, industries that make carpet cushions and adhesives have not adopted such a certification program.
- Be sure that you can exchange or return the carpet if you develop symptoms because of its chemical emissions.
- Allow maximum ventilation before, during, and for forty-eight to seventy-two hours after installation of a new carpet. If possible, leave doors and windows open and use fans to increase the flow of outdoor air.

- To reduce exposure to pollutants in homes, leave during the installation of a new carpet. In the office, ask building managers to consider installing a new carpet when the area is not in use.
- Request that the dealer or installer leave the new carpet unrolled in a well-ventilated area for one or two days before delivering it to your premises for installation.
- Be sure to vacuum the old carpet well before its removal to reduce the amount of dust generated.
- Use low-emission adhesives. Remember that the carpet is part of your total floor-covering system, which may include the cushion and installation adhesives. The cushion and adhesives are also sources of emissions. New low-emission adhesives are available that can greatly reduce emissions from new carpet installations.
- New carpet is usually installed during home or office decoration, building construction, or renovation. Interior decorating usually includes the use of new materials such as wall treatments (painting, wallpapering, paneling), floor covering (carpet, vinyl, wood, ceramic), window covering (fabric, wood, plastic), and furniture. Any or all of these materials may produce chemical emissions and odors.
- A carpet sealer can be applied to carpet that prevents off-gassing of toxic fumes. Before application, shampoo the carpet first, then apply a product like AFM Enterprises's Carpet Guard. Let the carpet dry for about six hours. See under *Cleaning Products* in Appendix A for the company's address.
- If you have suffered health problems because of exposure to new carpet, you may want to alert the federal Consumer Product Safety Commission, which is studying the potential health effects of carpet chemical emissions. Write to Carpet Complaints, Room 529, U.S. Consumer Product Safety Commission, Washington, DC 20207.

Recommended Alternatives

- Use rugs that are made of cotton, cotton/wool blend, sheepskin, or unmothproofed wool without jute or latex backing.
- Use hardwood flooring, tile, and natural linoleum.
- Use woven carpet, which does not have latex adhesives to hold the fibers together.
- For carpet padding, try synthetic jute, felted wool, or other natural material with low toxic binders and backings.

CORRECTION FLUIDS

Product Type

Liquid.

Safe Use Tips

If you *must* use brands containing solvents such as 1,1,1-trichloroethane, use in a well-ventilated area. Avoid direct inhalation.

Correction Fluids

Product				Acute Health Advisory				Chronic Health Advisory		
🛒 Little to No Risk	🛒 Minimal Risk	🛒 Caution	✔ Recommended	Flammability	Causticity	Irritants	Allergens and Strong Sensitizers	Carcinogens	Neurotoxins	Reproductive Effects
Liquid Paper 48, 83, 151				🛒	🛒	🛒	🛒	🛒	🛒	🛒
Mead Correction Fluid 151				🛒	🛒	🛒	🛒	🛒	🛒	🛒
PENTEL Pocket Correction Pen 63, 151				🛒	🛒	🛒	🛒	🛒	🛒	🛒
Wite-out ✔				🛒	🛒	🛒	🛒	🛒	🛒	🛒

COTTON CLOTHING

Clothing made with conventionally grown cotton is contaminated with a wide array of pesticides and dyes, which can be absorbed through the skin, especially when you perspire.

The good news is that major cotton growers throughout the nation, especially in California, have recently decided to grow their crops organically, despite increased costs. They are making this transition because of growing consumer concerns about the use of pesticides and its consequences on water quality, worker safety, and their health. Interestingly, organic cotton farmers are achieving virtually the same yields as their chemically dependent neighbors. And they are finding a huge demand for their cotton among some of the nation's leading clothing companies. Organic, natural clothing is made from unsprayed, undyed cotton. Instead of using solvents at the factories that process the cotton, organic cotton manufacturers use water or beeswax. And instead of using formaldehyde for shrink-proofing garments, they now use a mechanical process. Furthermore, cotton can be grown in colors such as green and brown. For additional colors, natural dyes, derived from renewable plant and insect sources, are used and processed with water only. The availability of organic cotton clothing is increasing dramatically, and you can now find it through mail-order suppliers or in stores in major cities.

Chronic Health Advisory

Pesticides

One of the most heavily sprayed crops in agriculture is cotton; in the United States alone, approximately thirty-five million tons of pesticides are applied to the cotton crop, and the textile industry is the sixth most polluting industry in the world. Many of the pesticides used to grow cotton are carcinogenic, neurotoxic, and teratogenic.

Industrial Chemicals

Sizing, which is any of various gelatinous or glutinous preparations made from glue or starch for filling the pores of cotton materials, can contain formaldehyde, which is carcinogenic. The ginning process, which removes seeds from cotton, also uses petroleum-based solvents. Synthetic dye processes use heavy metals, alkalies, and salt. Some heavy metals such as arsenic and lead are carcinogenic, neurotoxic, or teratogenic.

Safe Shopping Tips

- You might be wearing organic clothing right now and not even know. A wide range of organic clothing is available, ranging from pants, jumpsuits, sweatshirts, parkas, baby's and children's clothing, skirts, shirts and blouses, and undergarments.
- Levi's Naturals brown denim jeans and jackets are made with naturally colored cotton called Fox Fibre, which grows in brown, cream, and green, needing no bleaching and fewer, if any, pesticides, because of its natural pest resistance.
- Environmentally friendly clothing is now offered by firms as large as Levi Strauss & Co., VF Corp (owner of Lee and Wrangler), Esprit, and Nike.
- One brand to look for is O Wear, available in Los Angeles and San Francisco, Chicago, and New York City. The company is also considering markets in Seattle, Denver, and Atlanta.
- An excellent brand is Esprit, which uses not only organic cotton, but also environmentally friendly zippers, snaps, and buttons. The usual way of making standard zippers and other metal fasteners for clothing involves electroplating, which creates millions of tons of hazardous waste.

- See Appendix A for addresses of organic cotton clothing suppliers.

ELECTROMAGNETIC FIELDS

Electricity is everywhere. It is important to our well-being and comfort. The walls of homes and offices are filled with electrical wires. The nation's streets and highways are intertwined with power lines. Electricity creates biologically active, long waves of radiation called electromagnetic fields (EMFs), and EMFs are associated with virtually all buildings that we reside in. The human body generates electrical impulses that are controlled by the nervous system, a process by which every living cell is regulated.

Modern research is now realizing that EMFs interfere with the body's electrical field and can have damaging effects on the immune system and health in general, especially as cancer agents. But exposures created by EMFs need not necessarily be from high-voltage power lines that crisscross the American landscape. In fact, much of your exposure to EMFs results from everyday appliances such as hair dryers and televisions, and even grounding connections to metallic water pipes.

There is growing evidence that EMFs exert a powerful effect on our health. Recently, the Special Epidemiology Studies Program of the California Department of Health Services noted that these fields do, in fact, change biological tissue, although all their health effects remain unknown. Also, studies in the last twenty years have found possible associations between EMFs and miscarriages, birth defects, leukemia, brain cancers, breast cancers, and lymphomas.

Little of what is known by government and industry has been made public. As a result, standards of safety for electrical appliances are spotty at best and almost completely voluntary. For example, the United States has set no standards for magnetic fields from video display terminals (VDTs), one of the most common sources of EMFs in the workplace, whereas, in contrast, the Swedish government has already set up exposure standards. Its standard of 2.5 milligauss (mG) at a distance of fifty centimeters (about twenty inches) from the VDT has become a de facto standard in the VDT industry worldwide.

Health Advisory

Carcinogens

Much of the evidence on the carcinogenicity of EMFs stems from occupational and power line studies.

Although most studies to date have focused on occupational exposures, some household appliances provide greater exposure than do power lines, because of the proximity at which appliances are used. We know a little about cancer hazards stemming from EMFs generated by everyday appliances, thanks to two studies on electric blankets, which create a continuous exposure for seven to eight hours.

A recent study found that prenatal electric blanket exposure was associated with a small increase in the incidence of childhood cancers, especially leukemia and brain cancer, while postnatal exposure to electric blankets also was weakly associated with childhood cancer, especially lymphocytic leukemia. A small statistically nonsignificant increase in breast cancer has been reported among postmenopausal women who used electric blankets continuously throughout the night.

Neurotoxins

We know very little about the neurotoxic effects of EMFs. We do know that exposure to radiation from television has been shown to alter the sodium balance of various brain regions and that this could result in subtle neurotoxic effects. But if you protect yourself from the cancer hazard posed by EMFs, you probably will end up protecting yourself from any central nervous system effects.

Reproductive Effects

There is growing evidence that EMFs affect pregnancy outcomes.

Television: Exposure to radiation from television has been found to cause lower birth weight, as well as slower than normal growth rates in offspring in experimental animal studies. It is difficult to apply this information to human exposures. But we would urge some caution in the distance from which you watch television.

VDTs/computers: Exposure to radiation from VDTs may possibly be a cause of miscarriages. One study of some sixteen hundred pregnant women found that those using computers more than twenty hours per week had twice the miscarriage rate of female workers who did similar work but did not use computers. Finnish researchers found a miscarriage increase of three times among women exposed to VDT magnetic fields of 3 mG or more.

Electric heat cables: Miscarriage incidence is increased among women living in houses with electric heat cables installed in ceilings.

Safe Shopping/Use Tips

- Avoid any unnecessary EMF exposure. Obviously you're not going to get rid of your refrigerator, stove, or television, all of which are sources of EMFs. But where you can conveniently reduce exposures to EMFs, you probably should. In general, replace electrical appliances with nonelectrical appliances whenever possible and feasible. Of particular importance is replacement of those appliances that are both regularly used and have the highest emissions of EMFs.

- Use a hand can opener instead of an electric can opener; a hand whisk instead of an electric whisk; a hand beater instead of an electric beater. Use two blankets instead of a single electric blanket. Hand dry your hair instead of using an electric hair dryer.
- Always maintain distance from electrical appliances whenever possible, as EMFs rapidly drop off in intensity with increasing distance. For example, neither you nor your children should sit close to the television, and you can keep your electric digital alarm clock a few feet away from your head while you sleep at night. When possible arrange electrical appliances so that they will be six feet or more from your body during their normal operation.
- Before buying new appliances, ask for information on EMF emissions. If your sales representative does not have such information, get the telephone number of the manufacturer and call it. Talking with the manufacturer about this issue will provide you with important consumer information—and place pressure on industry to make changes that are better for your health.
- Turn appliances off when you are finished.

Consider buying the videotape, *Current Switch: How to Reduce or Eliminate Electromagnetic Pollution in the Home and Office,* available for $49.95 from Baubiologie Hardware, 207B 16th Street, Pacific Grove, CA 93950; (408) 372-8626.

GLUES

Product Types
Aerosol; liquid; paste; squeeze tube.

Safe Use Tips
- Use in well-ventilated areas.
- For prolonged use with glues that contain carcinogenic, neurotoxic, or teratogenic ingredients, wear a respirator.
- Wear nonpermeable gloves.
- Avoid use of glues with reproductive effects during pregnancy.
- Store glues in childproof area.
- Should there be a fire when using adhesive products containing solvents, do not use water, as its use may spread the fire because solvents float on water. Use a fire extinguisher.

Glues

Product				Acute Health Advisory				Chronic Health Advisory		
(Little to No Risk)	(Minimal Risk)	(Caution)	✓ Recommended	Flammability	Causticity	Irritants	Allergens and Strong Sensitizers	Carcinogens	Neurotoxins	Reproductive Effects
Biofa Wood Glue ✓				○	○	○	○	○	○	○
Conros Kid's Natural School Glue ✓				○	○	○	○	○	○	○
Conros Kwik-Set Epoxy Glue 152				○	○	●	●	○	○	○
Conros Woodworker's Glue ✓				○	○	○	○	○	○	○
Duco Spray Adhesive (aerosol) 63, 81, 112				●	○	●	○	●	●	○
Duro Clear Formula Vinyl Adhesive 1, 48, 124, 146				●	○	●	○	●	●	●
Duro E-Pox-E Repair Kit 10				○	○	○	●	○	○	○
Duro Master Mend E-Pox-E System Quick Set 93				○	○	●	●	○	○	○
Duro Plastic Mender 1, 48, 69, 115, 124				●	○	●	○	●	●	●
Duro Quick Gel Super Glue 109, 124				○	○	●	○	○	○	○
Duro White Plastic Rubber Adhesive 35, 80				●	○	●	○	●	●	●
Kid's Natural School Glue ✓				○	○	○	○	○	○	○
3M Photo Mount Spray Adhesive 35, 63, 68, 112				●	○	●	○	●	●	○
3M Super 77 Spray Adhesive 63				●	○	●	○	●	●	○
Macklanburg-Duncan Craft & Hobby Glue ✓				○	○	○	○	○	○	○
Macklanburg-Duncan Professional Carpenter's Glue ✓				○	○	○	○	○	○	○
Ross Arts and Crafts Glue ✓				○	○	○	○	○	○	○
Ross Colored Playtime Glue ✓				○	○	○	○	○	○	○
Ross Contact Cement 63, 150				●	○	●	○	○	●	●
Ross Glue Stick ✓				○	○	○	○	○	○	○

Product				Acute Health Advisory				Chronic Health Advisory		
Little to No Risk	Minimal Risk	Caution	Recommended ✓	Flammability	Causticity	Irritants	Allergens and Strong Sensitizers	Carcinogens	Neurotoxins	Reproductive Effects
Ross Household Cement 18				(Caution)	(Minimal)	(Caution)	(Minimal)	(Minimal)	(Caution)	(Minimal)
Ross Kidstik ✓				(Minimal)	(Minimal)	(Minimal)	(Minimal)	(Minimal)	(Minimal)	(Minimal)
Ross Paper Fix ✓				(Minimal)	(Minimal)	(Minimal)	(Minimal)	(Minimal)	(Minimal)	(Minimal)
Ross Rubber Cement 63				(Caution)	(Minimal)	(Caution)	(Minimal)	(Minimal)	(Caution)	(Minimal)
Ross School Glue ✓				(Minimal)	(Minimal)	(Minimal)	(Minimal)	(Minimal)	(Minimal)	(Minimal)
Ross Snif Proof Plastic Cement #65 ✓ 111				(Little to No Risk)	(Minimal)	(Minimal)	(Minimal)	(Minimal)	(Minimal)	(Minimal)
Ross Super Glue 34				(Caution)	(Minimal)	(Caution)	(Minimal)	(Minimal)	(Minimal)	(Minimal)
Ross Ultra Super Glue 34				(Caution)	(Minimal)	(Caution)	(Minimal)	(Minimal)	(Minimal)	(Minimal)
Ross White Glue—Durafix ✓				(Minimal)	(Minimal)	(Minimal)	(Minimal)	(Minimal)	(Minimal)	(Minimal)
Ross White Glue ✓				(Minimal)	(Minimal)	(Minimal)	(Minimal)	(Minimal)	(Minimal)	(Minimal)

MOTH REPELLENTS

Product Types

Chips; solid.

Health Advisory

Naphthalene, used in the old-style moth repellents, is neurotoxic and can cause blood damage to the fetus because it is transported across the placenta.

Also, naphthalene is highly volatile, so products containing it should never be used near newborn babies and children. Skin exposure is most dangerous for newborns.

Safe Use Tips

- Some products may contain 1,4-dichlorobenzene, which is carcinogenic. If the label states that a product contains this ingredient, do not use it.
- Also avoid products that contain naphthalene.

Recommended Alternatives

- Cedar blocks, chips, and sachets work well for repelling moths. You can buy cedar in many forms, from blocks for dresser drawers to bagged chips for hanging in closets, at hardware stores and drugstores.
- Line closets with cedar.
- Store seasonal clothing in plastic bags that you can zip. Put in a cedar block. This will provide them with excellent protection and save you from having to replace moth-eaten clothing.

Moth Repellents

Product				Acute Health Advisory				Chronic Health Advisory		
Little to No Risk	Minimal Risk	Caution	Recommended	Flammability	Causticity	Irritants	Allergens and Strong Sensitizers	Carcinogens	Neurotoxins	Reproductive Effects
Cedar Blocks, Chips, or Sachets ✓				●	●	●	●	●	●	●
Enoz Moth Blok 41				●	●	●	●	●	●	●
Enoz Moth Cake 41				●	●	●	●	●	●	●
Moth Repellent (naphthalene)				●	●	●	●	●	●	●

POOL, SPA, AND HOT TUB CHEMICALS

Product Types

Powder; tablet.

Health Advisory

Pool chlorine (i.e., calcium hypochlorite) is both highly caustic and strongly irritating to your eyes and mucous membranes. A recent Canadian survey found that chlorinated pool water causes respiratory distress such as wheezing and difficulty breathing. Prolonged exposure to chlorine can cause sensitization, including asthma.

Pool chlorine can also burst its container if it gets too hot. It can burst into flames if it comes in contact with oils and solvents.

Safe Use Tips

- Never mix chlorine with ammonia-based compounds and products.
- Always store separately from other chemicals, especially acids, oils, and paints.
- Never repack into another container.
- Always wear gloves when handling pool chlorine.
- Handle containers carefully, as friction can ignite pool chlorine.
- If pool chlorine gets on the skin or in the eyes, flush well with water.
- If spilled on clothing, immediately remove your clothing, or literally jump in the pool, as pool chlorine can ignite spontaneously.
- Test kits are used to measure the acidity and the amount of free chlorine in the pool and to help in maintaining the correct levels. These kits often contain highly toxic ingredients. They should be used with caution.
- In general, many pool chemicals are highly corrosive and should be handled with extreme caution.
- Pregnant women should avoid saunas and hot tubs. Heat exposure during pregnancy from sauna and hot tub use increases the risk of neural tube birth defects. A study evaluating over twenty-three thousand women found that women who had exposure to saunas or hot tubs in early pregnancy had a risk of neural tub birth defects that was nearly three times normal for hot tub use and two times higher than normal for saunas. The combination of two of these sources of heat raised the risk of birth defects to more than six times above normal. The authors of the study concluded that exposure to heat in the form of a hot tub or sauna in the first three months of pregnancy is associated with an increased risk of neural tube defects.

Recommended Alternatives

Several nontoxic pool products are now available. In addition, the following guidelines will help reduce the need for pool chemicals:

- Use electrolytic chlorinators, which generate chlorine directly from water, to which salt has been added.
- Reduce chemical use by keeping the pool clean with regular upkeep and an efficient filter system.
- Insist that people shower before swimming.
- People with oil in their hair should wear bathing caps.
- Babies in diapers should not be allowed in pools.

Pool, Spa, and Hot Tub Chemicals

Product	Acute Health Advisory				Chronic Health Advisory		
(🛒 Little to No Risk · 🛒 Minimal Risk · 🛒 Caution · ✓ Recommended)	Flammability	Causticity	Irritants	Allergens and Strong Sensitizers	Carcinogens	Neurotoxins	Reproductive Effects
Natural Chemistry Pool Formula ✓	Little	Little	Little	Little	Little	Little	Little
Natural Chemistry Spa/Hot Tub Formula ✓	Little	Little	Little	Little	Little	Little	Little
Pool chlorine (generic) 26	Caution	Caution	Caution	Minimal	Little	Little	Little

SHOE POLISHES AND RELATED PRODUCTS

Product Types

Aerosol; brush-on; pump; roll-on.

Safe Use Tips

- Always wear nonpermeable gloves.
- Work in a well-ventilated area.

Shoe Polishes and Related Products

Product	Acute Health Advisory				Chronic Health Advisory		
(🛒 Little to No Risk · 🛒 Minimal Risk · 🛒 Caution · ✓ Recommended)	Flammability	Causticity	Irritants	Allergens and Strong Sensitizers	Carcinogens	Neurotoxins	Reproductive Effects
Auro/Tapir Leather Balm ✓	Little	Little	Little	Little	Little	Little	Little
Auro/Tapir Shoe Polish ✓	Little	Little	Minimal	Minimal	Little	Minimal	Little
Kiwi Cream Shoe Polish 156	Little	Little	Minimal	Caution	Little	Minimal	Little
Kiwi Cream Shoe Polish (White) 156	Little	Little	Minimal	Caution	Little	Minimal	Little
Kiwi Elite 55	Little	Little	Caution	Little	Little	Little	Caution
Kiwi Elite (White) 149	Little	Little	Minimal	Little	Minimal	Little	Little
Kiwi Heel & Sole Edge Dressing 49, 55	Little	Little	Caution	Little	Little	Caution	Caution
Kiwi Leather Balm 83	Little	Little	Minimal	Little	Little	Caution	Little

Product				Acute Health Advisory				Chronic Health Advisory		
Little to No Risk	Minimal Risk	Caution	Recommended ✓	Flammability	Causticity	Irritants	Allergens and Strong Sensitizers	Carcinogens	Neurotoxins	Reproductive Effects
Kiwi Leather Dye 55										
Kiwi Liquid Wax 55										
Kiwi Neatsfoot Oil ✓										
Kiwi Saddle Soap ✓										
Kiwi Scuff Magic 55										
Kiwi Scuff Magic (water-based White shoe dressing) 149										
Kiwi Shoe Creme (except White) 85, 87										
Kiwi Shoe Polish (except White) 138, 140										
Kiwi Shoe Stretch Spray 68, 71, 112										
Kiwi Shoe White 149										
Kiwi Sneaker Shield 22, 61, 68, 83, 112										
Kiwi Sneaker White 149										
Kiwi Twist 'N Shine Soft Wax Shoe Polish 138, 156										
Kiwi Twist 'N Shine Soft Wax Shoe Polish (White) 149, 156										
Kiwi White Shoe Creme 87, 140, 149										
Kiwi White Shoe Polish 140, 149										

TOYS

Toys pose acute hazards such as accidental choking, lacerations, contusions, and abrasions, as well as chronic hazards from unlabeled toxic chemicals. One out of six toys sampled in 1992 by the CPSC was found to be so dangerous that it should not have been offered for sale. Yet, 99 percent of children's toys are never even inspected for their safety.

According to *The 1992 Toy Safety Report* published by the Institute for Injury Reduction, "Toy injuries continue to climb . . . and the increase is much greater than the child population increase." In 1992, more children were killed or injured by toys than in any year prior. Compounding both acute and chronic health hazards for toys is that product labels all too often mislead parents into believing a product is safe when its hazards are simply hidden by inadequate and vague disclosure requirements. Many product labels do not provide clear information on possible hazards such as choking. A product that claims to be "nontoxic" certainly could pose delayed health effects. Products ranging from artificial snow to nail polish can pose unacceptable chronic hazards.

Health Advisory

Acute

An estimated 123,000 children under age fifteen were treated in U.S. hospital emergency rooms for toy-related injuries in 1989. More than one-third of these injuries resulted from children falling off of or being hit by riding toys such as scooters, tricycles, and wagons. While most injuries reported were minor, primarily lacerations, contusions, and abrasions, several toy-related deaths occur annually because of choking. These deaths are caused primarily by choking on balloons, small toys such as balls, marbles, and blocks, or parts of toys. Often, toys that kill *passed all legal size requirements of the government's small parts regulation that addresses choking hazards associated with products that are intended for children under three years of age.*

Safe Shopping Tips

After you have bought a toy—even if you have checked it out against the hazards that follow—watch your child when using the toy. See whether he or she dismantles it, eats it, throws it, or stabs with it. Every time a new toy is introduced to your child—even if just for a moment while being shared through another child—repeat the whole process before letting your child use the toy alone. Never assume that toys used safely by one child—even a hand-me-down—will be used safely by another child.

Here are further suggestions from the Institute for Injury Reduction:

Choking Hazards

- When buying a toy, anticipate that the child will use that toy in the most injurious way possible. Children may dismantle it, eat its smallest, sharpest, and most toxic components, throw or jab its sharp edge and points, blast it close to their eyes and ears, and wrap its cords and strings around their necks. As a result, a child could choke, strangle, lacerate, deafen, blind, or otherwise harm himself, herself, or other children with a toy that might seem completely safe to you. Never assume that a toy is safe for a child just because that child is within the recommended age range shown on the label.

- Before buying a toy of any kind, buy an inexpensive small part cylinder, called the "choke test tube," from your toy store. Carry it with you when you shop, so that you can put every toy or potentially dismantled toy part into the cylinder. If the toy or part fits or even comes close to fitting within the cylinder, do not buy it. Your child could choke trying to swallow it. If you can't find a choke test tube from your toy store, look for the No Choke Tube from Safety First, on sale at such stores as Kmart and Wal-Mart for about $2, or call Safety First at (800) 962-7233. Better yet, see if the toy fits inside an empty toilet paper roll. This item is cheaper, and the larger diameter of the paper roll test will give your child a better margin of safety.

- Some small parts pose more obvious hazards than others. These include marbles, small balls and dolls, blocks, and balloons. Small parts are particularly deceptive when they are attached to larger toys that your child may dismantle. Examples of detachable small parts are toy vehicle tires; doll hands, limbs, and apparel; pacificier components; toy house fixtures; and building blocks.

Strangulation Hazards

- Any toy that consists of or contains a rope, chain, string, elastic band, or other cord long enough to encircle your child's neck could strangle the child.
- Crib toys that dangle to be reached at and stretched by babies have caused strangulations. Toys containing hidden cords, which are released only when pulled and then retracted, create the same hazard. Pacifiers and other items should never be looped or tied around your child's or baby's neck.

Toy Chests

- The lid on any compartment such as a suitcase, chest, trunk, or box can close on a curious child who leans over the edge or crawls inside. When a lid closes, the blow can strangle or injure the children leaning over the edge, or the children inside the compartment can suffocate.

Toxic Hazards

- Learn about the product before you buy. Read labels, but you should know that labels often provide little, if any, disclosure of hazardous ingredients. Label precautions such as *Warning, Caution, Danger,* or *Toxic* should alert you to possibly dangerous toys.
- Do not buy toys with artificial colors.
- Toys that mimic adult products such as nail polish and paints may well contain the same hazardous chemicals found in adult versions.

For more information on toy safety, see Appendix A.

WATER FILTERS

Most people take their tap water for granted. But contamination of public drinking water supplies is widespread, and this contamination has dangerous consequences. The federal Centers for Disease Control and Prevention estimate that yearly some 940,000 people become ill from consuming contaminated water and 900 people die. A recent report noted (italics in original): "Few members of the public are aware, for example, that according to the most recent published review of studies of actual cancer cases in the United States, a single class of drinking water contaminants [known generally as trihalomethanes] is associated with *10,700 or more bladder and rectal cancers per year*—about *thirty cancers per day.* That is twice as many people as die from fires, and more people than are killed by handguns."

Both federal and state regulations legally allow contaminants in drinking water, ranging from commonly occurring by-products of chlorination to industrial chemicals, arsenic, lead, pesticides, radiation, and harmful bacteria and viruses. Your water may meet all state and federal standards established by law and yet still be unfit to drink. But water filtration can overcome many of these hazards. For further details on drinking water contamination, see also "Beverages" in part III of *The Safe Shopper's Bible.*

Contaminants found in drinking water fall into three major categories: chemicals, radiation, and microorganisms.

Chemicals include both nonorganic minerals and metals such as fluoride, arsenic, and lead; VOCs such as trihalomethanes (THMs), trichloroethylene, and perchloroethylene, which become gaseous at room temperature; and nonvolatile organic chemicals such as dieldrin and polychlorinated biphenyls.

Affecting some fifty million Americans and a documented cause of cancer, most of the specific contaminants that fall under the category of *radiation* are not effectively regulated by federal rules. Common forms of radiation include radon and radium.

Microorganisms include bacteria, protozoans, and viruses. Each year nearly one million people become sick from contaminated drinking water. At greatest risk are people with AIDS, those who have had cancer or liver disease, children, and others with weakened immune systems.

Testing Your Water

There are two steps to determining whether or not your drinking water requires filtration. These include finding out if your water is contaminated and by what, then figuring out what filtration methods will be the best in removing these contaminants.

The first step in determining the contaminants in your drinking water is to call or request in writing water analysis results from your local water supplier. Ask for analyses for all possible contaminants. In many states, such as California, public water suppliers are legally required to provide this information. But you should presume that you will only receive what you ask for. If you do not design your request broadly and specifically enough, then your water supplier may leave out key information on your water quality.

In writing or speaking with your water supplier, mention key words to ensure that you will receive *all* pertinent information on your tap water quality. Be sure to mention the following: total coliform count; inorganic chemicals (including metals and minerals); inorganic chemicals and physical factors such as suspended solids and particulates; volatile organic chemicals (including THMs, perchloro-ethylene, trichloroethylene, and many other industrial chemicals); non-volatile organic chemicals such as polychlorinated biphenyls (PCBs); radiation (gross, alpha, beta) as well as radium and radon; and pesticides.

Following is a sample letter.

(Date)

(Your name)
(Street address)
(City, state, zip code)

Dear Sir or Madam:

Please send me your most recent monitoring reports covering the last twelve months for water supplied to the above address.

These reports should specify weekly and/or monthly average measurements for the following:

Volatile organic chemicals and other industrial chemicals	Radiation, radium, radon, and uranium
Bacteria	Trihalomethanes and chloroform
Total dissolved solids	Metals
Nitrates	Minerals (including fluoride)
Pesticides	Alkalinity

My request is supported by public right-to-know laws in this state. If you choose not to deliver this information, please notify me where I can get the information. I request a timely delivery of the requested information.

Sincerely,

But we must warn you that you cannot rely exclusively on what your public water supplier tells you about your water quality. Their results may reflect several statistical manipulations that make *your* water appear to be less contaminated than it really is. For example, even a small city of only several thousand population may draw water from a variety of sources. The water supplier may average high-contaminant values from one well delivering water to your home with low-contaminant values from another well that delivers water elsewhere. Furthermore, concentrations of some contaminants such as lead vary from home to home, depending on the kind of plumbing pipes, water hardness, and municipal service connectors.

That is why you should also have your tap water independently analyzed by a third party. This is easily done, with costs ranging from $12 for a simple lead-contamination test to $150 to $200 for a complete screening of all possible contaminants. We have listed water test companies under *Beverages* in Appendix A.

Buying a Water Filter

If your water is contaminated, then buying a good-quality water filtration system may be one of the most important things you do for your health.

Buying a water filter can seem like a daunting task. There are many different kinds, ranging from those filtering water from the tap to others that filter *all* the water that enters your home. Some fit under your sink; others fit like lids over pitchers, or cover the end of the faucet. Some filters use blocks of solid activated carbon; others rely on reverse osmosis, distillation, or a combination of these and other methods. Each performs some filtration tasks well, and others poorly.

That is why it is important to understand your drinking water's contamination before buying a water filter: Certain types of filters excel at screening various contaminants, and you should be sure to match the filtration method to the type of contamination that you will want to remove from your drinking water.

Where Filters Are Used

Point of Use (POU)

Attached to the water faucet or installed under the sink, point-of-use filters are among the most popular. The types that fit at the end of the faucet are useless, as the water does not stay in contact with the carbon filter long enough to make a significant difference. Those that fit under the sink can work quite effectively. But a point-of-use system is not always adequate for your health; in some cases, you will need to filter *all* the water coming into your home.

Point of Entry (POE)

Systems that filter all the water coming into your home are especially important if your water is significantly polluted with volatile organic chemicals (VOCs) or radon, as only a small amount of your exposure actually comes from drinking water. Indeed, drinking and cooking account for only about one-third of your exposure to VOCs. Another one-third of exposure results from showering, inhalation, and skin absorption, and another one-third of exposure results from volatilization of chemicals from dishwashers, washing machines, and toilets. A point-of-entry filter removes contaminants before they even enter your home, reducing your exposure from other sources such as bathing and using appliances.

Countertop

Some countertop filters work just like a coffee filter. You pour the water into the filter and it trickles through. Others fit over the tops of pitchers, such as the Brita water filter. These are not quite as effective as a POU or POE system.

Types of Filters

Screen Filters

Important for the removal of bacteria, screen filters are really very fine membranes. Screen filters are rated for the size of bacteria they remove. Lower-rated screen filters are better at the removal of bacteria than higher-rated screen filters. Medical professionals generally use screen filters with a 2 micron rating. The use of a screen filter is especially important in areas where there is known or suspected contamination with microorganisms such as bacteria or some other pathogens. For example, if your public water supplier has reported past problems with the protozoan *Giardia lamblia,* you probably should have a screen filter. Many of the best water filter systems contain screen filters together with other kinds of filters. Cost for replacement of screen filters can be $100 or more.

Depth Filters

Adept at removal of suspended solids and particulates, depth filters are rated by the size of substances they remove from the water. A 10 micron filter will remove many solids but not bacteria, which range in size from 1 to 10 microns. A 100 micron filter will remove particles about the diameter of human hair, which is about 100 microns in diameter. Depth filters are often combined with the other filters discussed below.

Activated Carbon Filters

One of the oldest types of water filters, activated carbon absorbs organic substances that contaminate drinking water, including the radioactive contaminant radon. Activated carbon filters are excellent for removing VOCs and THMs, as well as some nonvolatile chemicals. But they are no good at all for removing inorganic contaminants such as lead, arsenic, and other metals, or other forms of radioactive contaminants such as strontium 90, uranium, radium, and other man-made products of nuclear fission. The best filtration systems incorporate activated carbon filters as part of their system but do not rely exclusively on activated carbon, combining it with depth or screen filters as well as reverse osmosis (RO) or distillation.

Activated carbon systems can be mounted on the faucet or under the sink. A study has found that under-the-sink models remove up to 99 percent of contaminants, whereas faucet models removed only 76 percent. We recommend against faucet-mounted models.

Activated carbon systems are rated on their ability to remove iodine and phenols. The best systems will have an iodine removal number of at least 1,000. On the other hand, the phenol removal rating is best if under thirty parts per million. Always demand to know the iodine and phenol removal numbers.

Furthermore, you should make sure that the filter has a life span rated for the removal of at least two thousand gallons of water. Most people use approximately four gallons of water daily for consumption and cooking, meaning that a system at two thousand gallons will last two people approximately 250 days and four people 125 days. You should always change the filter long before the recommended amount of usage to ensure optimum performance. Replacement filter costs range from $10 to $100, depending on the model.

Activated carbon filters are made from natural substances, including lignite and bituminous coal. Your choice of materials will make a difference in how well the filter works. Experts agree that those filters made from bituminous coal are most effective at removing the widest range of contaminants.

Also, make sure that the carbon filter you choose is a structured carbon block or *granulated* activated carbon. In the past, *powdered* carbon systems have been sold, but they were not long-lasting and they quickly became ineffective.

Always make sure that your system contains a depth filter to remove suspended particles in the water. If your water has a lot of particles, the effectiveness of the activated carbon will be compromised. A sediment prefilter should cost under $50; replacement filters generally run less than $10.

Finally, activated carbon filters provide a fertile breeding ground for pathogenic microorganisms. The first flush of your water will generally be most contaminated. You should allow water to run for one to two minutes when it has been sitting overnight or a few hours before drinking it.

We strongly recommend that when buying a filter you combine activated carbon filters with reverse osmosis filters as both together will remove a wide range of possible contaminants.

Reverse Osmosis

One of the best all-around methods for removing a wide variety of contaminants, RO is especially important if your drinking water contains lead, other metals, radioactive contaminants such as strontium 90, uranium, and radium, or pesticides including chlorinated hydrocarbons and organophosphates such as DDT, heptachlor, dieldrin, aldrin, malathion, and parathion. RO systems also are effective at removal of microorganisms. However, reverse osmosis is very poor for the removal of THMs and nitrates, which are commonly found in drinking water supplies in agricultural regions.

When buying an RO system, make sure that your filter membrane is made from cellulose acetate if your drinking water is chlorinated, since chlorine will quickly destroy thin-film (polyamide) composite membranes.

Be aware that RO systems work slowly and may produce only about two gallons of water daily, and they waste water. One report notes that for every gallon of water produced, some four to nine gallons go down the drain.

Many of the best filtration systems combine RO with activated carbon and screen filters. Their cost ranges from $200 to $700.

Consumers should look for several features when buying an RO unit. These include making sure the model has a warranty on the membrane; a prefilter to remove suspended solids that would plug the membrane; automatic backflush capability for cleaning the membrane, enabling it to be used longer; a method for disinfection; instructions that tell how to disinfect units; and an automatic shutoff when the storage tank is full.

We strongly recommend that you buy RO units with activated carbon filtration for more thorough removal of a wide range of contaminants. Remember, RO membranes must be changed regularly.

Distillation

Adept at removal of a wide range of contaminants by boiling water and then condensing the purified steam into another reservoir, distillation works best when combined with activated carbon. Distillation, for example, does not remove THMs or other VOCs, since these have lower boiling points than water and will condense along with the water. This is a serious flaw, since THMs and other VOCs are common drinking water contaminants. However, distillation will do an adequate job of removing man-made nuclear fission products such as strontium 90. Also, because distillation removes minerals such as calcium and magnesium, people have complained that distilled water is tasteless. Thus, before committing to distillation, you should taste the water and see whether or not you like it. Costs range from $200 to $2,000.

Ultraviolet

Excellent for destroying many bacteria, ultraviolet treatment is not always effective against protozoans such as *Giardia,* parasites, or viruses and should therefore be combined with a highly selective screen filter. Furthermore, if water contains a great deal of suspended solids, its effectiveness will also be limited. Cost is around $500.

Water Softeners

Adept at removing minerals such as calcium and magnesium and even man-made nuclear fission products such as strontium 90, *a water-softening system is not intended, however, for the removal of contaminants.* We mention water softeners primarily because many consumers, especially new home owners, are approached by salespeople from water softener companies who offer to perform tests on their tap water, are told that their water is "hard" (i.e., containing high amounts of minerals such as calcium and magnesium), and then are given a sales pitch explaining that hard water causes kidney stones, gallstones, and even heart disease, all pointed at convincing you to spend a lot of money on a device that allegedly will "solve" your water's "problems." Well, folks, water softeners will not solve your water problems, and may cause unwelcome problems. Water softeners add back a great deal of sodium to the water. Too much sodium can be harmful, particularly for people who are borderline hypertensive. It can also kill your grass. Furthermore, minerals in hard water such as calcium and magnesium have been shown to protect against heart disease, yet water softeners end up removing them. *If you buy a water-softening unit, then be sure that it has both reverse osmosis and activated carbon post-filters that will also remove the excess sodium.*

Table 3. Filtration Methods for Common Drinking Water Contaminants

Contaminant	Best Filtration Method
Bacteria	ultraviolet light, screen filter
Lead	distillation, reverse osmosis

continued

Contaminant	Best Filtration Method
Nuclear fission products (strontium 90)	reverse osmosis, water softeners
Particulates	depth filter
Pesticides	activated carbon, reverse osmosis
Radium	reverse osmosis
Radon	activated carbon
Uranium	reverse osmosis
Volatile organic chemicals	activated carbon, reverse osmosis

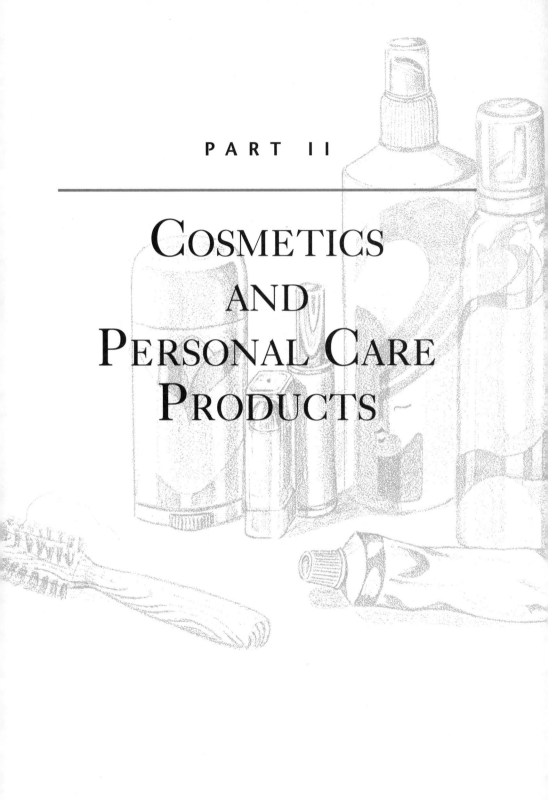

PART II

COSMETICS AND PERSONAL CARE PRODUCTS

Healthy Beauty

Throughout time—even before written history—cosmetics have been used for beauty, power, and heightened sexuality. Through their use, men and women attracted lovers, disguised both real and imagined effects of aging and physical imperfections, and intimidated enemies.

Cosmetic formulae were discussed in great detail in the Egyptian papyri, and, indeed, many of today's cosmetics trace their origins as far back as the women of ancient Egypt, Greece, and Rome.

The Egyptians, for example, lived in the Nile valley, rich in natural resources for making cosmetics. Egyptian women wore eye makeup made from a variety of minerals and other natural compounds. Especially important was an antimony compound called *kohl* that women used to darken their lashes and brows. Egyptian women also used lead sulfate for painting their upper lids black and powdered stone for painting their lower lids green or for the blue coloring between the upper lid and the eyebrow. They used ivory or wooden sticks as applicators. Cleopatra was known for her exquisite use of kohl and her tinted nails and palms.

The ancient Hebrews used oils of olives, almonds, sesame seeds, and gourds as well as fatty materials from animals and fish, both as emollients and for sun protection.

Centuries later in ancient Athens, the use of cosmetics and number of cosmeticians increased dramatically. Women applied powder to their faces, colored their lips, and painted their eyebrows with charcoal pencils.

By Roman times, cosmetics were sometimes causing larger problems than they solved. Although women used safe, gentle walnut extracts to darken their hair, they also used toxic mercury compounds for tinting and white lead to whiten their skin. The Romans were among the first people to recognize the dangers of cosmetics. "This coated face which is covered with so many drugs and where unfortunate husbands press their lips, is it a face or a sore?" mused Juvenal.

Even in the 1990s, cosmetic safety remains an ideal, and not a reality. Cosmetics are the least regulated products under the Federal Food, Drug, and Cosmetic Act (FFDCA). The FFDCA does not require premarket safety testing, review, or approval for cosmetics; the FDA pursues enforcement action only after the cosmetic enters into the stream of commerce or sometimes after it is on the shelf. Because of minimal regulation, products plainly dangerous to your health can be, and are being, sold. Far more to the point, the FDA has never sought legislative amendment of the FFDCA that would allow it to regulate cosmetics in keeping with its overall mandate to protect consumer health and safety.

For example, one widely used fragrance throughout the 1970s was acetylethyltetramethyltetralin (AETT). Tests on laboratory animals found that AETT was readily absorbed through the skin and not only dyed the inner organs of these animals blue but also damaged the brain and spinal cord. Although the FDA would neither ban the chemical nor remove products with AETT from the shelves, the cosmetic industry imposed its own ban—but only after these products had been widely distributed and used by consumers for many years.

And then there are the hair-coloring products that are used by up to 40 percent of women in the United States. The use of these products places women at increased risk of cancer, particularly non-Hodgkin's lymphoma, multiple myeloma, and Hodgkin's disease. In fact, the evidence is strong that the use of hair-coloring products accounts for up to 20 percent of all non-Hodgkin's lymphoma cases in all U.S. women. There is also suggestive evidence, from both animal and human studies, that women who use hair dyes may be at increased risk for breast cancer.

Yet few women know about the dangers of hair-coloring products. Thanks to special interests' lobbyists, hair dyes are among the most loosely regulated of all consumer products. The FFDCA requires no warning on the label to inform consumers that the use of hair-coloring dyes is a cause of human cancer. In fact, the hair-coloring industry has consistently gone to great lengths to assure consumers their products are completely safe.

A recent government investigation of the cosmetics industry provides strong evidence of how poorly regulated it is:

- FDA officials have found that many cosmetic manufacturers lack adequate data on safety tests and have generally refused to disclose the results of these tests.
- The FDA estimates that only a tiny percentage—3 percent—of the 4,000 to 5,000 cosmetic distributors have filed reports with the government of injuries to consumers.
- The FDA believes that less than 40 percent of the nation's 2,000 to 2,500 cosmetic manufacturers are even registered.
- Despite the cosmetic industry's reliance on its voluntary program of self-regulation, industry participation has actually declined slightly in the last decade.
- The National Institute of Occupational Safety and Health found that 884 of the chemicals available for use in cosmetics have been reported to the

government as toxic substances. A General Accounting Office report notes that the FDA has committed no resources for assessing the safety problems of those chemicals that have been found to cause genetic damage, biological mutations, and cancer.

The FDA acknowledges that it is difficult to remove unsafe ingredients—unless the administration can "convincingly demonstrate before a court of law that such a product is harmful when used according to label direction or under customary conditions of use." For example, nail polish remover contains an ingredient that turns into cyanide when accidentally ingested; it has caused many serious poisonings, especially of children, and the product is clearly a threat to children. But since its customary use does not include ingestion, the FDA, even if it wanted to, would be unable to remove such products from the marketplace.

Furthermore, even if an ingredient is carcinogenic, as in the case of some nitrosamines that contaminate cosmetic products, the available evidence may be insufficient to establish risk to the user in the manner prescribed by law.

This multi-billion-dollar industry can urge millions of Americans to apply chemicals to their bodies daily yet not be held accountable. In 1990, there were some 38,000 cosmetic-related injuries that required medical treatment in the United States. That figure does not include the many people who use cosmetics and suffer from allergies, irritation, and photosensitization yet accept these uncomfortable complications as the normal cost of grooming. They never visit their doctor or a hospital emergency room, and they rarely connect their allergies or irritated eyes to the cosmetics they use.

None of this would be so important if the skin were not so permeable. But cosmetic ingredients most certainly are absorbed through the skin. Some chemicals may penetrate the skin in significant amounts, especially when left on the skin for long periods, as in the case of facial makeup. One study showed that 13 percent of the cosmetic preservative butylated hydroxytoluene (BHT) and 49 percent of the carcinogenic pesticide DDT (which is found in some cosmetics containing lanolin) is absorbed through the skin. The question people concerned about their health must ask is what the adverse effects might be of so many chemicals that are absorbed through the skin every day, including carcinogens and neurotoxins.

The cosmetic industry will not tell you that some of the ingredients used in its products are health hazards. But that is no reason to remain uninformed. Who wants stinging eyes, reddened skin, or allergic contact dermatitis, not to mention an increased cancer risk? Nobody does, of course, and you should know about the hazards that might be present from your use of cosmetics and personal care products so that you can make better shopping choices.

Today, effectiveness, coupled with safety, gentleness, environmental awareness, and humane testing of animals, should be the trademark qualities of the best cosmetics and personal care products. That means banning or avoiding the use of toxic chemicals and offering products that work without causing minor irritation and allergies or placing consumers at increased risk of cancer. Many companies, in fact, sell good products, and they are listed in the following pages. Other companies do not and we will show you these products, too. But because most consumers know so little about the chemicals used in cosmetics, they do not know how to tell the difference. Thus, they are at risk for allergies, irritation, photosensitization, and cancer, in addition to other acute and chronic maladies.

Presenting this information is meant to empower you. Yes, beauty and health can go hand in hand. You *can* find safe cosmetics and personal care products. That's what *The Safe Shopper's Bible* is all about.

CONTACT DERMATITIS HAZARDS:
ALLERGENS, SENSITIZERS, AND IRRITANTS

Cosmetics and personal care products may pose a wide array of health hazards, ranging from allergic reactions, sensitization, and irritation to cancer.

Experts estimate that as many as two million people in the United States suffer from contact dermatitis in the form of allergies, sensitization, or irritation. These figures are probably underestimated, for many consumers who have had adverse reactions to cosmetics do not know that their problem was caused by a cosmetic or personal care product. Others who use cosmetics simply chalk up their watery eyes, skin irritation, and other symptoms to the cost of beauty, enduring these minor discomforts.

The symptoms of contact dermatitis—such as swelling, itching, and inflammation—can all be caused by the allergy-causing, sensitizing, and irritating ingredients in the cosmetics and personal care products that you use on your body. Here are the differences:

Irritation is a nonallergic inflammatory reaction that occurs at the site of exposure to a substance. The irritation may occur on first exposure or after repeated exposure to the same site. Generally, the inflammation appears within minutes to hours of the first contact, and its severity depends on the concentration of the irritant in the substance. Symptoms diminish when you stop using the product.

Unlike irritants, *allergens* and *sensitizers* involve the immune system. The effects of allergens and sensitizers can be similar to irritation, but typically the reaction appears from twenty-four to forty-eight hours after exposure, and the symptoms often increase in intensity over two to three days following the exposure.

Sensitizing chemicals can be particularly troubling for consumers. The first use of a sensitizer may not trigger a reaction, but subsequent or repeated use can cause a person to develop an allergic reaction to very low levels of the original chemical *or related substances*. Furthermore, the allergic reaction may show up not only in the original area of exposure, but also anyplace else on the skin, and may persist for several days or even weeks after exposure. People who have suffered such reactions may have to avoid using products containing the allergen or other related chemicals.

Fragrances, Scents, and Perfumes

The two leading causes of allergy, sensitization, and irritation in cosmetics are fragrances and preservatives. If you suffer watery eyes, reddened skin, irritation, or allergic reactions, the culprit could be the fragrance added to cosmetics and personal care products. Other commonly reported symptoms include spaciness, nausea, mood changes, depression, lethargy, restlessness, irritability, anger, memory lapses, and inability to concentrate.

Many chemicals found in fragrances are designated as hazardous, including methylene chloride, toluene, methyl ethyl ketone, methyl isobutyl ketone, ethyl alcohol, and benzyl chloride. Yet manufacturers are not required to list on product labels the ingredients used in formulating their fragrances, scents, and perfumes. In other words, if these products are carried to a hazardous waste site in your community, you have the right to know, but if you are going to apply them to the skin, you do not.

A considerable number of fragrance materials have been found to have sufficient sensitization potential to warrant a recommendation by the International Fragrance Association to severely curtail their use. Among some of the most popular sensitizing scents are cinnamon, vanilla, lemon, and citrus (see table 4).

Table 4: Fragrance Ingredients That Cause Contact Dermatitis

Ingredient	*Scent*
Cinnamon bark oil	Cinnamon
Clove oil	Cloves
Vanillin	Vanilla
Hydroxycitronellal	Linden blossoms
Eugenol	Cloves
Citral	Lemony, citrus
Diethyl maleate	Green apples
Fennel oil	Bitter
Peruvian balsam	Pine

Once, fragrances did not pose the same degree of hazard that they do today. For thousands of years herbs, flowers, and animals such as the Asian musk deer, beaver, and sperm whale have been sources of fragrances. However, expanding consumer demand and scarcity of these resources—coupled with advanced technology—led to a whole new area of synthetic fragrances, and today some 95 percent of the mix in most fragrances is made from synthetic chemicals. *If you are sensitive to cosmetics, one of the simplest methods of self-protection is to avoid using products containing fragrances.*

Many major cosmetic brands that you see advertised in fashion magazines contain fragrances derived from mixtures of six hundred or more raw materials and synthetic chemicals. Few have been tested for their safety. A recent government report targeted fragrances as one of the six categories of chemicals that should be given highest priority for neurotoxicity testing—along with insecticides, heavy metals, solvents, food additives, and air pollutants. In fact, some 84 percent of the ingredients used in fragrances have never been tested for human toxicity, or tested only minimally. Meanwhile, the National Institute of Occupational Safety and Health reports that 884 toxic substances were identified in a list of 2,983 chemicals used in the fragrance industry as capable of causing breathing difficulty, allergic reactions, multiple chemical sensitivities, and other serious maladies, including neurotoxicity. The FDA acknowledges that the incidence of adverse reactions to perfume products appears to be increasing and that these reactions involve the immune system and cause neurotoxic reactions. Yet the FDA has declined to take any action, in part because it claims "the number of people experiencing adverse reactions to perfume is still very small and consumers not adversely affected by these fragrances should not be deprived of their enjoyment." In fact, consumers have the right to full disclosure of the ingredients used to formulate fragrances that they apply to their bodies on a daily basis.

Asthma

Scents may be particularly troubling for the nation's ten million asthmatics. For example, toluene was detected in every fragrance sample collected by the EPA for a report in 1991. Toluene not only triggers asthma attacks, but it is also known to cause asthma in previously healthy people. (To make matters more troubling for chemically sensitive individuals, toluene is also neurotoxic; furthermore, toluene-laced products have become increasingly pervasive in the last ten years and are used not only in perfumes, but also in furniture waxes, plastic garbage bags, inks, hair gel, hair spray, and cat litter.) In one study, nearly three-fourths of asthma patients suffered adverse reactions to perfume. A Danish toxicological journal reports that the perfume used in cat litter gravel is a cause of asthma in humans. You can imagine the peril faced by fragrance-sensitive persons bombarded daily by scents worn by office workers and other individuals, as well as exposure from magazines that carry perfumed advertising, and even the scents from fragranced laundry detergents. For such people, fragrances are truly a serious health threat.

Photosensitivity

Sometimes when fragrances are exposed to the sun, they can adversely affect the skin, causing rashes, burns, swelling, and unsightly splotches. The result can be either irritation or allergic reaction and is called either *phototoxicity* (irritation) or *photosensitization* (allergy). Experts believe that it takes about an hour of sun exposure within about a half hour of putting on a fragrance for photosensitization to occur. If you plan to be in the sun and are concerned about this problem, avoid applying these substances to your body.

Fragrance ingredients that cause photosensitization include:

Bergamot oil
Marigold oil
Cumin oil
Orange bitter/essence/oil
Lemon essence/juice/oil
Rue oil
Lime essence/juice/oil
Verbena oil

Natural Fragrances

Are fragrances made with natural ingredients safer and less prone to cause irritation than those made from synthetic ingredients? Not necessarily. For example, bergamot oil is classified as a strong sensitizer on the same order as formaldehyde. This natural ingredient, as well as patchouli oil, civet, galbanum, and asafetida, can pose problems for the chemically sensitive cosmetic user, even though each is natural. So there is no blanket assurance that natural fragrances are safer.

That said, however, you are less likely to suffer allergic reactions and irritation if you consistently use one oil or a blend of no more than two or three than if you use synthetic fragrances. As noted earlier, synthetic fragrances can be made up of six hundred or more raw ingredients. Common sense says that the probability of a fragrance causing allergic reactions or irritation increases as its list of ingredients lengthens. Therefore, a simple combination of essential oils means fewer ingredients thrown into the pot.

And don't think that just because a company has a reputation for producing "natural" cosmetics, the fragrances in the product are also natural. Anita Roddick, founder of the Body Shop, notes that natural musk (which is extracted from the glands of the male musk deer) isn't used in one of her best-selling fragrances. Rather, a synthetic fragrance is used.

Preservatives

Cosmetics and personal care products require preservatives or they will become contaminated with bacteria, and it would be irresponsible for companies not to use preservatives. The choice of preservatives is especially important because this family of ingredients is, like fragrances, one of the leading causes of contact dermatitis.

Some of the most allergenic and irritating preservatives release small amounts of formaldehyde, which is an irritant and sensitizer as well as a carcinogen and neurotoxin. Many cosmetic companies do not use such ingredients because they can make the eyes sting and irritate the skin. But many companies do, and you should be able to identify these ingredients so you can avoid products containing them.

The following ingredients contain formaldehyde, may release formaldehyde, or may break down into formaldehyde:

- 2-bromo-2-nitropropane-1,3-diol
- Diazolidinyl urea
- DMDM hydantoin
- Imidazolidinyl urea
- Quaternium 15

Seekers of the most gentle yet effective cosmetics should limit their exposure to these chemicals. On the other hand, one of the arts of manufacturing cosmetics and personal care products is in formulating products to achieve an effective yet gentle balance of ingredients; so some of these chemicals may be used at such low concentrations that they are not allergenic or irritating to most people.

Other preservatives do not contain formaldehyde. Still, studies have shown that they can have greater than normal potential for causing allergic reactions or irritation. These include:

- Methylchloroisothiazolinone
- Methylisothiazolinone
- Parabens (butyl, ethyl, methyl, propyl)

The following ingredients—which research shows are both extremely gentle and effective—can also be used as preservatives and seem to cause the least irritation and fewest allergic reactions:

- Grapefruit seed extract
- Phenoxyethanol
- Potassium sorbate

- Sorbic acid
- Tocopherol (vitamin E)
- Vitamin A (retinyl)
- Vitamin C (ascorbic acid)

These are the preservatives that you should prefer whenever possible.

CANCER RISKS

Cancer is one of the few massive killers of Americans that is rapidly increasing. It is important for consumers to be informed of which brands of cosmetics and personal care products contain carcinogens or carcinogenic precursors. In this section carcinogens are discussed in general; more limited and specific issues have been reserved for discussion under appropriate product categories.

DEA, TEA, Bronopol, and Padimate-O

Many cosmetics, both natural and from mainstream companies, contain either diethanolamine or triethanolamine (used as wetting agents), abbreviated on labels as DEA and TEA, and sometimes shown bound to other compounds as in cocamide DEA or TEA sodium lauryl sulfate.

Neither DEA nor TEA is carcinogenic. However, if products contain nitrites (used as a preservative or present as contaminants and not disclosed on cosmetics labels), their presence (especially DEAs) in cosmetics can cause a chemical reaction during formulation or even as products sit on store shelves. This reaction leads to the formation of *nitrosamines*. Most nitrosamines, including those formed from DEA or TEA, are carcinogenic.

Not all products containing DEA or TEA contain nitrosamines. Some may; others will not. Yet because of the failure of the FDA to request Congress to enact adequate label disclosure legislation, the consumer has no way of knowing which products are contaminated with nitrosamines. That leaves the consumer to play cancer roulette and hurts the entire cosmetic industry, making all products suspect.

The FDA accepts that the presence of DEA and TEA in cosmetics can pose a significant consumer health threat. In the 1970s it published a notice in the *Federal Register* in which it urged the industry to remove these products from cosmetics. The industry has made some progress by using higher quality control standards in its selection of raw materials. But an FDA report from the late 1980s noted that some 37 percent of the products tested contained carcinogenic nitrosamine impurities. It is unfortunate that low-level to high-level nitrosamine contamination is so prevalent, because this is a problem that could be easily eliminated.

German cosmetics, for example, are unlikely to contain nitrosamines. This is because of official recommendations by the German Federal Health Office in 1987 that discouraged manufacturers from using DEA and TEA. Thus, German cosmetics would make a good choice for concerned consumers.

Your best self-protection is to boycott products containing DEA or TEA. That will send a clear message to the cosmetic industry.

Two more chemicals pose similar hazards for nitrosamine formation. The chemical 2-bromo-2-nitropropane-1,3-diol (also known as Bronopol) may break down in products into formaldehyde and also cause the formation of carcinogenic nitrosamines under certain conditions. One of the most expensive lines of cosmetics today, Chanel, often uses this chemical. So do many leading brands of baby products. And the Body Shop, whose product sales are built on a reputation of containing natural ingredients, also offers products containing this chemical. There are many safer yet equally effective products available.

Padimate-O (also known as octyl dimethyl PABA) is found in cosmetics, especially sunscreens. It can also cause formation of nitrosamines. At present it is not known whether the particular nitrosamine formed in this product is carcinogenic. Some experts have recommended that consumers continue to use sunscreens with padimate-O. The jury, however, is still out on the nitrosamine formed from padimate-O, and nobody knows for sure whether it will prove carcinogenic. So the most prudent consumer will prefer sunscreens without padimate-O, until the industry proves that the nitrosamine by-product that may be formed is not carcinogenic.

Although many products contain DEA, TEA, 2-bromo-2-nitropropane-1, 3-diol, or padimate-O, some manufacturers have added ingredients such as antioxidants that may slow or retard, but do not prevent, formation of nitrosamines. It is always better to avoid buying products with potential nitrosamine-forming ingredients.

Ethoxylated Alcohols and 1,4-Dioxane

Cosmetics containing ethoxylated wetting agents (e.g., detergents, foaming agents, emulsifiers, and solvents) may be contaminated with 1,4-dioxane, which is carcinogenic. Studies show that dioxane readily penetrates human skin. It can be removed from cosmetics through vacuum stripping during processing without an unreasonable increase in raw material cost. Doing so is not mandatory but should be. At present, there is not enough information shown on product labels to enable you to determine whether products are contaminated. The best way to protect yourself is to recognize ingredients most likely to be contaminated with 1,4-dioxane. These include ingredients with the prefix, word, or syllable *PEG, Polyethylene, Polyethylene Glycol, Polyoxyethylene, eth* (as in sodium laur*eth* sulfate), or *oxynol*. Both polysorbate 60 and polysorbate 80 may also be contaminated with 1,4-dioxane.

We provide this information as a general caution. It is impossible to determine which products are contaminated and which have gone through vacuum stripping, so some products we recommend may contain ingredients that possibly are contaminated with 1,4-dioxane.

Artificial Colors

Some artificial colors, such as Blue 1 and Green 3, are carcinogenic. Impurities found in commercial batches of other cosmetic colors such as D&C Red 33, FD&C Yellow 5, and FD&C Yellow 6 have been shown to cause cancer not only when ingested, but also when applied to the skin. Some artificial coal tar colors contain heavy metal impurities, including arsenic and lead, which are carcinogenic. Nevertheless, the FDA maintains that these color additives, impurities notwithstanding, do not pose a hazard when used in cosmetics and personal care products. We have recommended against many products containing artificial colors when clear evidence of their carcinogenic hazard is available. In some cases, products with artificial colors have been recommended in the absence of such information. Many consumers may simply want to avoid products containing artificial colors. Most alternative brands, sold in health food stores, do not contain them.

Hair Dyes

The use of permanent or semipermanent hair color products, particularly black and dark brown colors, is associated with increased incidence of human cancer. As stated earlier, the use of these products places women at increased risk of non-Hodgkin's lymphoma, multiple myeloma, and Hodgkin's disease. In fact, there is growing evidence that the use of hair-coloring products accounts for 20 percent of all non-Hodgkin's lymphoma cases in all U.S. women. These products should be banned. Until that happens, they should be clearly labeled for their cancer hazard. We found several brands of natural hair-coloring products that are relatively effective and safe. These are listed in the shopping charts and should be your preferred choices.

Lanolin

Lanolin itself is perfectly safe, and its presence in cosmetics is generally beneficial to your skin, especially when it is sore and cracked (although some people develop allergic reactions to this ingredient). But cosmetic-grade lanolin can be contaminated with carcinogenic pesticides such as DDT, dieldrin, and lindane, in addition to other neurotoxic pesticides. Some sixteen pesticides were identified in lanolin sampled in 1988 (including the neurotoxic organophosphate pesticide diazinon, which was found in twenty-one out of twenty-five samples and readily penetrates the skin).

These chemicals *are* likely to migrate through the skin into the bloodstream. The National Academy of Sciences has expressed concern over the frequency of contamination of cosmetics containing lanolin with pesticides. The FDA recognizes that the contamination of lanolin is a problem, especially in the case of skin products used by nursing mothers directly on their nipples, because their infants may end up ingesting these carcinogenic impurities. Furthermore, lanolin is often applied to children's and babies' skin with the potential for significant absorption of pesticides.

The FDA has done nothing to improve the quality of cosmetic lanolin, though the industry has voluntarily reduced, but not removed, the contamination of these carcinogens. The fact that labels need not disclose this information leaves the consumer unsure of which products are pure and which are contaminated with carcinogenic pesticides. Again, the lack of full label disclosure causes the entire industry to be suspect, rather than limiting the problem to those companies that are not purifying their lanolin-based ingredients.

Although the FDA believes the risk to consumers is small, interestingly, Dr. Stan Milstein, special assistant to the director of the FDA Office of Cosmetics and Colors, adds this caution: "Given all the carcinogens in the environment that the consumer is bombarded with, do we really need to be increasing our exposure even incrementally?"

Information on which products contain lanolin is provided as a general caution but cannot be used as a criterion for evaluating carcinogenic hazards of individual products in the following charts, as it is impossible to determine which products will be free from such contaminants and which will, in fact, contain pesticide contaminants in lanolin ingredients. Some recommended products do contain lanolin. The cautious among you will want to eliminate lanolin-based compounds from your shopping carts.

Talc

Cosmetic talc is carcinogenic. Powdered products containing talc and used around the face must be assumed to expose the consumer or professional cosmetologist via inhalation. Inhaling talc and using it in the genital area, where its use is associated with increased risk of ovarian cancer, are the primary ways this substance poses a carcinogenic hazard. In most cases, we have designated a "minimal risk" rating to products containing talc. However, products containing talc that are used in the genital region are given the "caution" rating because of clear evidence that talc causes ovarian cancer. Although some recommended products contain talc, these are generally liquid formulations and pose minimal, if any, carcinogenic risk.

(Talc should never be used on babies both because of its carcinogenicity and acute respiratory distress from inhalation that often results in death.)

Silica

Some silica used in cosmetics, especially amorphous hydrated silica, may be contaminated with small amounts of crystalline quartz. Crystalline silica is carcinogenic. We simply cannot tell whether the silica used in specific cosmetics and personal care products contains small amounts of crystalline quartz, or none. Furthermore, exposure via inhalation is assumed to be limited to special use situations; for example, people who use facial makeup, especially powders, may inhale the silica. The situation is obviously more perilous for beauty care professionals, as they may end up inhaling contaminants continuously. There are inadequate data to determine that amorphous silica is not carcinogenic; therefore we have assigned products containing silica the minimal risk rating. The hazard of silica is primarily via inhalation. As with talc, although some recommended products contain silica they are still better than their competitors.

Synthetic Fragrances

As noted earlier, fragrances are made up of hundreds of chemicals. Some, such as methylene chloride, are carcinogenic. Because manufacturers are not required to disclose hazardous chemicals used in manufacturing fragrances, consumers have no way of knowing whether their brands' fragrances contain carcinogens. The wise consumer will make the assumption that all synthetic fragrances contain carcinogens. However, in the absence of such information we are unable to evaluate fragrances for their presence. Although some brands containing synthetic fragrances are recommended in the absence of available information, some consumers may simply wish to avoid such products.

Formaldehyde-Releasing Preservatives

As we mentioned earlier, some fragrances contain or release formaldehyde. We have occasionally recommended such products in the absence of available data on the preservative's carcinogenicity. Once again, many readers will want to avoid using products that contain formaldehyde-based preservatives. See page 188 for a listing.

The government should ban carcinogenic chemicals used in cosmetics, and industry should implement safer alternatives. Until that happens, concerned consumers will want to reduce exposure whenever alternatives are available. And while it may not be possible to avoid every carcinogenic exposure, you should still do the best you can. Plenty of good choices are available, as the following charts show.

HOW WE EVALUATED COSMETICS
AND PERSONAL CARE PRODUCTS

Contact Dermatitis: Allergens, Sensitizers, and Irritants

We identified the chemicals contained in cosmetics and personal care products from their labels. The more chemicals a product contains that are major allergens, sensitizers, and irritants, the more likely it is to cause reactions in a large number of consumers.

We also based our evaluations on the results of a major five-year study of cosmetic reactions conducted by the North American Contact Dermatitis Group, a task force of the American Academy of Dermatology, from 1977 to 1983 with FDA funding. Before this study, data on reactions to cosmetics consisted almost exclusively of information obtained from published case studies, complaints consumers reported to manufacturers or the FDA, and a three-month consumer survey from 1974. The task force conducted one of the most extensive cosmetic reaction studies ever undertaken in the United States and Canada. In evaluating cosmetic and personal care products, we used the study's findings to identify those ingredients that caused allergies, sensitization, and irritation. We assigned each ingredient a numeric value, depending on the number of people in the study who reported an adverse reaction. In this way we were able to come up with a listing that reflects the potential for products to cause contact dermatitis.

Table 5 on page 198 presents the leading contact dermatitis problem ingredients in cosmetics and personal care products along with their identifying number, which you will find listed in the charts. The numeric value assigned to each ingredient represents the number of people who reported reactions in the major five-year study. Ingredients are listed only if they caused reactions in at least two participants in the study. Just about any ingredient can cause an allergic reaction in *somebody*. Those listed in the table are *major* allergens, sensitizers, and irritants. By the way, fragrances are assumed to be synthetic—unless product labels specifically state they are naturally derived.

We assigned a "little to no risk" rating to products with a numeric score of 64 or less, and "minimal risk" to products with a numeric score between 65 and 131. Products with a numeric value of 132 or greater were rated for "caution."

Here are some examples of how the system works:

- Almay Matte Classic Duo Eyeshadow contains no ingredients likely to cause an allergic reaction. Its total numeric value would therefore be 0, and its rating would be little to no risk.

- L'Oréal Performing Preference Permanent Creme-In Hair Color contains propylene glycol (numeric value 29), phenylenediamine (41), resorcinol (3), and fragrance (67), for a total numeric value of 140. It should be used with caution.
- Neutrogena Shampoo contains fragrance (67), imidazolidinyl urea (21), and parabens (19), for a numeric value of 107. It presents a minimal risk.
- Pantene Progressive Treatment Vitamin Therapy Shampoo (for normal hair) contains fragrance (67), octyl dimethyl PABA (5), and toco-pherol (2). Its numeric value is 74. This product presents a minimal risk.

Very simply, those products with ingredients most likely to cause allergic sensitization or irritation have higher scores and demand greater caution in their use.

Carcinogens

We assigned a caution rating to products that contain chemicals classified as probable or known human carcinogens or chemicals that are animal carcinogens and possible human carcinogens, as determined by the International Agency for Research on Cancer, other recognized bodies of experts, and the scientific literature.

We assigned a minimal risk rating to products containing chemicals that are not necessarily carcinogenic themselves but are carcinogenic precursors (e.g., DEA and TEA). We also used the minimal risk rating for products containing ingredients about which the data are inadequate to determine their human cancer risk. A product may contain more than one problem ingredient, of course; obviously the more it contains, the greater its hazards. We have evaluated products based on their most hazardous carcinogenic ingredient.

As for products containing DEA, TEA, octyl dimethal PABA (padimate-O), or 2-bromo-2-nitropropane-1,3-diol, to some people, particularly those in the cosmetic industry, it may seem unduly alarmist that we have rated products containing these ingredients for minimal caution. However, we believe that it should not be left to the consumer to play cancer roulette. The burden of safety should be on the manufacturer. If a product contains DEA, TEA, octyl dimethyl PABA, or 2-bromo-2-nitropropane-1,3-diol, the manufacturer should certify that it does not contain carcinogenic nitrosamines or formaldehyde by stating so on the label or in accompanying literature. You can easily find products without these ingredients, and you would be wise to assume all such products are contaminated until the cosmetic industry provides greater documentation of their safety.

Products have *not* been evaluated for containing lanolin, ethoxylated alcohols, polysorbate 60 or 80, or other similar ingredients that might be contaminated with carcinogenic impurities such as 1,4-dioxane. But you can read the label and make your own decision.

SAFE USE RECOMMENDATIONS

- Choose cosmetics and personal care products that contain the fewest ingredients, yet are still effective. As the list of a product's ingredients grows, so does the possibility that it will cause adverse reactions, including allergy, irritation, and cancer.
- Handle all cosmetics in a way that prevents bacterial contamination. This is especially important for products preserved with milder ingredients and those used near the eyes. Do not leave product containers uncapped. Do not share them; do not use your fingers instead of applicators. Do not store them in heated areas or leave them in the sun, which could create a breeding ground for bacteria.
- Some experts suggest that consumers perform their own patch tests if they want to know whether or not they are allergic to a cosmetic product. You can do this by applying a small amount to the inner arm, covering the area with a bandage, and leaving it on twenty-four hours. Redness or soreness may mean you are sensitive to an ingredient in the product. If no redness or soreness occurs, you can use the product with some degree of confidence that it will not cause an allergic reaction or irritation.

HOW TO USE THE CHARTS

You can determine the safety of your present brand or any brand that you are thinking of buying by checking its evaluation in the shopping charts under each category. In the sample chart below, the first column lists shampoos in alphabetical order and includes numbers representing their hazardous ingredients. A table of hazardous ingredients appears on pages 198–99 that will be used to determine the contact dermatitis–causing, carcinogenic, and inadequately tested ingredients for each product in the charts that follow.

For example, to determine which problem ingredients are present in Neutrogena Shampoo, look in column one, where you'll see the numbers 6, 7, and 14, meaning that this product contains fragrance (6), imidazolidinyl urea (7), and parabens (14). It also contains DEA as you can see by the number 28. In column two you can see that it poses a minimal risk for contact dermatitis. In column three you can see that it poses a minimal cancer risk.

On the other hand, Neutrogena Shampoo for Permed or Color-Treated Hair contains fragrance (6), imidazolidinyl urea (7), parabens (14), and propylene glycol (16), making it a higher-risk product for contact dermatitis, as you can see in column two where it is rated as deserving caution. Furthermore, the product contains DEA (28), D&C Red 33 (27), and FD&C Blue 1 (29); its rating in column three is minimal risk.

Contact Dermatitis, Carcinogens

Column One				Column Two	Column Three
Product				Acute Health Advisory	Chronic Health Advisory
Little to No Risk	Minimal Risk	Caution	Recommended	Contact Dermatitis	Carcinogens
Neutrogena Shampoo 6, 7, 14, 28				Caution	Minimal Risk
Neutrogena Shampoo for Permed or Color-Treated Hair 6, 7, 14, 16, 27, 28, 29				Caution	Minimal Risk

You can see that Neutrogena Shampoo is the slightly safer of the two products. Of course, even safer choices are available, as you will see when you look at the full chart for shampoos.

One last word. As with household products, for acute health effects, the difference between a minimal risk or caution rating and little to no risk may be small and, in some cases, even negligible. A caution rating for contact dermatitis should not be construed as a blanket condemnation of a product. Many people will be able to use products rated with caution notices with complete comfort. There is definitely an interplay between the skills of the product formulator, the percentage of the chemical in the formula, and individual skin types. Based on these facts, even products with seemingly irritating ingredients may well provide an agreeable experience for consumers.

On the other hand, products that seem as though they should pose absolutely no dermatological hazards may cause allergies or irritation in a few people. There will always be exceptions to the guidelines detailed in this book.

Also, please note that some recommended products are not perfect. Even so, they are preferred, and we include them to provide consumers with as wide a range of choices as possible.

Table 5 lists chemicals that are carcinogens or precursors to carcinogens (e.g., DEA), or that have not been adequately tested. The first column lists the chemical and its identifying number. The second and third columns note the degree of risk. Please note that a handful of carcinogenic chemicals also cause allergic reactions or irritation; these chemicals have dual ratings for both categories but will be listed under those ingredients posing contact dermatitis hazards.

Table 5: Ingredients in Cosmetics and Personal Care Products that Cause Dermatitis and Cancer

Ingredients	Number of People with Contact Dermatitis Reactions	Cancer Risk

Ingredients Causing Contact Dermatitis

Ingredients	Number of People with Contact Dermatitis Reactions	Cancer Risk
1. Allantoin	2	
2. Benzyl alcohol	3	
3. 2-bromo-2-nitropropane-1,3-diol (Bronopol) (carcinogen precursor)	16	Minimal Risk
4. Butylated hydroxyanisole (BHA)/(carcinogenic)	3	Caution
5. Formaldehyde (carcinogenic)	16	Caution
6. Fragrance (excluding naturally derived fragrances when disclosed)	67	
7. Imidazolidinyl urea	21	
8. Lanolin	15	
9. Lanolin alcohol	12	
10. Lanolin oil	2	
11. Oak moss	3	
12. Octyl dimethyl PABA (padimate-O) (inadequately tested to establish noncarcinogenicity)	5	Minimal Risk
13. Para-aminobenzoic acid (PABA)	3	
14. Parabens	19	
15. Phenylenediamines (found in permanent and semi-permanent hair coloring products)	41	Caution
16. Propylene glycol	29	
17. Quaternium-15	65	

continued

Ingredients	Number of People with Contact Dermatitis Reactions	Cancer Risk
18. Resorcinol	3	
19. Tocopherol	2	
20. Toluenesulfonamide/ formaldehyde resin	23	
21. Triethanolamine (TEA)/ (carcinogen precursor)	3	Minimal Risk

Carcinogenic, Carcinogen Precursors, and Inadequately Tested Ingredients

22. Butylated Hydroxytoluene (BHT)		Minimal Risk
23. Coal tar		Caution
24. D&C Green 5		Minimal Risk
25. D&C Orange 17		Minimal Risk
26. D&C Red 19		Minimal Risk
27. D&C Red 33		Minimal Risk
28. Diethanolamine (DEA)		Minimal Risk
29. FD&C Blue 1		Minimal Risk
30. FD&C Green 3		Minimal Risk
31. FD&C Red 4		Minimal Risk
32. FD&C Red 40		Minimal Risk
33. FD&C Yellow 5		Minimal Risk
34. FD&C Yellow 6		Minimal Risk
35. Fluoride		Minimal Risk
36. Lead acetate		Caution
37. Methyl methacrylate		Minimal Risk
38. Saccharin		Caution
39. Silica		Minimal Risk
40. Talc		Minimal Risk–Caution (depending on area of use)

CHAPTER 8

Eye and Face Makeup

BLUSHES

Product Types

Liquid; powder.

Health Advisory

Contact Dermatitis

For some highly sensitive people, fragranced products can be a problem. Other ingredients to avoid include formaldehyde and quaternium 15. Propylene glycol and imidazolidinyl urea can irritate sensitive skin. Acrylate compounds can be strong irritants.

Carcinogens

Avoid using products containing BHA and formaldehyde. If looking for a natural product, also avoid brands containing D&C Red 33, FD&C Yellow 5, FD&C Yellow 6, and other artificial colors.

Talc is commonly used in blushes. If this concerns you, choose liquid products, which significantly reduce the inhalation of talc.

Blushes

Product				Health Advisory	
(Little to No Risk)	(Minimal Risk)	(Caution)	✓ Recommended	Contact Dermatitis	Carcinogens
Almay Cheek Color 7, 14, 40				🛒	🛒
Bare Escentuals Beginning & Finishing Powders ✓				🛒	🛒
Bare Escentuals Blushing & Highlighting Powders ✓				🛒	🛒
Bare Escentuals Bronzing & Contouring Powders ✓				🛒	🛒
Bare Escentuals Glimmer Powders ✓				🛒	🛒
Beauty Without Cruelty Blusher Powder 4, 14, 16, 23, 40				🛒	🛒
Borghese Blush Milano 14, 29, 33, 34, 40				🛒	🛒
Clarion Face Enhancing Blush 4, 14, 17, 23, 33, 40				🛒	🛒
Coty Dual Pan Bare Blusher 6, 7, 14, 40				🛒	🛒
Cover Girl Classic Color Brush-On Blush 4, 5, 6, 14, 33, 40				🛒	🛒
Cover Girl Moisture Wear Nourishing All-Day Blush 4, 5, 6, 14, 17, 33, 40				🛒	🛒
Cover Girl Oil Control Fresh Blush 4, 6, 14, 17, 33, 40				🛒	🛒
Cover Girl Professional Contouring Blush 4, 6, 14, 17, 33, 40				🛒	🛒
Cover Girl Replenishing Creamy Powder Blush 4, 6, 14, 17, 40				🛒	🛒
Cover Girl Sheer Blush Mates 5, 6, 14, 17, 22, 33, 40				🛒	🛒
Dr. Hauschka Burgundy Cheek & Lip (Red) ✓				🛒	🛒
Dr. Hauschka Rose Cheek & Lip (Pink) ✓				🛒	🛒
Dr. Hauschka Cheek & Lip (Apricot) ✓				🛒	🛒
Ecco Bella Eyeshadow/Blush ✓				🛒	🛒
Flame Glow Sheer Cheekcolor 9, 17, 19, 33, 34, 40				🛒	🛒
Ida Grae Creme Rouge ✓				🛒	🛒
Ida Grae Earth Rouge ✓				🛒	🛒
Ida Grae Translucent Powder ✓				🛒	🛒

Product				Health Advisory	
Little to No Risk	Minimal Risk	Caution	✓ Recommended	Contact Dermatitis	Carcinogens
Lancôme Blush Subtil Delicate Powder Blush 6, 33				🛒	🛒
L'Oréal Microblush Softly Sheer Cheekcolor 6, 9, 14, 22, 23				🛒	🛒
Max Factor New Definition 9, 14, 33, 34, 39				🛒	🛒
Max Factor Satin Blush 14, 33, 40				🛒	🛒
Maybelline Advanced Color Fresh Formula Natural Bristle Brush ✓ 14, 17, 40				🛒	🛒
Maybelline Brush/Blush III 4, 7, 9, 10, 14, 40				🛒	🛒
Maybelline Brush/Blush III Advanced Color Fresh Formula ✓				🛒	🛒
Maybelline Shine Free Oil Control Blush ✓ 7, 14, 40				🛒	🛒
Nature Cosmetics Nature Blush 14, 19, 29, 34				🛒	🛒
Paul Penders Blushers ✓ 19				🛒	🛒
Rachel Perry Earth Blush ✓ 6, 7, 9, 10, 14, 19, 40				🛒	🛒
Revlon Naturally Glamorous Blush-On 14, 33, 40				🛒	🛒
Revlon Powder Creme Blush 4, 14, 33, 39				🛒	🛒
Revlon Sheer Face Color 9, 14, 27, 33, 34, 39, 40				🛒	🛒
Revlon Springwater Blush Oil Free for Sensitive Skin 14, 16, 33, 37, 39				🛒	🛒

CONCEALERS

Product Types

Brush-on; stick.

Health Advisory

Contact Dermatitis

The two most irritating ingredients people are likely to encounter are imidazolidinyl urea and propylene glycol. Some people are sensitive to lanolin alcohol and lanolin oil; both are commonly used in concealers. The parabens are also quite widely used; they are not bothersome for most people, but occasionally cause allergies or irritation.

Carcinogens

Avoid using products containing DEA and TEA. Since concealers remain on all day, nitrosamines that have formed in products will be absorbed through the skin. Products containing BHA should not be used; this carcinogen also is absorbed through the skin.

Although many brands contain silica and talc, most products come in liquid or stick, reducing inhalation. Thus, talc and silica probably are not hazardous in this context of usage.

Concealers

Product				Health Advisory	
🛒 Little to No Risk 🛒 Minimal Risk 🛒 Caution ✓ Recommended				Contact Dermatitis	Carcinogens
Almay Cover-Up Stick 4, 14, 16				🛒 Little to No Risk	⚫ Caution
Almay Under Eye Cover Cream 4, 14, 22				🛒 Little to No Risk	⚫ Caution
Almay SPF8 Extra Protection Concealer 7, 14, 16, 28				🛒 Minimal Risk	🛒 Minimal Risk
Beauty Without Cruelty Cover Up Stick 4				🛒 Little to No Risk	⚫ Caution
Cover Girl Moisture Wear All-Day Perfecting Concealer 4, 9, 10, 14, 16, 19, 22				🛒 Minimal Risk	🛒 Little to No Risk
Cover Girl Replenishing Concealer ✓ 14, 16, 19, 40				🛒 Little to No Risk	🛒 Minimal Risk
La Formule Aromatherapy Blemish Pen ✓				🛒 Little to No Risk	🛒 Little to No Risk
Logona Concealer Pen ✓ 19, 40				🛒 Little to No Risk	🛒 Minimal Risk
Maybelline Shine Free Blemish Concealer 7, 9, 14, 16, 21				🛒 Minimal Risk	🛒 Minimal Risk
Maybelline Shine Free Cover Stick 4, 14				🛒 Little to No Risk	⚫ Caution
Revlon New Complexion Concealer 7, 9, 14, 16, 21, 28, 37, 39				🛒 Minimal Risk	🛒 Minimal Risk

FOUNDATIONS

Product Types

Cream; liquid.

Health Advisory

Contact Dermatitis

Foundation and other facial makeup are the third leading cause of contact dermatitis among cosmetics users. So it is especially important that consumers stay with those products with the least number of problem ingredients. Furthermore, foundations contain a wide range of allergens and irritants and your exposure will be all day. So make sure you select brands carefully.

Brands containing 2-bromo-2-nitropropane-1,3-diol or quaternium 15 could expose you to formaldehyde, a problem ingredient for a lot of people. Furthermore, people with sensitive skin may have problems with fragrances and propylene glycol; both can sting. For some people, triethanolamine can be irritating. A few people will have problems with lanolin, padimate-O, and parabens, but for most these ingredients are not a problem.

Foundations often cause a condition known medically as cosmetic acne, characterized by very small pimples that occur intermittently. Cosmetic acne affects about one-third of all women in their twenties through fifties at one time or another. This is not the kind of acne associated with puberty. It is the result of acnegenic ingredients in foundations. If you are suffering from small blemishes, especially pimples, and are not sure why, try switching products. Choose one of our recommendations. If the situation is troubling and nothing seems to work, you might want to stop using face creams such as foundation altogether.

The following ingredients have various degress of potential to cause cosmetic acne.

Ingredient	Cosmetic Acne Potential
Butyl stearate	Moderate-strong
Cocoa butter	Strong
Corn oil	Weak-moderate
Isopropyl myristate	Weak
Lauryl alcohol	Weak
Linseed oil	Strong

Ingredient	*Cosmetic Acne Potential*
Margarine	Weak
Methyl oleate	Weak-moderate
Mineral oil	Varies from weak to moderate
Oleic acid	Strong
Olive oil	Moderate-strong
Peanut oil	Moderate-strong
Petrolatum	Varies greatly from weak to strong
Safflower oil	Weak
Sesame oil	Moderate-strong
Stearic acid	Weak

Carcinogens

Stay away from products containing 2-bromo-2-nitropropane-1,3-diol, which can break down into formaldehyde or, under certain circumstances, cause the formation of nitrosamines. DEA and TEA should also be avoided.

Many products today contain the inadequately tested ingredient padimate-O as a sunscreen. But if you are searching for a really effective and safe sunblock, titanium dioxide in a cream or liquid foundation is a better choice. A full-spectrum sunblock, titanium dioxide shields the skin from both ultraviolet A (UVA) and ultraviolet B (UVB) rays. It is also less allergenic and irritating.

Products containing silica and talc have been evaluated for minimal risk; these substances are carcinogenic when inhaled or dusted. But as long as you use cream or liquid foundation, they will not be a problem.

Foundations

Product				Contact Dermatitis	Carcinogens
🛒 Little to No Risk	🛒 Minimal Risk	🛒 Caution	✓ Recommended		
Almay Fresh Glow Moisture Renew Make-up 7, 14, 16, 21				🛒	🛒
Almay Matte Finish Make-Up 1, 7, 14, 19, 21, 40				🛒	🛒
Almay Moisture Balance Make-Up for Normal Skin 7, 14, 16, 21, 40				🛒	🛒
Almay Moisture Tint Sports Formula ✓ 7, 14, 40				🛒	🛒
Aubrey Natural Translucent Base ✓ 1				🛒	🛒

Product			Health Advisory	
	Little to No Risk	Minimal Risk	Caution	Recommended ✓
			Contact Dermatitis	Carcinogens
Avon Advanced Foundation Enhancing Liquid 6, 7, 14, 21			● Caution	● Minimal
Bare Escentuals Beginning & Finishing Powders ✓			Little	Little
Bare Escentuals Bronzing & Contouring Powders ✓			Little	Little
Bare Escentuals Rice Powder–Pink ✓			Little	Little
Bare Escentuals Rice Powder–White ✓			Little	Little
Beauty Without Cruelty Makeup Base 7, 14, 16, 28, 40			Minimal	Little
Chanel Teint Naturel Liquid Makeup Base SPF8 3, 6, 9, 12, 14, 16, 21			● Caution	Little
Chanel Teint Pur Matte Makeup SPF8 3, 14, 16			Little	Little
Chanel Teint Pur Matte Satin Makeup SPF8 3, 14, 16, 19, 21, 40			Little	Little
Clarins Matte Finish Foundation 6, 14, 16, 19, 39			Little	Little
Clarion Face Perfect Complexion Lightweight Make-up 14, 16, 19, 28, 40			Minimal	Little
Clarion Moisturizing Liquid Make-Up 14, 16, 28, 40			Minimal	Little
Clarion Natural Finish Liquid Make-Up 14, 16, 28			Minimal	Little
Clarion Oil-Free Liqiud Make-Up 4, 14, 16, 28, 40			Minimal	● Caution
Clarion Protection 15 Liquid Make-Up 14, 16, 19, 28, 40			Minimal	Minimal
Clinique Extra-Help Makeup 7, 9, 14, 16, 19, 21, 40			Little	Little
Clinique Pore-Minimizer Makeup ✓ 16, 40			Minimal	Little
Clinique Stay-True Makeup Oil-free Formula 7, 14, 16, 21			Little	Little
Corn Silk Oil Absorbent Liquid Make-Up 6, 14, 16, 17, 28, 40			● Caution	Little
Cover Girl Clarifying Make-Up ✓ 6, 14, 16, 40			Little	Little
Cover Girl Clean Make-Up 6, 14, 16, 21, 40			Little	Little
Cover Girl Extremely Gentle Make-Up 14, 16, 28, 40			Minimal	Little
Cover Girl Moisture Wear Moisturizing Cream Make-Up 6, 14, 16, 21, 40			Little	Little

Product	Health Advisory	
Legend: 🛒 Little to No Risk · 🛒 Minimal Risk · 🛒 Caution · ✓ Recommended	Contact Dermatitis	Carcinogens
Cover Girl Moisture Wear Moisturizing Liquid Make-up 4, 6, 8, 9, 14, 16, 21, 22, 40	Caution	Caution
Cover Girl Oil Control Make-Up 6, 14, 16, 21, 40	Minimal Risk	Minimal Risk
Cover Girl Replenishing Natural Finish Liquid Make-Up 4, 6, 8, 9, 14, 16, 21, 22, 40	Caution	Caution
Cover Girl Replenishing Ultra-Finish Creme Make-Up 6, 14, 16, 21, 40	Minimal Risk	Minimal Risk
Dr. Hauschka Catechu Day Cream (Dark Foundation Color) ✓	Little to No Risk	Little to No Risk
Dr. Hauschka Day Cosmetic (Bronze) ✓	Little to No Risk	Little to No Risk
Dr. Hauschka Ratanhia Day Cream (Medium Foundation Color) ✓	Little to No Risk	Little to No Risk
Estée Lauder Demi-Matte Oil-free Makeup	Minimal Risk	Minimal Risk
Estée Lauder Lucidity Light-Diffusing Makeup SPF8 7, 14, 16, 19, 21, 37, 40	Minimal Risk	Minimal Risk
Estée Lauder Polished Performance Liquid Makeup 6, 7, 9, 14, 16, 21, 28, 40	Caution	Minimal Risk
Ida Grae Creme Foundation ✓ 8, 19	Little to No Risk	Little to No Risk
Logona Tinted Day Cream Beige-Gold ✓ 9, 19	Little to No Risk	Little to No Risk
Lagona Tinted Day Cream Beige-Rose ✓ 9, 19	Little to No Risk	Little to No Risk
L'Oréal Illuminating Matte Make-Up 14, 16, 19, 21	Little to No Risk	Minimal Risk
L'Oréal Visuelle Invisible Coverage Make-Up 9, 12, 14, 16, 21	Minimal Risk	Minimal Risk
la prairie Cellular Oil-free Treatment Foundation 6, 7, 14, 16, 19, 21	Caution	Minimal Risk
Max Factor New Definition Make-Up ✓ 14, 39, 40	Little to No Risk	Minimal Risk
Max Factor Pan-Stik Ultra Creamy Make-Up ✓ 6, 14	Minimal Risk	Caution
Max Factor Satin Splendor Flawless Complexion Make-Up 4, 12, 14	Little to No Risk	Caution
Max Factor Whipped Creme Make-Up 6, 9, 14, 16, 17, 21, 39, 40	Caution	Minimal Risk
Max Factor Active Protection Make-Up 4, 7, 8, 9, 12, 14, 40	Minimal Risk	Minimal Risk
Maybelline Active Wear Liquid Make-Up 7, 14, 16, 19, 28	Minimal Risk	Minimal Risk
Maybelline Finish Matte Water-Based Liquid Make-Up 6, 7, 14, 16, 21, 40	Caution	Minimal Risk
Maybelline Long Wearing Liquid Make-Up 6, 7, 9, 14, 16, 21, 40	Caution	Minimal Risk

Product		Health Advisory	
(icons row)		Contact Dermatitis	Carcinogens
Maybelline Moisture Whip Liquid Make-up 6, 9, 14, 16, 19, 21, 40		Minimal Risk	Minimal Risk
Maybelline Shades of You Liquid Water-Based Make-Up 7, 9, 14, 16, 21, 40		Minimal Risk	Minimal Risk
Maybelline Sheer Essentials Liquid Make-Up 9, 14, 16, 19, 21, 40		Minimal Risk	Minimal Risk
Maybelline Shine Free Normal to Combination Skin Liquid Make-Up 6, 7, 9, 14, 16, 21, 40		Caution	Minimal Risk
Maybelline Shine-Free Oil Control Liquid Make-up 7, 14, 16, 21, 40		Minimal Risk	Minimal Risk
Maybelline Ultra Performance Pure Liquid Make-Up 7, 14, 16, 28, 40		Minimal Risk	Minimal Risk
Monteil Habitat Natural-Light Makeup 7, 14, 16, 19, 21, 39, 40		Minimal Risk	Minimal Risk
Nature Cosmetics Nature Face Foundations 12, 14, 16, 19, 21		Little to No Risk	Minimal Risk
Origins Natural Color Matte Makeup 1, 14, 16, 21, 39, 40		Minimal Risk	Minimal Risk
Origins Natural Color Moisture Makeup 7, 14, 16, 28, 40		Minimal Risk	Minimal Risk
Paul Penders Make-Up Cream ✓ 14		Little to No Risk	Little to No Risk
Physician's Formula Le Velvet Film Make-Up ✓ 14, 40		Little to No Risk	Minimal Risk
Physician's Formula Oil Control Matte Make-Up 4, 14, 17, 40		Minimal Risk	Caution
Prescriptives Custom Blended Foundation 1, 14, 19, 21, 39, 40		Little to No Risk	Minimal Risk
Rachel Perry Bee Pollen-Jojoba Nutrient Make-Up #1–#7 6, 7, 14, 16, 19, 21		Minimal Risk	Minimal Risk
Revlon Springwater Make-Up 7, 14, 16, 21, 40		Minimal Risk	Minimal Risk
Revlon Touch & Glow Moisturizing Make-Up 6, 9, 14, 16, 21, 40		Minimal Risk	Minimal Risk

Icon legend: Little to No Risk · Minimal Risk · Caution · Recommended ✓

FACIAL POWDERS

Product Types

Compressed; loose.

Health Advisory

Contact Dermatitis

Problem ingredients include 2-bromo-2-nitropropane-1,3-diol, formaldehyde, and quaternium 15; all expose you to formaldehyde. Some people have problems with fragrance, lanolin, imidazolidinyl urea, and parabens.

Carcinogens

Many of the Cover Girl facial powders contain formaldehyde. Chanel's Sheer Pressed Powder contains 2-bromo-2-nitropropane-1,3-diol, which catalyzes formation of nitrosamines and may break down into formaldehyde. Stay away from both!

Don't use products that list formaldehyde, DEA, TEA, or padimate-O as ingredients. Because facial powders are worn for extended periods, if nitrosamines are formed, there is ample opportunity for them to be absorbed. As for silica and talc, avoid use of loose-powder products, which can be inhaled. With compressed powder, there is less inhalation.

Facial Powders

Product	Health Advisory	
🛒 Little to No Risk 🛒 Minimal Risk 🛒 Caution ✓ Recommended	Contact Dermatitis	Carcinogens
Almay Luxury Finish Loose Powder 39, 40	🛒	🛒
Almay Matte Finish Pressed Powder 40	🛒	🛒
Almay Oil-Blotting Pressed Powder 40	🛒	🛒
Aubrey Deep Tone Silken Earth Make-Up Powder ✓ 1	🛒	🛒
Aubrey Light Tone Silken Earth Make-Up Powder ✓ 1	🛒	🛒
Aubrey Medium Silken Earth Make-Up Powder ✓ 1	🛒	🛒
Aubrey Rose Tone Silken Earth Make-Up Powder ✓ 1	🛒	🛒
Bare Escentuals Beginning & Finishing Powders ✓	🛒	🛒
Bare Escentuals Blushing & Highlight Powders ✓	🛒	🛒
Bare Escentuals Bronzing & Contouring Powders ✓	🛒	🛒
Bare Escentuals Glimmer Powders ✓	🛒	🛒
Beauty Without Cruelty Face Powder/Compressed 4, 14, 16, 40	🛒	🛒
Beauty Without Cruelty Translucent Powder 14, 40	🛒	🛒
Borghese Molto Bella Liquid/Powder Makeup with Sunscreen 4, 14, 39, 40	🛒	🛒
Chanel Joues Contraste Powder Blush 3, 6, 9, 14, 29, 33, 34	🛒	🛒
Chanel La Poudre Pressée De Chanel Sheer Pressed Powder 3, 6, 9, 14, 19, 34	🛒	🛒

Legend:
- 🛒 Little to No Risk
- 🛒 Minimal Risk
- 🛒 Caution
- ✓ Recommended

Product	Contact Dermatitis	Carcinogens
Chanel La Poudre De Chanel Translucent Loose Powder 3, 6, 14, 33	Minimal Risk	Minimal Risk
Clarion Natural Finish Pressed Powder 14, 17, 22, 40	Minimal Risk	Minimal Risk
Clarion Oil Free Translucent Pressed Powder 14, 17, 22, 40	Minimal Risk	Minimal Risk
Clarion Perfect Complexion Refining Loose Powder 14, 17, 22	Minimal Risk	Minimal Risk
Clarion Silk Perfection Pressed Powder 14, 17, 22	Minimal Risk	Minimal Risk
Clinique Blended Face Powder and Brush 40	Little to No Risk	Minimal Risk
Corn Silk Oil Absorbent Loose Powder ✓ 6, 7, 14	Minimal Risk	Little to No Risk
Corn Silk Oil Absorbent Pressed Powder ✓ 6, 7, 14, 40	Minimal Risk	Minimal Risk
Cover Girl Clarifying Pressed Powder 6, 14, 17, 22, 39, 40	Caution	Minimal Risk
Cover Girl Clean Make-Up Pressed Powder 4, 6, 14, 17, 40	Caution	Caution
Cover Girl Extremely Gentle Make-Up Pressed Powder 4, 14, 17, 40	Minimal Risk	Caution
Cover Girl Moisture Wear Perfecting Pressed Powder 4, 6, 14, 17, 40	Caution	Caution
Cover Girl Oil-Control Make-Up Oil-Blotting Pressed Powder 4, 6, 14, 17, 40	Caution	Caution
Cover Girl Professional Finishing Loose Powder 4, 6, 14, 16, 33, 40	Caution	Minimal Risk
Cover Girl Replenishing Pressed Powder 4, 5, 6, 14, 17, 40	Caution	Minimal Risk
Ida Grae Translucent Powder ✓ 39	Little to No Risk	Minimal Risk
la prairie Cellular Complex Powder Blush 9, 14, 33, 40	Little to No Risk	Minimal Risk
Logona Translucent Powder ✓ 40	Little to No Risk	Minimal Risk
Max Factor Creme Puff Pressed Powder Make-Up 6, 7, 14, 33, 40	Minimal Risk	Minimal Risk
Max Factor Pan-Cake Water-Activated Make-Up 6, 8, 14, 21, 40	Minimal Risk	Minimal Risk
Max Factor Powder Pure Translucent Loose Powder 4, 6, 14, 33	Little to No Risk	Caution
Maybelline Moisture Whip Loose Powder 6, 7, 14, 40	Minimal Risk	Minimal Risk
Maybelline Moisture Whip Translucent Pressed Powder 6, 12, 14, 40	Caution	Minimal Risk
Maybelline Satin Complexion Pressed Powder 7, 14, 39, 40	Little to No Risk	Minimal Risk

Product	Health Advisory	
(icons) Little to No Risk / Minimal Risk / Caution / ✓ Recommended	Contact Dermatitis	Carcinogens
Maybelline Shades of You Oil-Free Pressed Powder 7, 14, 39, 40	🛒	🛒
Maybelline Shine Free Oil-Control Dual Powder Base (pressed) 7, 14, 40	🛒	🛒
Maybelline Shine Free Oil Control Loose Powder 7, 14, 39, 40	🛒	🛒
Maybelline Shine Free Oil Control Translucent Pressed Powder 7, 14, 39, 40	🛒	🛒
Monteil Silkpowder Blush Rouge à Joues 7, 14, 33, 37, 39, 40	🛒	🛒
Origins Loose Powder 14, 33, 40	🛒	🛒
Rachel Perry Chamomile Translucent Powder ✓ 6, 14, 19	🛒	🛒
Revlon Love Pat Moisturizing Pressed Powder 6, 8, 14, 21, 33, 40	🛒	🛒
Revlon New Complexion Loose Powder 12, 14, 39, 40	🛒	🛒
Revlon New Complexion Pressed Silky Light Powder Fragrance-free 12, 14, 39, 40	🛒	🛒
Revlon Pure Radiance Sunglow Effects Loose Powder 14, 40	🛒	🛒
Revlon Powdercreme Make-Up Pressed Powder Full Matte 4, 14	🛒	🛒
Revlon Springwater Pressed Powder ✓ 14, 39	🛒	🛒
Revlon Touch & Glow Translucent Pressed Powder 9, 14, 21, 40	🛒	🛒

MASCARAS

Product Types
Cake; cream; liquid.

Health Advisory

Contact Dermatitis

Mascara is one of those cosmetics most likely to cause health problems. In 1990, there were at least 1,964 emergency room admissions because of mascara-related injuries. A small but significant number of eye maladies that women suffer are caused by eye makeup. Conjunctivitis, for example, can be caused by use of mascara. The usual problem is not from ingredients in mascara but rather scratching the eyeball with the applicator, increasing the chance of bacterial infection.

Be wary of products containing the preservative quaternium 15, which is a direct eye irritant.

Some products may contain phenylmercuric acetate, which is both an allergen and a skin irritant. It should never be used around the eyes.

Carcinogens

Some products contain BHA and TEA, but absorption is minimal. Some contain silica but inhalation is unlikely.

Safe Use Tips

- Never use mascara if your eye is injured, irritated, infected, or scratched.
- Ulcers on the cornea (the outside covering of the eye) and the loss of lashes are symptoms of bacterial infection.
- Always handle and apply mascara in a careful and sanitary manner. Never add anything—not even tap water—to mascara. Do not share mascara with others.
- Mascara is likely to become contaminated with bacteria, in spite of the use of preservatives. Store mascara in the refrigerator, which will help reduce bacterial contamination.
- Do not keep mascara longer than four months; even substantial amounts of preservatives break down over time and with use.
- Never apply eye makeup immediately after putting on nail polish or using nail polish remover as their ingredients can be irritating to the eyes with direct contact.

Mascaras

Product				Health Advisory	
🛒 Little to No Risk	🛒 Minimal Risk	🛒 Caution	✓ Recommended	Contact Dermatitis	Carcinogens
Almay Longest Lashes Mascara ✓ *7, 14, 17*				🛒	🛒
Bare Escentuals Mascara ✓ *7, 14, 40*				🛒	🛒
Beauty Without Cruelty Mascara *14, 21*				🛒	🛒
Chanel Cils Magiques Aqua Resistant Instant Waterproof Mascara ✓ *14, 16, 19*				🛒	🛒
Chanel Cils Magiques Instant Lash Mascara *14, 16, 19, 21*				🛒	🛒
Clinique Naturally Glossy Mascara *14, 21*				🛒	🛒

Product		Health Advisory	
		Contact Dermatitis	Carcinogens
Cover Girl Clean Lash Washable Waterproof Mascara 4, 9, 14, 16, 17		Minimal Risk	Caution
Cover Girl Extremely Gentle Sensitive Eyes Mascara 14, 16, 17, 21		Minimal Risk	Minimal Risk
Cover Girl Long 'N Lush Mascara ✓ 14, 17		Minimal Risk	Little to No Risk
Cover Girl Natural Lash Clear Mascara 14, 21		Little to No Risk	Minimal Risk
Cover Girl Professional Mascara 16, 17, 21		Minimal Risk	Minimal Risk
Ecco Bella Mascara ✓		Little to No Risk	Little to No Risk
Estée Lauder Luscious Creme Mascara ✓ 7, 14, 16		Minimal Risk	Little to No Risk
Estée Lauder More than Mascara Moisture-Binding Formula ✓ 7, 14, 16, 39		Minimal Risk	Minimal Risk
Estée Lauder Precision Lash Mascara 7, 14, 21		Little to No Risk	Minimal Risk
Flame Glow Mascara ✓ 7, 14, 17		Minimal Risk	Little to No Risk
Lancôme High Definition Mascara 7, 14, 21		Little to No Risk	Minimal Risk
la prairie Mascara Cellulaire Cellular Mascara ✓ 7, 14, 19		Little to No Risk	Little to No Risk
Logona Mascara (black, blue, brown) ✓		Little to No Risk	Little to No Risk
Maybelline Contact Lens Safe 4, 8, 14		Little to No Risk	Caution
Maybelline Illegal Lengths 14, 16, 17, 21		Minimal Risk	Minimal Risk
Maybelline Natural Look 7, 14, 16, 37, 39, 40		Minimal Risk	Little to No Risk
Maybelline Shine Free 7, 14, 16, 37		Minimal Risk	Minimal Risk
Monteil Luxe Premier Mascara 14, 21		Little to No Risk	Minimal Risk
Nature Cosmetics Thicklash Mascara 7, 14, 19, 21		Little to No Risk	Minimal Risk
Nature Cosmetics Waterproof Mascara ✓ 14, 17		Little to No Risk	Little to No Risk
Paul Penders Mascara ✓ 14		Little to No Risk	Little to No Risk
Prestige 7, 14, 21		Little to No Risk	Minimal Risk
Reviva Liquid Mascara ✓ 1, 7, 14, 16		Little to No Risk	Little to No Risk

EYE SHADOWS

Product Types

Powder; stick.

Health Advisory

Contact Dermatitis

No products containing quaternium 15 have been recommended, as this ingredient is a direct eye irritant. Also watch out for triethanolamine, another eye irritant.

Carcinogens

Avoid products with BHA, which is carcinogenic, and TEA, which can interact with nitrites in products to form carcinogenic nitrosamines.

Eye Shadows

Product	Contact Dermatitis	Carcinogens
Little to No Risk / Minimal Risk / Caution / ✔ Recommended		
Almay 8-House Eye Color ✔ *7, 14, 40*	Minimal Risk	Minimal Risk
Almay Eye Color Single ✔ *7, 14, 39, 40*	Minimal Risk	Minimal Risk
Almay Matte Classic Duo ✔ *39, 40*	Minimal Risk	Caution
Bare Escentuals Matte Eyeshadows ✔	Minimal Risk	Minimal Risk
Beauty Without Cruelty Eye Color Crayon ✔	Minimal Risk	Minimal Risk
Beauty Without Cruelty Eyeshadow Pressed Powder *4, 14, 16, 40*	Minimal Risk	Caution
Borghese Eye Accento Pencil *4, 14, 40*	Minimal Risk	Caution
Chanel Les Quatre Ombres Quadra Eye Shadow *3, 9, 14*	Little to No Risk	Minimal Risk
Clarion Captive Color *14, 19, 22, 39, 40*	Minimal Risk	Little to No Risk
Clarion Silk Palette Eye Shadow *14, 22, 39, 40*	Minimal Risk	Little to No Risk
Clinique Daily Eye Treat Moisturizing Shadow Color *14, 16, 21, 39*	Minimal Risk	Little to No Risk
Cover Girl Luminesse Shadow *4, 14, 17, 40*	Little to No Risk	Caution

Product	Health Advisory	
	Contact Dermatitis	Carcinogens
Little to No Risk *Minimal Risk* *Caution* ✓ *Recommended*		
Cover Girl Natural Eyes Breeze-On Shadow 14, 22, 39, 40	🛒	🛒
Cover Girl Pro-Colors 4, 14, 17, 40	🛒	🛒
Cover Girl Professional ColorMatch Frost Shades 5, 14, 17, 22, 40	🛒	🛒
Cover Girl Professional ColorMatch Matte Shades 14, 17, 22, 40	🛒	🛒
Cover Girl Soft Radiants Silky Matte Shadow 4, 5, 14, 40	🛒	🛒
Dr. Hauschka Saphir Eye Shadow (Blue) ✓ 8	🛒	🛒
Dr. Hauschka Smaragd Eye Shadow (Green) ✓ 8	🛒	🛒
Dr. Hauschka Topaz Eye Shadow (Beige) ✓ 8	🛒	🛒
Ecco Bella Eyeshadow/Blush ✓	🛒	🛒
Flame Glow Long-Wearing Sheer Eyeshadow 9, 17, 19, 22	🛒	🛒
Ida Grae Earth Eyes ✓	🛒	🛒
Ida Grae Earth Eye/Lip Cream ✓ 10, 19	🛒	🛒
la prairie Cellular Complex Eye Colour 4, 14, 40	🛒	🛒
Logona Cosmetic Eye Pencils ✓ 19, 40	🛒	🛒
L'Oréal Couleur ✓ 14, 40	🛒	🛒
Max Factor Visual Eyes ✓ 8, 14, 40	🛒	🛒
Maybelline Blooming Colors Eye Shadow ✓ 7, 14, 37, 40	🛒	🛒
Maybelline Ultra Brow 4, 8, 14, 40	🛒	🛒
Monteil Rich Powder Eyeshadow Grand Duo ✓ 7, 14, 37, 39, 40	🛒	🛒
Nature Cosmetics Brow Liner Pencil ✓ 39	🛒	🛒
Nature Cosmetics Eyeliner 14, 16, 19, 21	🛒	🛒
Nature Cosmetics Eyeshadow Pencil ✓ 14	🛒	🛒
Paul Penders Eyeshadows & Blushers ✓ 1, 19	🛒	🛒
Pavion Wet 'n' Wild ✓ 14	🛒	🛒

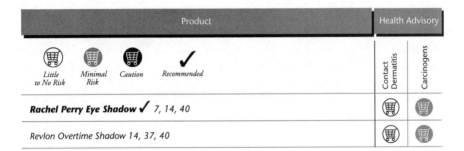

Product				Health Advisory	
				Contact Dermatitis	Carcinogens
🛒 *Little to No Risk*	🛒 *Minimal Risk*	🛒 *Caution*	✓ *Recommended*		
Rachel Perry Eye Shadow ✓ *7, 14, 40*				🛒	🛒
Revlon Overtime Shadow 14, 37, 40				🛒	🛒

LIPSTICKS, GLOSSES, AND LIP PENCILS

Product Type

Stick.

Health Advisory

Contact Dermatitis

Although contact dermatitis cases caused by cosmetic pigments (i.e., artificial colors) are uncommon, those that have occurred were due to the colors found in lipsticks. For the chemically hypersensitive, use of coal tar colors is said to cause nausea, headaches, skin problems, fatigue, mood swings, or other allergic symptoms.

Additional allergens commonly found in lipsticks include:

- Amyldimethylamino benzoic acid
- Castor oil
- Diisostearyl malate
- Glycerol diisostearate
- Microcrystalline wax
- Pigments
- Propyl gallate
- Ricinoleic acid
- Yellow 11

Eosin dyes, lanolin, and fragrances in lipsticks can cause drying or cracking of lips, a condition known as *cheilitis*.

Although eosin dyes are not used as much today as they once were, those that are (and may cause irritation) include:

- D&C Orange 5
- D&C Red 21
- D&C Red 27

Carcinogens

Applying carcinogens to your lips does not make sense! They are going to be absorbed into your body as you moisten your lips throughout the day. That is why you should avoid products containing BHA, sodium saccharin, and artificial colors such as D&C Orange 5, D&C Orange 17, D&C Red 9, D&C Red 19, FD&C Blue 1, FD&C Yellow 5, and FD&C Yellow 6. You will find many more colors than these or than those listed in the charts on lipstick labels. The bottom line is that there is probably no such thing as a safe coal tar color. Stay away!

Safe Use Tips

- If you have dry or cracking lips, use lipsticks without artificial colors or lanolin.
- Natural lipsticks require special handling. Because they are softer and more moist, care must be taken to twist up only a small amount; because they melt more easily than most commercial lipsticks, they should not be left in a hot car or in direct sunlight. Certain colors—the hot reds or bright oranges—cannot be produced from natural color pigments.

Lipsticks, Glosses, and Lip Pencils

Product				Health Advisory	
Little to No Risk	Minimal Risk	Caution	Recommended	Contact Dermatitis	Carcinogens
Almay Glossy Lip Shine 4, 14, 29, 33, 34				Little to No Risk	Caution
Almay Matte Cream Lipcolor 14, 29, 33, 34				Little to No Risk	Minimal Risk
Aubrey Natural Lips (Crystal Clear, Mocha Brown, Natural Red, Petal Pink) ✓				Little to No Risk	Little to No Risk
Bare Escentuals Conditioning Lip Glaze ✓ 10, 19				Little to No Risk	Little to No Risk
Bare Escentuals Lip/Eye Pencils 4, 14, 29, 34				Little to No Risk	Caution
Bare Escentuals Lip Glosses 4, 10, 14, 19				Little to No Risk	Caution
Beauty Without Cruelty Lipstick 4, 12, 16, 33, 34				Little to No Risk	Caution
Bonne Bell Bubble Gum Lip Smacker Flavored Lip Gloss ✓ 6, 16				Minimal Risk	Little to No Risk
Bonne Bell Dr. Pepper Lip Smacker Flavored Lip Gloss 6, 16, 29, 33, 38				Minimal Risk	Caution
Bonne Bell Grape Lip Smacker Flavored Lip Gloss 6, 16, 29, 38				Minimal Risk	Caution

Product				Health Advisory	
Little to No Risk	Minimal Risk	Caution	Recommended	Contact Dermatitis	Carcinogens
Bonne Bell Orange Pop Lip Smacker Flavored Lip Gloss 6, 16, 33, 38				Minimal Risk	Minimal Risk
Bonne Bell Peppermint Lip Smacker Flavored Lip Gloss ✓ 6, 16				Minimal Risk	Little to No Risk
Bonne Bell Red Raspberry Lip Smacker Flavored Lip Gloss 6, 16, 29, 38				Minimal Risk	Minimal Risk
Bonne Bell Strawberry Lip Smacker Flavored Lip Gloss ✓ 6, 16				Minimal Risk	Little to No Risk
Bonne Bell Watermelon Lip Smacker Flavored Lip Gloss 6, 16, 33, 38				Minimal Risk	Minimal Risk
Bonne Bell Wild Raspberry Lip Smacker Flavored Lip Gloss 6, 16, 29				Minimal Risk	Minimal Risk
Borghese Perfetta Lip Pencil 4, 14, 33				Little to No Risk	Minimal Risk
Chanel Rouge A Lèvres Super Hydrabase Creme Lipstick 6, 8, 10, 14, 16, 27, 29, 33				Minimal Risk	Minimal Risk
Clarion Creme 14, 19, 29, 33				Little to No Risk	Minimal Risk
Cover Girl Continuous Color Lipstick 6, 14, 19, 29, 33				Minimal Risk	Minimal Risk
Cover Girl Lip Advance Lasting Lip Color 8, 10, 14, 19, 29, 33, 34				Little to No Risk	Minimal Risk
Cover Girl Lip Slicks Lip Gloss 6, 8, 10, 14, 16, 19, 29, 33				Caution	Minimal Risk
Cover Girl Luminesse Lipstick 6, 14, 19, 29, 33				Minimal Risk	Minimal Risk
Cover Girl Remarkable Lip Color 1, 8, 10, 14, 16, 19, 29, 33				Minimal Risk	Minimal Risk
Dana Lipstick (Acapulco, Argentine, Bar Harbour, Biarritz, Biscay, Casablanca & Grenada) 4, 6, 16, 29, 33, 34				Minimal Risk	Caution
Dana Lipstick (Kyoto Red, Las Brisas, Majorca Sun, Málaga, Monaco, Monte Carlo, Palm Beach & Valencia) 4, 6, 16, 29, 33, 34				Minimal Risk	Minimal Risk
Dana Lipstick (Lolita, Malibu, Marbella, Seville, Sun Valley, Tattoo & Torremolinos) 4, 6, 8, 16, 29, 33, 34				Minimal Risk	Caution
Dr. Hauschka Lipsticks ✓ 8				Little to No Risk	Little to No Risk
Ecco Bella Lip Colors ✓ 19				Little to No Risk	Little to No Risk
Flame Glow Natural Fruit Flavor Automatic Lip Gloss 14, 38				Little to No Risk	Caution
Flame Glow Natural Fruit Flavor Roll-On Lip Gloss 14, 38				Little to No Risk	Caution
Flame Glow Sheer Lipcolor 1, 6, 9, 10, 12, 14, 19, 29, 33, 34				Minimal Risk	Minimal Risk

Product				Health Advisory	
Little to No Risk	Minimal Risk	Caution	✔ Recommended	Contact Dermatitis	Carcinogens
Germaine Monteil Protective Lip Tint with Sunscreen SPF6 4, 9, 14, 29, 33, 34, 39				Minimal Risk	Caution
Ida Grae Earth Lip Creme ✔ 10, 19				Minimal Risk	Minimal Risk
Kiss My Face Kiss Colors ✔ 19				Minimal Risk	Minimal Risk
Lancôme Sorbet de Lancôme Fondant à lèvres Lip Gloss 6, 8, 14, 22, 33				Little to No Risk	Little to No Risk
la prairie Lip Pencil 4, 14, 29, 33, 34				Little to No Risk	Caution
Logona Lip Pencils (all colors) ✔ 9, 19, 40				Minimal Risk	Minimal Risk
Max Factor New Definition Lip Color 4, 6, 10, 14, 27, 29, 33, 34				Little to No Risk	Little to No Risk
Maybelline Kissing Koolers Flavored Lip Gloss 4, 10, 14, 16, 29, 33, 38				Minimal Risk	Caution
Maybelline Kissing Potion Flavored Roll-On Lip Gloss 4, 14, 38				Minimal Risk	Caution
Maybelline Lipstick 4, 6, 10, 14, 17, 29, 33				Little to No Risk	Caution
Maybelline Long Wearing Lipstick 4, 6, 10, 14, 16, 29, 33				Minimal Risk	Caution
Maybelline Moisture Whip Lipstick 4, 6, 10, 14, 16, 29, 33				Minimal Risk	Minimal Risk
Maybelline Revitalizing Color Lipstick 4, 6, 10, 14, 16, 19, 29, 33				Minimal Risk	Minimal Risk
Maybelline Sheer Accents Lipstick with SPF8 4, 6, 10, 14, 29, 33				Minimal Risk	Caution
Nature Cosmetics Nature Gloss 1, 8, 13, 14, 19, 24, 25, 33				Minimal Risk	Little to No Risk
Nature Cosmetics Nature Lips 1, 9, 13, 14, 19, 24, 25, 26, 34				Minimal Risk	Little to No Risk
Paul Penders Lip Colors ✔ 19				Minimal Risk	Minimal Risk
Pavion Wet 'n Wild Lipstick 19, 29, 33, 34				Minimal Risk	Little to No Risk
Rachel Perry Nutrient Lip Pencil 14, 24, 27, 29, 33, 34				Minimal Risk	Little to No Risk
Rachel Perry Nutrient Luster Lip Gloss 6, 10, 13, 14, 19, 24, 29, 33, 34				Little to No Risk	Little to No Risk
Rachel Perry Nutrient Luster Lipstick 14, 24, 27, 29, 33, 34				Minimal Risk	Little to No Risk
Reviva Lipstick 6, 8, 12, 19				Minimal Risk	Little to No Risk

CHAPTER 9

Hair Care

HAIR CONDITIONERS

Product Type

Liquid.

Health Advisory

Contact Dermatitis

Most mainstream and many alternative brands of conditioners rely on quaternary compounds for thickening the hair. Quaternary compounds can be irritating to the eyes and skin, depending on their concentration, the dose, and which specific members of the quaternary family of chemicals are in the conditioner. Benzalkonium chloride, cetrimonium bromide, quaternium 15, and quaternium 18 are all quaternary compounds; they all have potential for eye irritation.

Carcinogens

Products containing formaldehyde should not be used. Avoid products containing artificial colors such as D&C Red 33, FD&C Blue 1, FD&C Red 4, FD&C Red 40, and FD&C Yellow 6. Also be aware of products containing polysorbate 80 as they may be contaminated with the carcinogen 1,4-dioxane.

Hair Conditioners

Product				Health Advisory	
![Little to No Risk] Little to No Risk	![Minimal Risk] Minimal Risk	![Caution] Caution	✓ Recommended	Contact Dermatitis	Carcinogens
Agree Pro-Vitamin (Extra Body & Regular) ✓ 6, 16, 19				Minimal	Little to No Risk
Alberto VO5 Conditioner (Balsam and Protein, Collagen, Essence of Natural Henna & Extra Body) 5, 6, 31, 34				Minimal	Caution
Alberto VO5 Conditioner (Jojoba) 6, 31				Minimal	Minimal
Aloegen Biotreatment 22 Conditioner ✓ 14				Little to No Risk	Little to No Risk
Aloegen Biotreatment 22 Revitalizing Gel 1, 13, 16, 21				Little to No Risk	Minimal
Aloegen Biogenic Treatment Conditioner ✓ 6, 13, 14, 28				Minimal	Minimal
Aloegen Biogenic Perm Conditioner ✓ 6, 7, 13, 14				Minimal	Little to No Risk
Aloegen Tangle-Free Spray-On Conditioner ✓ 6, 13, 16				Minimal	Little to No Risk
Aloe Vera—Real Aloe Company Hair Conditioner ✓ 6, 14				Minimal	Little to No Risk
Aubrey Biotin Hair Repair ✓ 13, 19				Little to No Risk	Little to No Risk
Aubrey GPB Glycogen Protein Balancer ✓ 19				Little to No Risk	Little to No Risk
Aubrey Island Naturals Island Spice Cream Rinse ✓ 19				Little to No Risk	Little to No Risk
Aubrey Jojoba & Aloe Hair Rejuvenator & Conditioner ✓ 19				Little to No Risk	Little to No Risk
Aubrey Jojoba Oil ✓				Little to No Risk	Little to No Risk
Aubrey Polynatural 60/80 Hair Rejuvenating Conditioner ✓ 13, 19				Little to No Risk	Little to No Risk
Aubrey Rosa Mosqueta Rose Hip Conditioning Hair Cream ✓ 19				Little to No Risk	Little to No Risk
Aubrey Rosemary & Sage Hair & Scalp Rinse ✓ 19				Little to No Risk	Little to No Risk
Aubrey Swimmers Condition ✓ 13, 19				Minimal	Little to No Risk
Aussie Instant Daily Conditioner with Australian Sea Vegetable Extracts ✓ 6, 14				Minimal	Little to No Risk
The Australian 3 Minute Miracle Hair Reconstructor & Conditioner 6, 14, 34				Minimal	Minimal
Awapuhi Conditioner 6, 14, 17, 19				Caution	Little to No Risk
Beauty Without Cruelty Oil-Free Conditioner ✓ 1, 6, 14, 19				Minimal	Little to No Risk

Product	Health Advisory	
	Contact Dermatitis	Carcinogens
Beauty Without Cruelty Oil-Free Extra Body Conditioner ✓ *6, 14*	🛒 Little to No Risk	🛒 Little to No Risk
Beehive Botanicals Moisturizing Conditioner ✓ *6, 13, 14, 19*	🛒	🛒
Biopure Conditioner (Apple with Pectin, Jojoba) ✓ *6*	🛒	🛒
Bold Hold Salon Formula Volumizing Conditioner with Collagen Protein *6, 30*	🛒 Minimal Risk	🛒 Minimal Risk
Bold Hold Salon Formula Replenishing Conditioner with Essential Nutrients & Emollients *6, 19, 29*	🛒 Minimal Risk	🛒 Minimal Risk
Breck Conditioner Number 3 Extra Body for Fine, Limp Hair *6, 14, 16, 31, 33*	🛒 Minimal Risk	🛒 Minimal Risk
Camo Care Camomile Conditioner *6, 7, 14, 16, 19*	🛒 Caution	🛒
Chica Bella Costa Rican Honey ✓ *6*	🛒 Minimal Risk	🛒
Chica Bella Herbal Forest ✓ *6*	🛒 Minimal Risk	🛒
Chica Bella Monteverde Aloe Vera ✓ *6*	🛒 Minimal Risk	🛒
Chica Bella Rare Orchid ✓ *6*	🛒 Minimal Risk	🛒
Chica Bella Tropical Bird of Paradise ✓ *6*	🛒 Minimal Risk	🛒
Chica Bella Wild Caribbean Seaweed ✓ *6*	🛒 Minimal Risk	🛒
Desert Essence Jojoba Conditioner ✓ *14, 19*	🛒	🛒
Earth & Body Vitamin Family Conditioner ✓ *6, 7, 19*	🛒 Minimal Risk	🛒
Earth Preserv Hair Vitalizer (all scents; JCPenney) ✓	🛒	🛒
Earth Science Citresoft Conditioner ✓ *1*	🛒	🛒
Earth Science Fragrance Free Conditioner ✓ *1, 19*	🛒	🛒
Earth Science Intensicare Conditioner ✓ *1, 19*	🛒	🛒
Earth Science Herbal Astringent Conditioner ✓ *1, 6*	🛒 Minimal Risk	🛒
Ecco Bella 60 Second Conditioner ✓ *14, 19*	🛒	🛒
Emerald Forest Conditioner ✓ *6, 14*	🛒 Minimal Risk	🛒
Faith in Nature Aloe Vera Conditioner ✓ *6*	🛒 Minimal Risk	🛒

Legend: 🛒 Little to No Risk, 🛒 Minimal Risk, 🛒 Caution, ✓ Recommended

Product	Health Advisory	
	Contact Dermatitis	Carcinogens
Little to No Risk · Minimal Risk · Caution · Recommended		
Faith in Nature Jojoba Conditioner ✓ 6	Minimal Risk	Minimal Risk
Faith in Nature Rosemary Conditioner ✓ 6	Minimal Risk	Minimal Risk
Faith in Nature Seaweed Conditioner ✓	Little to No Risk	Minimal Risk
Finesse Conditioner Extra Moisturizing For Dry or Overstyled Hair ✓ 6	Minimal Risk	Minimal Risk
Finesse Conditioner (Regular for Normal Hair) ✓ 6, 16	Minimal Risk	Minimal Risk
Flex Hair Conditioner (Balsam & Protein, Dry/Damaged, Extra Body & Regular) 6, 14, 33, 34	Minimal Risk	Caution
Giovanni Direct Conditioner–White ✓ 6	Minimal Risk	Minimal Risk
Giovanni Morebody–Blue ✓ 6	Minimal Risk	Minimal Risk
Giovanni Nutrafixx–Yellow ✓ 6	Minimal Risk	Minimal Risk
Giovanni 50/50 Balanced Remoisturizer–Green ✓ 6	Minimal Risk	Minimal Risk
Golden Lotus Rosemary & Lavender Conditioner ✓ 14	Little to No Risk	Minimal Risk
Head Original Conditioner ✓ 6, 14	Minimal Risk	Minimal Risk
Head Pure & Basic Lite Conditioning Rinse ✓ 6, 14	Minimal Risk	Minimal Risk
Home Health Oliva Olive & Aloe Conditioner 33	Minimal Risk	Minimal Risk
Infinity Camomile Conditioning Rinse ✓ 6	Little to No Risk	Minimal Risk
Infinity Rosemary Conditioning Rinse ✓ 6	Little to No Risk	Minimal Risk
Ivory Conditioner (Dry/Permed Hair, Fine Hair, & Normal Hair) ✓ 6	Minimal Risk	Minimal Risk
Jason Aloe Vera Gel Conditioner 1, 6, 7, 14, 16, 19	Caution	Minimal Risk
Jason Biotin Conditioner ✓ 1, 6, 7, 14, 19	Minimal Risk	Minimal Risk
Jason EFA Primrose Oil Conditioner ✓ 1, 6, 7, 14, 19	Minimal Risk	Minimal Risk
Jason Henna Highlights Conditioner 6, 16, 17	Caution	Minimal Risk
Jason Herbal Conditioner ✓ 6, 7, 14, 19	Minimal Risk	Minimal Risk
Jason Jojoba Conditioner ✓ 6, 16, 19	Minimal Risk	Minimal Risk

Product	Health Advisory — Contact Dermatitis	Health Advisory — Carcinogens
Jason Keratin Conditioner ✓ *1, 14, 16, 19*	Little to No Risk	Little to No Risk
Jason Sea Kelp Conditioner ✓ *6, 7, 14, 19*	Minimal Risk	Little to No Risk
Jason Vitamin E Conditioner ✓ *6, 7, 14, 19*	Minimal Risk	Little to No Risk
Jhirmack E.F.A. Moisturizing Conditioner (Dry, Permed, & Color Treated Hair) ✓ *6, 14*	Minimal Risk	Little to No Risk
Jhirmack Nutri-Body Extra Body Conditioner (Fine, Thin Hair) 6, 14, 16, 17, 29, 33	Caution	Minimal Risk
Johnson's Baby Conditioner 6, 32	Minimal Risk	Minimal Risk
Kiss My Face Conditioner ✓ *6, 14*	Minimal Risk	Little to No Risk
Logona Burdock Root Hair Treatment ✓	Little to No Risk	Little to No Risk
Logona Rosemary Conditioner ✓ *19*	Little to No Risk	Little to No Risk
L'Oréal Ultra Rich Conditioner (Normal & Extra Body) ✓ *6*	Minimal Risk	Little to No Risk
Mera Conditioner for Normal Hair ✓	Little to No Risk	Little to No Risk
Mera Conditioner for Oily Hair ✓	Little to No Risk	Little to No Risk
Naturade Aloe Vera Conditioner ✓ *1, 13, 14*	Little to No Risk	Little to No Risk
Nature's Gate Aloe Vera Conditioner 6, 14, 19	Minimal Risk	Little to No Risk
Nature's Gate Awapuhi Conditioner ✓ *6, 14*	Minimal Risk	Little to No Risk
Nature's Gate Biotin Conditioner ✓ *14, 19*	Little to No Risk	Little to No Risk
Nature's Gate Jojoba Conditioner ✓ *14*	Little to No Risk	Little to No Risk
Nature's Gate Keratin Conditioner ✓ *14, 19*	Little to No Risk	Little to No Risk
Nature's Gate Rainwater Conditioner ✓ *14*	Little to No Risk	Little to No Risk
Nirvana Cherry Bark/Almond Hair Conditioner ✓ *14, 16, 19*	Little to No Risk	Little to No Risk
Nirvana Rosemary/Mint Hair Rinse ✓ *14*	Little to No Risk	Little to No Risk
O'Naturel Lavender Intensive Conditioning Pack 14	Little to No Risk	Little to No Risk

Legend: 🛒 Little to No Risk · 🛒 Minimal Risk · 🛒 Caution · ✓ Recommended

Product				Health Advisory	
Little to No Risk	Minimal Risk	Caution	✓ Recommended	Contact Dermatitis	Carcinogens
Original Apple Pectin Instant Protein Creme Conditioner 6, 14				🛒	🛒
Pantene Progressive Treatment Creme Conditioner de Pantene Dry Hair Moisture Replenishing Formula 6, 12, 33, 34				🛒	🛒
Pantene Progressive Treatment Creme Conditioner de Pantene Extra Body Fine Hair Thickening Formula ✓ 6				🛒	🛒
Pantene Progressive Treatment Creme Conditioner de Pantene (Normal Hair Bodifying Formula) 6, 12				🛒	🛒
Pantene Progressive Treatment Creme Conditioner de Pantene Permed Hair Revitalizing Formula 6, 12, 19				🛒	🛒
Pantene Progressive Treatment Creme Conditioner de Pantene Vitamin Therapy for Overworked or Damaged Hair 6, 12				🛒	🛒
Pantene Pro-V Pro-Vitamin Treatment Conditioner (Regular & Deep Conditioning) ✓ 6				🛒	🛒
Paul Penders German Herbal Hair Repair ✓ 6, 14				🛒	🛒
Paul Penders Lemon Yarrow Cream Rinse Conditioner ✓ 14				🛒	🛒
Paul Penders Color Conditioners ✓ 14				🛒	🛒
Perma Soft Body Building Conditioner ✓ 6, 16				🛒	🛒
Perma Soft Curl Maintenance Conditioner 6, 14, 16, 27, 31				🛒	🛒
Perma Soft Deep Moisturizing Conditioner ✓ 6, 14, 16				🛒	🛒
Prell Conditioner (Balanced Formula for Normal Hair & Moisturizing Formula for Dry, Damaged Hair) ✓ 6				🛒	🛒
Rainbow Research Henna & Biotin Conditioner ✓ 14, 19				🛒	🛒
Rave Conditioner (Extra Body, Moisturizing & Normal) 6, 22, 32				🛒	🛒
Reviva Seaweed Conditioner ✓ 6, 14, 16				🛒	🛒
Salon Selectives Conditioner Type B Body Building 6, 16, 32				🛒	🛒
Salon Selectives Conditioner (Type F Fortifying) ✓ 6, 16				🛒	🛒
Salon Selectives Conditioner (Type H Highlighting) ✓ 6, 16				🛒	🛒
Salon Selectives Conditioner (Type M Moisturizing) ✓ 6, 16				🛒	🛒

Product				Contact Dermatitis	Carcinogens
🛒 Little to No Risk	🛒 Minimal Risk	🛒 Caution	✓ Recommended		
Salon Selectives Conditioner (Type P Protective) 6, 16, 32				🛒	🛒
Salon Selectives Conditioner (Type S Sheer) ✓ 6, 16				🛒	🛒
Salon Selectives Leave-On Conditioning Treatment (Type L) ✓ 6, 16				🛒	🛒
Shi Kai Amla Conditioner ✓ 6, 7				🛒	🛒
Shi Kai Henna Gold Conditioner ✓ 6, 7				🛒	🛒
Shi Kai Moisture Plus Conditioner ✓ 6, 14				🛒	🛒
Shi Kai Spray-On Conditioner ✓ 6, 10, 14				🛒	🛒
Stony Brook Oil-Free Conditioner (Scented with Natural Fragrance) ✓ 14				🛒	🛒
Stony Brook Oil-Free Conditioner (Unscented) ✓ 14				🛒	🛒
Style Conditioner (Dry or Damaged Hair) 6, 14, 16, 33				🛒	🛒
Style Conditioner with Pro-Vitamin Complex for Fine, Limp Hair 6, 14, 16, 24, 33, 34				🛒	🛒
Suave Balsam & Protein Conditioner 6, 29, 33				🛒	🛒
Suave Extra Gentle Conditioner ✓ 6				🛒	🛒
Suave Full Body Conditioner ✓ 6				🛒	🛒
Suave Moisturizing Conditioner 6, 33				🛒	🛒
Suave Perm & Color ✓ 6				🛒	🛒
Suave Salon Formula Conditioner Nourishing Formula with Vitamins ✓ 6, 16, 19				🛒	🛒
Swiss Formula Conditioner Aloe Vera and Vitamin E 1, 6, 14, 19, 29, 33				🛒	🛒
Swiss Formula Conditioner Jojoba and Panthenol Conditioner 6, 14, 19, 27, 29, 31, 33				🛒	🛒
Swiss Formula Silk Protein Conditioner 6, 14, 27, 29, 31, 33				🛒	🛒
Thick Stuff Through & Through Conditioner ✓ 6, 14, 16				🛒	🛒
Thursday Plantation Tea Tree Conditioner ✓ 6, 7, 14				🛒	🛒

Product				Health Advisory	
				Contact Dermatitis	Carcinogens

Little to No Risk	Minimal Risk	Caution	Recommended

Product	Contact Dermatitis	Carcinogens
Tropical Botanicals Rainflowers Conditioner ✔ 6, 14	Minimal	Little
Unicure Jojoba Hair and Skin Conditioner ✔ 14	Little	Little
Vibrance Conditioner (Moisture Rich for Dry/Damaged Hair & Revitalizing for Permed/Colored Hair) 6, 14, 19, 32, 33	Minimal	Minimal
Vibrance Conditioner (Regular for Normal Hair & Body Building for Fine, Limp Hair) 6, 16, 19, 32, 33	Little	Minimal
Vidal Sassoon Deep Moisturizing Conditioner ✔ 6	Little	Little
Weleda Rosemary Conditioner (with Natural Fragrance) ✔	Little	Little
Weleda Chamomile Hair Conditioner (with Natural Fragrance) ✔	Little	Little
White Rain Conditioner (Regular & Extra Body) ✔ 6	Minimal	Little

SHAMPOOS

Product Type

Liquid.

Health Advisory

Contact Dermatitis

All shampoos are irritating. Shampoos rank among the products most often reported to the FDA for association with scalp irritation, stinging eyes, and tangled, split, and fuzzy hair. Shampoos contain synthetic detergents for cleaning hair and are so effective that they may remove some of the skin's or hair's natural oils. Furthermore, detergent suds may get into your eyes and sting them.

To make sure you are buying the mildest shampoo, stay away from brands containing 2-bromo-2-nitropropane-1,3-diol, coal tar (used in products for dandruff, psoriasis, and seborrheic dermatitis), formaldehyde, fragrance, propylene glycol, and quaternium 15. Also watch out for polyethylene glycol and DMDM hydantoin, either of which can degrade in the product during storage into formaldehyde.

Among other miscellaneous ingredients likely to be eye, skin, or mucous membrane irritants are:

- EDTA (ethylene diamine tetracetic acid)
- D&C Green 5
- Selenium sulfide (used in antidandruff shampoos)

Look for the mildest cleansing agents. Common cleansing ingredients contain the word *lauryl* or *laureth* in their names. Laur*yl* compounds are slightly more aggressive cleansers. Laur*eth* compounds are known for being slightly milder with equivalent cleansing but can contain 1,4-dioxane, which is carcinogenic. We have listed milder cleaners that are alternatives to laureth compounds.

The following ingredients provide the most *aggressive* cleansing action:

- Ammonium laur*yl* sulfate
- Diethanolamine (DEA) laur*yl* sulfate
- Monoethanolamine laur*yl* sulfate
- Sodium laur*yl* sulfate
- Triethanolamine (TEA) laur*yl* sulfate

Milder cleansers with good conditioning properties include:

- Cocoyl sarcosine
- Disodium oleamide sulfosuccinate
- Lauroyl sarcosine
- Potassium cocohydrolyzed animal protein
- Sodium cocoyl sarcosinate
- Sodium dioctyl sulfosuccinate
- Sodium laur*yl* isoethionate
- Sodium lauroyl sarcosinate

Gentle cleansers, nonirritating to the eyes, especially for baby shampoos and damaged and delicate hair, include:

- Amphoteric-2
- Amphoteric-6
- Amphoteric-20
- Cocamide diethanolamide
- Cocamide monoethanolamide
- Cocamido betaine
- Cocamidopropyl betaine
- Lauramide diethanolamide
- Lauramide monoethanolamide
- Polysorbate 20

- Polysorbate 40
- Sodium lauraminopropionate
- Sorbitan laurate
- Sorbitan palmitate
- Sorbitan stearate
- Stearamide diethanolamide
- Stearamide monoethanolamide

For oily hair try these mild cleansers:

- Disodium oleamide sulfosuccinate
- Sodium dioctyl sulfosuccinate

Carcinogens

A wide range of ingredients in shampoos break down to form formaldehyde. These include 2-bromo-2-nitropropane-1,3-diol, polyethylene glycol, and DMDM hydantoin.

Products containing coal tar (used in dandruff and related shampoos) or formaldehyde should not be used.

Be wary of products containing laureth compounds, as well as polysorbates 60 and 80. Each of these ingredients may be contaminated with 1,4-dioxane, which is carcinogenic.

Products containing D&C Red 33, FD&C Blue 1, FD&C Green 3, FD&C Red 4, FD&C Red 40, FD&C Yellow 6, DEA, and TEA should not be used.

The application of hot water and detergents to the scalp enhances the absorption of product contaminants. Be sure to be a selective shopper; buy only the safest, highest quality shampoo.

Shampoos

Product				Health Advisory	
Little to No Risk	Minimal Risk	Caution	Recommended	Contact Dermatitis	Carcinogens
Agree Extra Body Shampoo 6, 14, 34				Little to No Risk	Little to No Risk
Agree Moisture Rich Shampoo 6, 14, 16, 33				Little to No Risk	Little to No Risk
Agree Regular 6, 14, 30				Little to No Risk	Little to No Risk
Alberto VO5 Balsam & Protein Shampoo 6, 14, 28, 34				Little to No Risk	Little to No Risk

Product	Contact Dermatitis	Carcinogens
Health Advisory		
🛒 *Little to No Risk* 🛒 *Minimal Risk* 🛒 *Caution* ✓ *Recommended*		
Alberto VO5 Collagen Extra Body Shampoo 6, 14, 28, 29, 32	🛒	🛒
Alberto VO5 Essence of Natural Henna Shampoo 6, 14, 28	🛒	🛒
Alberto VO5 Extra Body Shampoo 6, 14, 28, 29, 32, 33	🛒	🛒
Alberto VO5 Jojoba Shampoo 6, 14, 27, 28, 31	🛒	🛒
Alberto VO5 Moisturizing Shampoo 6, 14, 24, 28	🛒	🛒
Alberto VO5 Normal Shampoo 6, 14, 28, 34	🛒	🛒
Aloegen Biogenic Treatment Shampoo 6, 14, 28	🛒	🛒
Aloegen Biotreatment 22 Shampoo 14, 28	🛒	🛒
Aloegen Biotin 60/80 Treatment Shampoo 14, 28	🛒	🛒
Aloe Vera–Real Aloe Company Shampoo 6, 28	🛒	🛒
Aubrey Blue Camomile Shampoo ✓ 19	🛒	🛒
Aubrey Camomile Luxurious Herbal Shampoo ✓ 19	🛒	🛒
Aubrey Egyptian Henna Shampoo ✓ 19	🛒	🛒
Aubrey Island Naturals Island Butter Shampoo ✓ 19	🛒	🛒
Aubrey J.A.Y. Desert Herb Shampoo ✓ 19	🛒	🛒
Aubrey Mandarin Magic Ginkgo Leaf & Earth Smoke Shampoo ✓ 19	🛒	🛒
Aubrey Men's Stock Ginseng Shampoo ✓ 19	🛒	🛒
Aubrey Polynatural 60/80 Hair Rejuvenating Shampoo ✓ 13, 19	🛒	🛒
Aubrey Primrose & Lavender Herbal Shampoo ✓ 19	🛒	🛒
Aubrey QBHL Qillaya Bark Hair Lather ✓ 19	🛒	🛒
Aubrey Rosa Mosqueta Rose Hip Herbal Shampoo ✓ 19	🛒	🛒
Aubrey Saponin A.A.C. Therapeutic Shampoo ✓ 1, 19	🛒	🛒
Aubrey Selenium Natural Blue Shampoo ✓ 1, 19	🛒	🛒
Aubrey Swimmers Shampoo ✓ 1, 13, 19	🛒	🛒

Product		Health Advisory	
		Contact Dermatitis	Carcinogens

Little to No Risk   Minimal Risk   Caution   ✓ Recommended

Product	Contact Dermatitis	Carcinogens
Aussie Mega Shampoo 6, 27, 28, 33	🛒	🛒
Aussie Moist Shampoo 6, 14, 27, 28, 33	🛒	🛒
Awapuhi Shampoo 6, 14, 17, 28	🛒	🛒
Beauty Without Cruelty Oil-Free Shampoo 6, 14, 28	🛒	🛒
Beauty Without Cruelty Oil-Free Extra Body Shampoo 6, 14, 28	🛒	🛒
Beehive Botanicals Conditioning Shampoo 6, 13, 14, 28	🛒	🛒
Bindi Hair Wash ✓	🛒	🛒
Breck #1 Dry Hair Shampoo 6, 14, 28, 31, 33	🛒	🛒
Breck #2 Normal Hair Shampoo 6, 14, 28, 31, 33	🛒	🛒
Camocare Shampoo 7, 14, 19, 28	🛒	🛒
Chica Bella Costa Rican Honey 28	🛒	🛒
Chica Bella Herbal Forest 6, 28	🛒	🛒
Chica Bella Monteverde Aloe Vera 6, 28	🛒	🛒
Chica Bella Rare Orchid 6, 28	🛒	🛒
Chica Bella Tropical Bird of Paradise 6, 28	🛒	🛒
Chica Bella Wild Caribbean Seaweed 6, 28	🛒	🛒
Citré Shine Revitalizing Shampoo 14, 28	🛒	🛒
Clinique Daily Wash Shampoo 7, 14, 24, 29	🛒	🛒
Clinique Extra Benefits Shampoo 14, 17, 21, 24, 28	🛒	🛒
Desert Essence Jojoba Spirulina Shampoo 14, 19, 28	🛒	🛒
Desert Essence Tea Tree Oil Shampoo ✓ 14	🛒	🛒
Earth & Body Care Herbal Family Shampoo 6, 7, 28	🛒	🛒
Earth Preserv Shampoo (all scents; JCPenney) ✓ 1, 14	🛒	🛒

Product				Contact Dermatitis	Carcinogens
(🛒) Little to No Risk	(🛒) Minimal Risk	(🛒) Caution	✓ Recommended		
Earth Science Chamopure Shampoo 28				🛒	🛒
Earth Science Citress Shampoo 28				🛒	🛒
Earth Science Fragrance-Free Shampoo 28				🛒	🛒
Earth Science Hair Treatment Shampoo ✓				🛒	🛒
Earth Science Herbal Astringent Shampoo ✓ 6				🛒	🛒
Ecco Bella Wake-Me-Up Shampoo ✓ 19				🛒	🛒
Emerald Forest Shampoo 6, 14, 28				🛒	🛒
Faith In Nature Aloe Vera Shampoo ✓ 6				🛒	🛒
Faith In Nature Jojoba Shampoo ✓ 6				🛒	🛒
Faith In Nature Rosemary Shampoo ✓ 6				🛒	🛒
Faith In Nature Seaweed Shampoo ✓ 6				🛒	🛒
Finesse Shampoo Extra Body 6, 16, 29, 28				🛒	🛒
Finesse Shampoo Extra Moisturizing for Dry or Overstyled Hair 6, 16, 28				🛒	🛒
Finesse Shampoo Plus Conditioner 6, 16, 28, 34				🛒	🛒
Finesse Shampoo Regular 6, 27, 28, 29				🛒	🛒
Flex Shampoo Dry/Damaged; Balsam & Protein 6, 14, 19, 28, 31, 33				🛒	🛒
Flex Shampoo (Extra Body, Frequent Use, Oily—Balsam & Protein, & Normal to Dry Hair) 6, 14, 19, 27, 28, 31				🛒	🛒
Giovanni 50/50 Balanced Shampoo–Peach 6, 16, 28				🛒	🛒
Giovanni Golden Wheat Shampoo 6, 16, 28				🛒	🛒
Golden Lotus Lemongrass Shampoo for Normal Hair 21, 28				🛒	🛒
Golden Lotus Shampoo for Normal Hair 6, 14, 21, 28				🛒	🛒
Halsa Moisture Revitalizing Shampoo 6, 19, 32				🛒	🛒
Head Dandruff Shampoo 6, 14, 19, 28				🛒	🛒

Product				Health Advisory	
⊞ *Little to No Risk*	⊞ *Minimal Risk*	⊞ *Caution*	✓ *Recommended*	Contact Dermatitis	Carcinogens
Head Original Shampoo 6, 14, 28				⊞	⊞
Head Pure and Basic Lite Shampoo ✓ *6*				⊞	⊞
Healthy Times Baby Shampoo 6, 19, 28				⊞	⊞
Home Health Chamovera Shampoo 19, 28				⊞	⊞
Home Health Oliva Olive & Aloe Shampoo 6, 21, 28				⊞	⊞
Infinity Golden Camomile Shampoo 28				⊞	⊞
Infinity Radiant Rosemary Shampoo 28				⊞	⊞
Ivory Shampoo Dry/Permed Hair ✓ *6*				⊞	⊞
Ivory Shampoo Fine Hair ✓ *6*				⊞	⊞
Ivory Shampoo Mild Formula ✓ *6*				⊞	⊞
Ivory Shampoo Normal Hair ✓ *6*				⊞	⊞
Ivory Shampoo Normal to Oily Hair ✓ *6*				⊞	⊞
Jason Aloe Vera Gel Shampoo 1, 7, 14, 19, 28				⊞	⊞
Jason Biotin Shampoo 6, 7, 14, 28				⊞	⊞
Jason E.F.A. Primrose Oil Shampoo 6, 7, 14, 19, 28				⊞	⊞
Jason Herbal Shampoo 6, 7, 14, 19, 28				⊞	⊞
Jason Henna Highlights Shampoo 6, 14, 17				⊞	⊞
Jason Jojoba Shampoo 1, 14, 28				⊞	⊞
Jason Sea Kelp Shampoo 6, 7, 14, 19, 28				⊞	⊞
Jason Vitamin E Shampoo 1, 6, 7, 14, 19, 28				⊞	⊞
Jhirmack Lite Frequent Use Shampoo For All Hair Types ✓ *6, 14*				⊞	⊞
Jhirmack Geláve Revitalizer Shampoo For Normal Hair 6, 14, 29				⊞	⊞
Jhirmack Nutri-Body Extra Body Shampoo For Fine, Thin Hair 6, 14, 28, 29, 33				⊞	⊞

Product	Health Advisory	
🛒 *Little to No Risk* 🛒 *Minimal Risk* 🛒 *Caution* ✓ *Recommended*	Contact Dermatitis	Carcinogens
Jhirmack Salon E.F.A. Moisturizing Shampoo For Dry, Permed & Color-Treated Hair ✓ *6, 14*	🛒	🛒
Johnson's Baby Shampoo 6, 17	🛒	🛒
Johnson's Baby Conditioning Shampoo 6, 17, 32	🛒	🛒
Kiss My Face Shampoo 6, 14, 28	🛒	🛒
Logona Algae Extra Care Shampoo ✓	🛒	🛒
Logona Avocado & Neem Shampoo ✓	🛒	🛒
Logona Chamomile & Lemon Regular-Care Shampoo ✓	🛒	🛒
Logona Color-Care Shampoo ✓	🛒	🛒
Logona Henna Regular-Care Shampoo ✓	🛒	🛒
Logona Honey & Wheat Germ Extra-Care Shampoo ✓	🛒	🛒
Logona Marigold Regular-Care Shampoo ✓	🛒	🛒
Logona Men's Shampoo & Shower Gel ✓	🛒	🛒
Logona Nettles Regular-Care Shampoo ✓	🛒	🛒
Logona Rosemary Regular-Care Shampoo ✓	🛒	🛒
L'Oréal Ultra Rich Shampoo Extra Body 2, 6, 28	🛒	🛒
L'Oréal Ultra Rich Shampoo Normal 2, 6, 28	🛒	🛒
L'Oréal Colorvive Technicare Gentle Shampoo For Color-Treated Hair 6, 14, 28	🛒	🛒
Mera Shampoo for Dry Hair ✓	🛒	🛒
Mera Shampoo for Normal Hair ✓	🛒	🛒
Mera Shampoo for Oily Hair ✓	🛒	🛒
Mountain Ocean Hair Maximum Shampoo 6, 14, 16, 17, 28	🛒	🛒
Naturade Aloe Vera Shampoo 13, 14, 19, 28	🛒	🛒
Naturade Baby Shampoo 14, 28	🛒	🛒

Product	Health Advisory	
	Contact Dermatitis	Carcinogens
Naturade Jojoba Shampoo 14, 28	(cart)	(cart)
Nature's Gate Aloe Vera Shampoo 16, 19, 28	(cart)	(cart)
Nature's Gate Awapuhi Shampoo 6, 14, 28	(cart)	(cart)
Nature's Gate Baby Shampoo 14, 21, 28	(cart)	(cart)
Nature's Gate Biotin Shampoo 14, 21, 28	(cart)	(cart)
Nature's Gate Henna Shampoo 6, 14, 28	(cart)	(cart)
Nature's Gate Herbal Hair Shampoo ✓ 14	(cart)	(cart)
Nature's Gate Jojoba Shampoo 14, 28	(cart)	(cart)
Nature's Gate Keratin Shampoo 1, 14, 28	(cart)	(cart)
Nature's Gate Rainwater Herbal Shampoo 10, 14, 228	(cart)	(cart)
Nature's Gate Rainwater Shampoo/Dry Hair 6, 14, 28	(cart)	(cart)
Nature's Gate Tea Tree Oil Shampoo 14, 28	(cart)	(cart)
Neutrogena Shampoo 6, 7, 14, 28	(cart)	(cart)
Neutrogena Shampoo Extra Mild Formula 6, 7, 14, 28	(cart)	(cart)
Neutrogena Shampoo for Permed or Color-Treated Hair 6, 7, 14, 16, 27, 28, 29	(cart)	(cart)
Nirvana Black Walnut Shampoo 14, 19, 28	(cart)	(cart)
Nirvana Blue Malva Shampoo 14, 19, 28	(cart)	(cart)
Nirvana Chamomile Shampoo 14, 19, 28	(cart)	(cart)
Nirvana Clove Shampoo 14, 19, 28	(cart)	(cart)
Nirvana Hibiscus Shampoo 14, 19, 28	(cart)	(cart)
O'Naturel Camomile Shampoo 14, 16, 28	(cart)	(cart)
O'Naturel Henna & Rosemary Shampoo 14, 16, 28	(cart)	(cart)
O'Naturel Honey & Sage Shampoo 14, 16, 28	(cart)	(cart)

Legend: (cart icons) Little to No Risk, Minimal Risk, Caution, ✓ Recommended

Product					Health Advisory	
🛒 *Little to No Risk*	🛒 *Minimal Risk*	🛒 *Caution*	✓ *Recommended*		Contact Dermatitis	Carcinogens
O'Naturel Lavender Conditioning Shampoo 14, 16, 28					🛒	🛒
Original Apple Pectin Shampoo Concentrate 6, 21, 28					🛒	🛒
Pantene Progressive Treatment For Color-Treated Hair 6, 12, 19					🛒	🛒
Pantene Progressive Treatment For Dry Hair 6, 12, 31, 33					🛒	🛒
Pantene Progressive Treatment Extra Body 6, 12					🛒	🛒
Pantene Progressive Treatment For Normal Hair 6, 12, 33					🛒	🛒
Pantene Progressive Treatment for Permed Hair 6, 12, 19					🛒	🛒
Pantene Progressive Treatment Vitamin Therapy 6, 12					🛒	🛒
Paul Penders Jasmine Chamomile Shampoo ✓ 14					🛒	🛒
Paul Penders Peppermint Hops Shampoo ✓ 14					🛒	🛒
Paul Penders Rosemary Lavender Shampoo ✓ 14					🛒	🛒
Paul Penders Walnut Oil Shampoo ✓ 14					🛒	🛒
Permavive Technique for Permed Hair, Extra Body, Gentle Shampoo for Dry/Damaged Hair 6, 14, 28					🛒	🛒
Rainbow Research Henna Shampoo 14, 28					🛒	🛒
Rainbow Research Kids Shampoo 14, 28					🛒	🛒
Reviva Brewer's Yeast Shampoo 28					🛒	🛒
Reviva Seaweed Shampoo 6, 28					🛒	🛒
Salon Selectives Shampoo Level 1 Frequent Use 6, 16, 28					🛒	🛒
Salon Selectives Shampoo Level 3 Gentle for Permed, Color-Treated or Heat-Styled Hair 6, 16, 27, 28, 33					🛒	🛒
Salon Selectives Shampoo Level 4 for Dry, Damaged or Over-Styled Hair 6, 16, 28					🛒	🛒
Salon Selectives Shampoo Level 5 Regular for Normal, Fuller Healthy Hair 6, 16, 28, 33					🛒	🛒

Product	Health Advisory	
Little to No Risk Minimal Risk Caution Recommended	Contact Dermatitis	Carcinogens
Salon Selectives Shampoo Level 6 Extra Body for Fine, Thin or Unmanageable Hair 6, 16, 27, 28, 33	Caution	Minimal Risk
Salon Selectives Shampoo Level 7 Deep for Normal to Oily Hair or Regular Users of Mousse, Gel or Hair Spray 6, 16, 27, 28, 33	Minimal Risk	Minimal Risk
Shi Kai Dry Hair Shampoo 6, 7, 28	Minimal Risk	Minimal Risk
Shi Kai Fine Hair Shampoo 6, 14, 28	Caution	Minimal Risk
Shi Kai Henna Gold Shampoo 6, 14, 17, 21, 28	Caution (black)	Minimal Risk
Shi Kai Normal Hair Shampoo 6, 14, 28	Caution	Minimal Risk
Shi Kai Permed Hair Shampoo 6, 14, 28	Caution	Minimal Risk
Stony Brook Oil-Free Shampoo (Scented with Natural Fragrance) 14, 28	Little to No Risk	Minimal Risk
Stony Brook Oil-Free Shampoo (Unscented) 14, 28	Little to No Risk	Minimal Risk
Style Plus Shampoo & Conditioner In One Level 1 Light Conditioning 6, 21, 24, 33, 34	Minimal Risk	Minimal Risk
Style Plus Shampoo & Conditioner In One Level 2 Regular Conditioning 6, 21, 24, 33, 34	Minimal Risk	Minimal Risk
Style Plus Shampoo & Conditioner In One Level 3 Extra Conditioning 6, 21, 24, 33, 34	Caution	Minimal Risk
Style Shampoo For Dry or Damaged Hair 6, 19, 24, 32, 33	Caution	Minimal Risk
Style Shampoo For Fine, Limp Hair 6, 28	Minimal Risk	Minimal Risk
Style Shampoo For Frequent Use 6, 19, 24, 33	Minimal Risk	Minimal Risk
Suave Salon Formula Shampoo with Vitamins 6, 16, 19, 28	Minimal Risk	Minimal Risk
Suave Shampoo Balsam & Protein 6, 14, 27, 28, 33	Caution	Caution
Suave Shampoo/Conditioner Normal to Dry Hair 6, 28, 29	Caution	Caution
Suave Shampoo Extra Gentle 6, 16, 28	Caution	Caution
Suave Shampoo Moisturizing 6, 28, 32, 33	Caution	Caution

Product				Health Advisory	
Little to No Risk	Minimal Risk	Caution	Recommended	Contact Dermatitis	Carcinogens
Suave Shampoo Soft Highlights 6, 16, 27, 28, 33				Caution	Minimal Risk
Suave Shampoo Special Protection 6, 16, 28				Minimal Risk	Caution
Swiss Formula Aloe Vera & Vitamin E Shampoo 6, 14, 17, 19, 28, 29, 33				Caution	Minimal Risk
Thursday Plantation Dry Hair Shampoo ✓				Recommended	Recommended
Thursday Plantation Normal/Oily Hair Shampoo ✓				Recommended	Recommended
Tropical Botanicals Rainflowers Shampoo 6, 14, 28				Minimal Risk	Minimal Risk
Ultra Care Shampoo/Protein Conditioner/Finishing Rinse in One (Dry, Permed or Color-Treated Hair) 6, 34				Little to No Risk	Minimal Risk
Ultra Care Shampoo/Protein Conditioner/Finishing Rinse in One (Extra Body for Fine Hair) 6, 34				Minimal Risk	Caution
Ultra Care Shampoo/Protein Conditioner/Finishing Rinse in One (Normal Hair) 6, 34				Little to No Risk	Minimal Risk
Urtekram Camomile Shampoo ✓				Recommended	Recommended
Urtekram Children's Shampoo ✓ 8				Recommended	Recommended
Urtekram Desert Moments Shampoo ✓				Recommended	Recommended
Urtekram Gypsy Night Dream Shampoo ✓				Recommended	Recommended
Urtekram Ocean Mist Shampoo ✓				Recommended	Recommended
Urtekram Rose and Jasmine Shampoo Soft Highlights ✓ 8				Recommended	Recommended
Weleda Chamomile Shampoo 28				Recommended	Caution
Weleda Rosemary Shampoo 28				Recommended	Caution
White Rain Shampoo Conditioning 6, 14, 21, 28				Little to No Risk	Minimal Risk
White Rain Shampoo For Dry or Treated Hair 6, 28				Little to No Risk	Caution
White Rain Shampoo Extra Body 6, 28				Minimal Risk	Caution

Dandruff Shampoos

Product				Health Advisory	
🛒 Little to No Risk	🛒 Minimal Risk	🛒 Caution	✓ Recommended	Contact Dermatitis	Carcinogens
Ecco Bella Dandruff Therapy Shampoo ✓ 19				🛒	🛒
Head & Shoulders Dandruff Shampoo Fine or Oily Hair 6, 29				🛒	🛒
Head & Shoulders Dandruff Shampoo Normal or Dry Hair 6, 29				🛒	🛒
Head & Shoulders Intensive Treatment Dandruff Shampoo 2-in-1 Shampoo Plus Conditioner 6, 31				🛒	🛒
Head & Shoulders Intensive Treatment Dandruff Shampoo Conditioning 6, 31				🛒	🛒
Head & Shoulders Intensive Treatment Dandruff Shampoo Regular Formula 6,31				🛒	🛒
Home Health Everclean Antidandruff Shampoo 1, 21, 28				🛒	🛒
Neutrogena Therapeutic T/Gel Shampoo 23				*	🛒
Selsun Blue Dandruff Shampoo Extra Conditioning Formula with Aloe 6, 16, 28, 29				🛒	🛒
Selsun Blue Dandruff Shampoo Regular 6, 28, 29				🛒	🛒
Tegrin Advanced Formula Dandruff Shampoo Extra Conditioning 6, 14, 23, 28, 29				🛒	🛒
Tegrin Advanced Formula Dandruff Shampoo Fresh Herbal 6, 14, 23, 28, 29				🛒	🛒

HAIR-COLORING PRODUCTS FOR WOMEN

Product Types

Permanent; semipermanent; temporary; shampoo-in; streak; frost; tip; bleach.

Health Advisory

The bad news is that lifetime use of permanent and semipermanent hair dyes, particularly dark and black colors, is clearly a cancer risk. The good news is that several natural coloring products on the market now offer women a viable alternative to dangerous petrochemical products. One line that is becoming widely popular in the finest New York salons is Igora Botanic from Schwarzkopf. These plant-based hair colors are composed exclusively of raw materials found in nature such as indigo, chamomile, walnut, logwood, cochineal, and guar gum. The line

---

Information not available.

offers eight shades for a variety of fashionable color results. For more information call (800) 234-4672. Several other additional brands from Logona and Rainbow Research also are available.

Contact Dermatitis

The phenylenediamine compounds in hair dyes can be extremely irritating and cause blindness if applied to the eyes.

Many hair-coloring products are highly alkaline. Consequently, they have significant potential to produce irritation.

Carcinogens

The use of permanent and semipermanent hair dyes is associated with significantly increased risk of non-Hodgkin's lymphoma, multiple myeloma, leukemia, and Hodgkin's disease; the evidence is also suggestive of an association with breast cancer. Women who use black, brown/brunette, and red hair dyes have higher risks than women who use lighter color dyes. There is little doubt that a significant percentage of the non-Hodgkin's lymphoma cases among women is due to use of hair dyes.

Any hair dye containing a phenylenediamine-based ingredient should immediately be considered able to induce human cancer.

Temporary hair dyes and rinses contain chemicals like Acid Orange 87, Solvent Brown 44, Acid Blue 168, and Acid Violet 73, which have shown evidence of carcinogenicity. Do not use these products, either.

The hair-coloring products that have been rated for caution have been done so based on epidemiological evidence of their cancer risk.

Safe Use Tips

- Never use any product with the following disclaimer on the package:

  CAUTION: THIS PRODUCT CONTAINS INGREDIENTS WHICH MAY CAUSE SKIN IRRITATION ON CERTAIN INDIVIDUALS AND A PRELIMINARY TEST ACCORDING TO ACCOMPANYING DIRECTIONS SHOULD FIRST BE MADE. THIS PRODUCT MUST NOT BE USED FOR DYEING THE EYELASHES OR EYEBROWS; TO DO SO MAY CAUSE BLINDNESS.

Such warnings on the label mean that the product contains ingredients that are exempt from provisions of the FFD&C Act and possibly contains carcinogenic dyes.

- Never use a product that lists a phenylenediamine compound on its label.
- Bleaches are much safer than dyes. They offer fewer, if any, long-term dangers, although they are potentially harsh.

- Hair colorings using pure henna, chamomile, and other herbs are safe from chronic effects. Botanical products are more sophisticated than they once were, and they can achieve a wider range of colors than ever before. They are especially good for adding sheen and lustre. They will darken and cover a small proportion of gray. They are worth exploring.
- Although the use of permanent and semipermanent hair dyes is not recommended, if you do use them, then do not leave on longer than necessary.
- Flood scalp thoroughly with water after use.
- Use a technique that involves minimum contact between the dye and scalp. Frosting, where a plastic cap is worn over the head and selected strands are pulled through holes in the cap, is better. Tipping, streaking, or painting involve less contact.
- There is some evidence that most of the carcinogenic risk of hair dyes is attributable to the black shades of hair dye.
- Put off using hair dyes as long as possible. Some experts claim the age at which women start to use hair dyes is an important factor determining risk. Women who start at age forty have a risk less than one-third of those who start at age thirty, while women who start at age twenty have a risk more than twice as great.
- Do not use hair dyes more often than necessary.

Hair-Coloring Products for Women

Product				Contact Dermatitis	Carcinogens
🛒 Little to No Risk	🛒 Minimal Risk	🛒 Caution	✓ Recommended		
Born Blonde No-Peroxide Lotion Toner (Blissfully Blonde) 6, 21, 22, 28				🛒	🛒
Clairesse Gentle Colors for Permed & Delicate Hair (Medium Ash Brown) 6, 15, 16, 17, 18, 28				🛒	🛒
Clairol Balsam Color Conditioning Shampoo-In Haircolor (Palest Blonde) 6, 15, 16, 28				🛒	🛒
Clairol Frost & Tip 6, 7, 14, 15, 28				🛒	🛒
Clairol Light Effects 6, 28				🛒	🛒
Clairol Loving Care Color Lotion 6, 21, 22, 28, 29				🛒	🛒

Risk legend:

🛒 Little to No Risk   🛒 Minimal Risk   🛒 Caution   ✓ Recommended

Product	Contact Dermatitis	Carcinogens
Clairol Nice 'n Easy 6, 14, 15, 16, 17, 18, 28	Caution	Caution
Clairol Maxi Blonde The Maximum Hair Lightener 6, 14, 39	Minimal Risk	Minimal Risk
Clairol Hairpainting Quiet Touch Brush-On Highlighting Kit Blonde to Light Brown Permed Hair 6, 7, 14, 28, 39	Minimal Risk	Minimal Risk
Clairol Quiet Touch Brush-On Highlighting Kit Hairpainting Original Formula for Blonde to Light Brown Hair 6, 7, 28, 39	Minimal Risk	Minimal Risk
Clairol Ultimate Blonde 6, 14, 15, 16, 18, 27, 28, 34	Caution	Caution
Clairol Ultress Gel Colourant (Dark Blonde) 6, 14, 15, 16, 18, 27, 28, 34	Caution	Caution
Igora Botanic ✓	Little to No Risk	Little to No Risk
Logona Henna Black ✓	Little to No Risk	Little to No Risk
Logona Henna Natural Red ✓	Little to No Risk	Little to No Risk
Logona Flame Red, Mahogany, Sahara, Walnut Brown ✓	Little to No Risk	Little to No Risk
L'Oréal Avantage (Light Ash Brown) 6, 14, 28, 33	Minimal Risk	Minimal Risk
L'Oréal Excellence Color Reliance (Dark Brown) 6, 15, 16, 18, 21, 28	Caution	Caution
L'Oréal Performing Preference Les Blondissimes 2, 15, 21, 28	Minimal Risk	Caution
L'Oréal Performing Preference Permanent Creme-In Haircolor 6, 15, 16, 18, 28	Caution	Caution
L'Oréal Summer Soleil Subtle Hair Lightener 6, 18, 28	Caution	Minimal Risk
L'Oréal Super Blonde Lightener Kit 6, 14, 16, 27	Minimal Risk	Minimal Risk
Miss Clairol (Sunny Blonde) 15, 16, 18, 28 34	Minimal Risk	Caution
Rainbow Research Henna ✓	Little to No Risk	Little to No Risk
Revlon Colorsilk Salon Formula Ammonia-Free Haircolor 6, 14, 15, 18, 21, 28	Caution	Caution
Salon Formula Sun-In ✓ 6	Minimal Risk	Little to No Risk
Wella Color Charm Liquid Creme Hair Color 6, 15, 18	Caution	Caution

HAIR-COLORING PRODUCTS FOR MEN

Product Types

Liquid.

Health Advisory

Men, if you want to add color to your hair, check out the botanical products recommended in hair-coloring products for women. None will completely cover the gray, but they will cover some (about 5 percent) and add highlights and sheen.

Contact Dermatitis

The major problem ingredient in men's hair colorants is phenylenediamine. It is very irritating. Do not apply near the eyes!

Carcinogens

Many products contain lead acetate and should not be used. Others containing DEA, TEA, or phenylenediamines should also not be used.

Hair-Coloring Products for Men

Product				Contact Dermatitis	Carcinogens
🛒 *Little to No Risk*	🛒 *Minimal Risk*	🛒 *Caution*	✓ *Recommended*		
Clairol Great Day Gray Control for Men Medium Brown 6, 22, 28				🛒	🛒
Clairol Option Instant Natural Black 6, 15, 16, 18, 28				🛒	🛒
Great Day Dark Brown/Black 6, 22, 28				🛒	🛒
Grecian Formula Cream with Groomer 6, 16, 36				🛒	🛒
Grecian Formula Liquid with Conditioner 6, 18, 36				🛒	🛒
Youthair Creme 6, 14, 36				🛒	🛒
Youthair Liquid 6, 36				🛒	🛒

HAIR SPRAYS AND STYLING PREPARATIONS

Product Types

Aerosol; gel; pump.

Health Advisory

Contact Dermatitis

Aerosols should never be used. Aerosol particles are highly respirable and so fine they penetrate to the deepest parts of the lungs, where they are transferred, like oxygen, into the bloodstream. Inhaling aerosol sprays also can cause allergic reactions. Symptoms include respiratory irritation and difficulty breathing.

Users of pump products also inhale a great deal of the product, and the ingredients are generally the same as aerosols. Of the two, prefer the pump. But try to avoid the use of both aerosols and pumps. All aerosols have been rated for caution.

Carcinogens

Avoid using products containing BHA, DEA, TEA, D&C Red 33, FD&C Blue 1, FD&C Green 3, FD&C Red 40, FD&C Yellow 5, FD&C Yellow 6, and padimate-O.

Some products contain ethoxylated alcohols, PEG compounds, or polysorbate 60 or 80, meaning that they might be contaminated with 1,4-dioxane. Avoid their use.

Safe Use Tips

- If you use aerosol or pump hair spray, be sure to follow all label directions and precautions and apply it in a well-ventilated area.
- Hair setting lotions are safest.

Hair Sprays and Styling Preparations

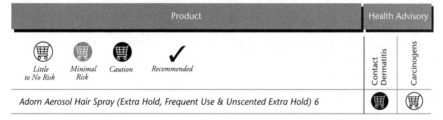

Product				Health Advisory	
🛒 Little to No Risk	🛒 Minimal Risk	🛒 Caution	✓ Recommended	Contact Dermatitis	Carcinogens
Adorn Aerosol Hair Spray (Extra Hold, Frequent Use & Unscented Extra Hold) 6				🛒	🛒

Product				Health Advisory	
🛒 Little to No Risk	🛒 Minimal Risk	🛒 Caution	✓ Recommended	Contact Dermatitis	Carcinogens
Alberto Moisturizing Styling Mousse Extra Control Aerosol 6, 17, 28, 33				Caution	Caution
Alberto Aerosol Styling Spray (Ultra Hold) 6				Caution	Minimal Risk
Alberto VO5 Aerosol Hair Spray (Conditioning Hard to Hold, Hard to Hold, & Unscented Hard to Hold) 6				Caution	Minimal Risk
Alberto VO5 Nonaerosol Hair Spray (Conditioning Hard to Hold, Extra Body Hard to Hold, Hard to Hold, & Unscented Hard to Hold) ✓ 6				Little to No Risk	Minimal Risk
Alberto VO5 Conditioning Hairdressing (Gray, White, Silver Blonde) 4, 6, 8				Little to No Risk	Minimal Risk
Alberto VO5 Conditioning Hairdressing (Normal/Dry Hair) 4, 6, 8				Minimal Risk	Minimal Risk
Alberto VO5 Conditioning Hairdressing (Unscented) 4				Minimal Risk	Minimal Risk
Alberto VO5 with Cholesterol Damaged Hair Treatment ✓ 6, 8, 14				Little to No Risk	Minimal Risk
Alexandra Avery Hair Oil ✓				Minimal Risk	Minimal Risk
Aloegen Hair Sculpting Setting Gel ✓ 6, 14, 16				Little to No Risk	Minimal Risk
Aloegen Styling Spritz ✓ 6				Little to No Risk	Minimal Risk
Aloegen Hair Spray ✓ 6, 13				Little to No Risk	Minimal Risk
Aquanet Aerosol Professional Hair Spray (All Purpose, Super-Hold, Unscented All-Purpose, Unscented Extra Super Hold, & Unscented Super Hold) 2, 6				Caution	Minimal Risk
Aquanet Aerosol Professional Hair Spray Ultimate Hold 6				Caution	Minimal Risk
Aquanet Nonaerosol Hair Spray (Extra Super Hold, Regular Hold, Unscented Regular Hold, Unscented Super Hold, & Super Hold) ✓ 6				Little to No Risk	Minimal Risk
Aubrey Chestnut Brown Natural Body Highliter Mousse ✓ 1, 13				Minimal Risk	Minimal Risk
Aubrey Design Gel ✓ 19				Minimal Risk	Minimal Risk
Aubrey Ginkgo Leaf & Ginseng Root Jelly ✓				Minimal Risk	Minimal Risk
Aubrey Ginseng Hair Control ✓				Minimal Risk	Minimal Risk
Aubrey Golden Chamomile Natural Body Highliter Mousse ✓ 1, 13				Minimal Risk	Minimal Risk
Aubrey Natural Missst Herbal Hairspray ✓				Minimal Risk	Minimal Risk
Aubrey Soft Black Natural Body Highliter Mousse ✓ 1, 13				Minimal Risk	Minimal Risk

Product	Contact Dermatitis	Carcinogens
Aussie Mega Styling Nonaerosol Spray (Aussie Sprunch Spray & Ultra Firm Working Spray) ✓ 6	🛒	🛒
Aussie Scould Spray Gel Nonaerosol Professional Sculpting and Molding Hair Fixture ✓ 6	🛒	🛒
Breck Aerosol Hair Spray (#1 Regular Hold, #2 Unscented Super Hold, #2 Superhold & #3 Ultimate Hold) 6	🛒	🛒
Clairol Final Net Nonaerosol Hair Spray (Extra Hold & Ultimate Hold) ✓	🛒	🛒
Condition Aerosol Hair Spray (Extra Hold Unscented) 6, 28	🛒	🛒
Condition 3-in-1 Aerosol Hair Spray (Extra Hold Unscented with Sunscreen) 28	🛒	🛒
Condition 3-in-1 Aerosol Hair Spray (Extra Hold with Sunscreen) 6, 28	🛒	🛒
Dep Mega Mousse Aerosol 6, 28	🛒	🛒
Dep Styling Gel Super Hold & Body 6, 14, 16, 21, 33, 34	🛒	🛒
Dippity-do Styling Gel 6, 14, 30	🛒	🛒
Earth Preserv ✓ 1, 14	🛒	🛒
Earth Science Silk Forte Hair Styling Mist ✓ 13	🛒	🛒
Earth Science Silk Lite Hair Styling Mist ✓ 6, 13	🛒	🛒
Finesse Extra Hold Aerosol Hair Spray 6	🛒	🛒
Finesse Nonaerosol Hair Spray (Extra Hold) ✓ 6	🛒	🛒
Giovanni Sunset Sculpset Lavender ✓ 6	🛒	🛒
Giovanni Vitapro Fusion-Orange ✓ 6	🛒	🛒
Giovanni L.A. Hold-Black ✓ 6	🛒	🛒
Giovanni L.A. Natural-Red ✓ 6, 16	🛒	🛒
Giovanni Natural Mousse ✓ 6	🛒	🛒
Jhirmack Nonaerosol Hair Spray ✓ 6	🛒	🛒
LA Looks Styling Gel Extra Super Hold 6, 14, 17, 27	🛒	🛒

Little to No Risk · Minimal Risk · Caution · Recommended ✓

Product		Health Advisory	
Little to No Risk / Minimal Risk / Caution / ✓ Recommended		Contact Dermatitis	Carcinogens
LA Looks Styling Gel Mega Hold Alcohol-Free 6, 14, 17, 29		🛒	🛒
Mera Hair Spray ✓ 6		🛒	🛒
Mera Misting Gel ✓ 6		🛒	🛒
Mera Sculpting Gel 6, 14, 21		🛒	🛒
Naturade Nonalcohol Styling Spray ✓		🛒	🛒
Naturade Hair Spray with Jojoba ✓		🛒	🛒
Nirvana Flax Sculpturing Gel 21		🛒	🛒
Pantene Aerosol Extra Firm Hold 6, 12		🛒	🛒
Pantene Nonaerosol Extra Firm Hold 6, 12		🛒	🛒
Perma Soft Aerosol Extra Hold Scented 6, 28		🛒	🛒
Rave Aerosol Hair Spray (Extra Hold, Mega Hold, Super Hold, & Ultra Hold) 6		🛒	🛒
Rave Aerosol All in One Hair Spray with Conditioning Nutrients (Ultra Hold) 6, 19		🛒	🛒
Rave Nonaerosol Hair Spray (Extra Hold, Super Hold, & Ultra Hold) ✓ 6		🛒	🛒
Rave Nonaerosol All in One Hair Spray with Conditioning Nutrients (Ultra Hold, Natural Hold, & Super Hold) ✓ 6, 19		🛒	🛒
Salon Selectives Aerosol Hair Spray (15 Max Control) 6, 16		🛒	🛒
Salon Selectives Nonaerosol (10 Extra Hold) ✓ 6, 16		🛒	🛒
Shi Kai Extra Hold Finishing Spray ✓ 6		🛒	🛒
Shi Kai Super Hold Styling Spray ✓ 6		🛒	🛒
Shi Kai Volume Plus Styling Gel 6, 7, 21		🛒	🛒
Style Aerosol Hair Spray (Natural Hold, Super Hold, Ultra Hold, & Unscented Super Hold) 6		🛒	🛒
Style Nonaerosol Hair Spray (Super Hold & Unscented Super Hold) ✓ 6		🛒	🛒
Style Aerosol Styling Mousse (Extra Hold with Aloe Vera and Jojoba Oil) 6, 16		🛒	🛒
Suave Aerosol Hair Spray (Extra Hold) 6		🛒	🛒

Product				Health Advisory	
🛒 Little to No Risk	🛒 Minimal Risk	🛒 Caution	✓ Recommended	Contact Dermatitis	Carcinogens
Suave Nonaerosol Styling Spray (Body Building) 6, 21				🛒	🛒
Suave Nonaerosol Hair Spray (Extra Hold) ✓ 6				🛒	🛒
Weleda Rosemary Hair Oil ✓				🛒	🛒
White Rain Aerosol (Extra Hold & Firm Hold) 6				🛒	🛒
White Rain Nonaerosol Hair Spray (Dry or Treated Hair) ✓ 6				🛒	🛒
White Rain Nonaerosol Hair Spray (Extra Hold) ✓ 6				🛒	🛒
White Rain Nonaerosol Hair Spray (Unscented Extra Hold) ✓ 6				🛒	🛒

Men's Hair Sprays and Styling Preparations

Product				Health Advisory	
🛒 Little to No Risk	🛒 Minimal Risk	🛒 Caution	✓ Recommended	Contact Dermatitis	Carcinogens
Alexandra Avery Hair Oil ✓				🛒	🛒
Aloegen Hair Sculpting Setting Gel ✓ 6, 14, 16				🛒	🛒
Aloegen Styling Spritz ✓ 6				🛒	🛒
Brylcreem Anti-Dandruff 6, 16, 21				🛒	🛒
Brylcreem Original 6, 22				🛒	🛒
Consort Aerosol Hair Spray (Extra Hold & Unscented) 6				🛒	🛒
Consort Fine Mist Pump Hair Spray (Extra Hold & Unscented) ✓ 6, 8				🛒	🛒
Consort Pump Hair Spray Super Hold Spritz ✓ 6				🛒	🛒
The Dry Look Aerosol Hair Spray (Extra Hold) 6				🛒	🛒
The Dry Look Pump Hair Spray (Max Hold) ✓ 6				🛒	🛒
Earth Science Sculpting Gel Glaze 6, 21				🛒	🛒
Groom & Clean 6, 16, 29				🛒	🛒

Product				Health Advisory	
🛒 *Little to No Risk*	🛒 *Minimal Risk*	🛒 *Caution*	✔ *Recommended*	Contact Dermatitis	Carcinogens
Score Hair Groom 6, 9, 28				🛒	🛒
Vaseline Hair Tonic and Scalp Conditioner ✔ 6				🛒	🛒
Vitalis Hair Tonic 6, 33				🛒	🛒
Vitalis The Pump Super Hold (Non-Aerosol) 6, 22				🛒	🛒

CHAPTER 10

Dental and Oral Hygiene

MOUTHWASHES

Product Type

Liquid.

Health Advisory

Contact Dermatitis

Sodium lauryl sulfate, which has a detergent action, may be slightly drying. Salicylate is allergenic.

Carcinogens

Do not use products with a high alcohol content. A 1991 survey of people with mouth, tongue, or throat cancers suggests that use of high-alcohol mouthwash contributes to increased risk of these tumors. Most of these individuals had used mouthwash at least daily for twenty or more years. The increased risk was seen only in people who used mouthwashes with 25 percent or higher alcohol content. This study corroborates an earlier report in the February 1983 issue of the *Journal of the National Cancer Institute* that found mouthwash to be associated with cancer of the mouth and throat among women who neither smoked nor drank.

Do not use products containing saccharin, FD&C Blue 1, FD&C Green 3, and FD&C Yellow 5. Avoid products containing polysorbate 60 or polysorbate 80 unless their labels specify they are free from 1,4-dioxane.

Mouthwashes

Product	Health Advisory	
🛒 Little to No Risk 🛒 Minimal Risk 🛒 Caution ✓ Recommended	Contact Dermatitis	Carcinogens
Cepacol 33, 38	🛒	🛒
Choice Clear Alcohol-Free 38	🛒	🛒
Desert Essence Tea Tree Mouthwash ✓	🛒	🛒
Listerine Cool Mint 38	🛒	🛒
Listerine Original (high alcohol content)	🛒	🛒
Listermint with Fluoride 30, 38	🛒	🛒
Logona Cistacea Oral Spray ✓	🛒	🛒
Logona Herbal Mouthwash Concentrate ✓	🛒	🛒
Merfluan Mouthwash Concentrate ✓	🛒	🛒
Oral Pure 38	🛒	🛒
Oral Pure Antiseptic Mouthwash (high alcohol content)	🛒	🛒
Oral Pure Mint Mouthwash & Gargle 29, 33	🛒	🛒
Plax 38	🛒	🛒
Scope Mint 29, 33, 38	🛒	🛒
Scope Peppermint 38	🛒	🛒
Tom's Cinnamint Mouthwash ✓	🛒	🛒
Tom's Spearmint Mouthwash ✓	🛒	🛒

Product					Health Advisory	
🛒 Little to No Risk	🛒 Minimal Risk	🛒 Caution	✓ Recommended		Contact Dermatitis	Carcinogens
Weleda Mouthwash ✓					🛒	🛒
Xylifresh Mouthwash ✓					🛒	🛒

TOOTHPASTES AND POWDERS

Product Types

Cream; gel; powder.

Health Advisory

Contact Dermatitis

Toothpastes do not generally pose a significant risk for allergic reactions except for among the most chemically hypersensitive. The amount of irritation caused by toothpaste is minimal but can include sore mouth and gums, wearing away tooth enamel, sore tongue, and sloughing of mucous membranes.

Carcinogens

Avoid using products containing saccharin and FD&C Blue 1. Also, the polysorbate 80 in some brands may be contaminated with 1,4-dioxane.

The use of fluoride in toothpastes is controversial because of suggestive evidence of its carcinogenicity.

Toothpastes and Powders

Product					Health Advisory	
🛒 Little to No Risk	🛒 Minimal Risk	🛒 Caution	✓ Recommended		Contact Dermatitis	Carcinogens
Arm & Hammer Dental Care The Baking Soda Gel 29, 35, 38					🛒	🛒
Arm & Hammer Tartar Control Dental Care The Baking Soda Toothpaste 35, 38					🛒	🛒
Arm & Hammer Dental Care The Baking Soda Tooth Powder 35, 38					🛒	🛒

Product				Health Advisory	
🛒 *Little to No Risk*	🛒 *Minimal Risk*	🛒 *Caution*	✔ *Recommended*	Contact Dermatitis	Carcinogens
Auromere Toothpaste ✔				🛒	🛒
Beehive Botanicals Propolis Toothpaste ✔				🛒	🛒
Bioforce Echinacea ✔				🛒	🛒
Colgate Toothpowder 35, 38				🛒	🛒
Colgate Fluoride Gel Toothpaste 35, 38				🛒	🛒
Colgate Tartar Control Fluoride Toothpaste 35, 38				🛒	🛒
Crest Tartar Control Toothpaste 29, 35, 38				🛒	🛒
Desert Essence Tea Tree Oil Toothpaste ✔				🛒	🛒
Herbal-Vedic Herbal Toothpaste ✔				🛒	🛒
Home Health Peri-Dent Herbal Gum Massage ✔				🛒	🛒
Home Health Salt 'N Soda Toothpowder ✔				🛒	🛒
Logona Children's Toothpaste ✔				🛒	🛒
Logona Peppermint & Clay Toothpaste ✔				🛒	🛒
Logona Rosemary & Sage Toothpaste ✔				🛒	🛒
Mer-Flu-An Anise Toothpowder ✔				🛒	🛒
Mer-Flu-An Cinnamon & Mint Toothpaste ✔				🛒	🛒
Mer-Flu-An Lemon Lime Toothpowder ✔				🛒	🛒
Mer-Flu-An Peppermint Toothpowder ✔				🛒	🛒
Nature's Gate Cherry Gel Toothpaste ✔				🛒	🛒
Nature's Gate Creme de Anise Toothpaste ✔				🛒	🛒
Nature's Gate Creme de Peppermint Toothpaste ✔				🛒	🛒
Nature's Gate Mint Gel Toothpaste ✔				🛒	🛒
Nature's Gate Wintergreen Gel Toothpaste ✔				🛒	🛒

Product	Health Advisory	
 ![Little to No Risk] Little to No Risk ![Minimal Risk] Minimal Risk ![Caution] Caution ✓ Recommended	Contact Dermatitis	Carcinogens
Peelu Toothpaste ✓	🛒	🛒
Peelu Toothpowder ✓	🛒	🛒
Rainbow Research Mint Toothpaste ✓	🛒	🛒
Tom's of Maine Baking Soda Toothpaste with Fluoride 35	🛒	🛒
Tom's of Maine Baking Soda Toothpaste (Peppermint) 35	🛒	🛒
Tom's of Maine Cinnamint Fluoride Toothpaste 35	🛒	🛒
Tom's of Maine Fennel Fluoride Toothpaste 35	🛒	🛒
Tom's of Maine Toothpaste for Children (nonfluoride) ✓	🛒	🛒
Tom's of Maine Toothpaste/Propolis and Myrrh/ Cinnamint (nonfluoride) ✓	🛒	🛒
Tom's of Maine Toothpaste/Propolis and Myrrh/ Fennel (nonfluoride) ✓	🛒	🛒
Tom's of Maine Toothpaste/Propolis and Myrrh/ Spearmint (nonfluoride) ✓	🛒	🛒
Ultra Brite Gel 38	🛒	🛒
Ultra Brite Toothpaste 38	🛒	🛒
Viadent Original Extra Strength Anti-Plaque Toothpaste 38	🛒	🛒
Vicco Pure Herbal Toothpaste ✓	🛒	🛒
Weleda Plant Toothpaste ✓	🛒	🛒
Weleda Pink Toothpaste ✓	🛒	🛒
Weleda Salt and Soda Toothpaste ✓	🛒	🛒
Xylifresh Cinnamon Toothpaste ✓	🛒	🛒
Xylifresh Peppermint Toothpaste ✓	🛒	🛒
Xylifresh Spearmint Toothpaste ✓	🛒	🛒

CHAPTER 11

Feminine Hygiene

DOUCHES, FEMININE DEODORANTS, AND HYGIENE PRODUCTS

Product Types

Liquid; powder; spray.

Health Advisory

Contact Dermatitis

Douches with highest potential for irritation contain essential oils such as eucalyptol, menthol, methyl salicylate, and chlorothymol.

Other problem ingredients include phenol, which can cause swelling, pimples, hives, and other skin rashes, and sodium lauryl sulfate, which is drying and can be irritating.

Citric acid can be an irritant if it is too concentrated; since some douches come in bulk form and must be measured and mixed by the user, it is possible that the concentration can become higher than recommended.

Symptoms of irritation from vaginal deodorants include burning, itching, swelling, rashes, and boils in the vaginal area; bladder infections; and blood in the urine.

Carcinogens

A study involving 674 women over three years found that those who used vaginal douches more than once a week experienced a four-fold risk for cervical cancer. The douching preparation used made no difference. The researchers concluded that frequent douching may alter the chemical environment, making the cervix more susceptible to pathologic changes.

Avoid using products containing FD&C Blue 1.

Safe Use Tips

- Women who experience itching, soreness, or genital odors should discontinue use of their douche and consult a physician.
- Seek products containing vinegar or baking soda, and stay away from those containing numerous essential oils or detergents. Those products with the fewest antiseptics, astringents, and essential oils will probably be the least irritating or sensitizing.

Douches, Feminine Deodorants, and Hygiene Products

Product	Health Advisory	
Little to No Risk • Minimal Risk • Caution • ✓ Recommended	Contact Dermatitis	Carcinogens
Bee Kind Disposable Douche ✓	🛒	🛒
Bio Botanica Douche Concentrate ✓	🛒	🛒
Camo Care Disposable Douche ✓	🛒	🛒
FDS Feminine Deodorant Spray with Powder (Baby Powder & Extra Strength) 2, 10	🛒	🛒
Massengill All Natural Extra Mild Vinegar & Water No Additives Disposable Douche ✓	🛒	🛒
Massengill Baking Soda & Water Disposable Douche ✓	🛒	🛒
Massengill Belle-Mai Fresh Baby Powder Scent Disposable Douche 29	🛒	🛒
Massengill Country Flowers Scent Disposable Douche 29	🛒	🛒
Massengill Douche Powder Packettes 33	🛒	🛒
Massengill Fresh Baby Powder Scent Disposable Douche 6, 14, 16, 29	🛒	🛒

Product				Health Advisory	
Little to No Risk	*Minimal Risk*	*Caution*	✓ *Recommended*	Contact Dermatitis	Carcinogens
Massengill with Natural Ingredients Extra Cleansing with Pura Clean Disposable Douche ✓				🛒	🛒
Massengill Fresh Mountain Breeze 6, 14, 16, 29				🛒	🛒
Summer's Eve Disposable Douche Vinegar & Water ✓				🛒	🛒
Summer's Eve Feminine Powder ✓ 6				🛒	🛒
Summer's Eve Feminine Wash The Intimate Cleanser 6, 29				🛒	🛒
Summer's Eve Fresh Scent ✓ 6				🛒	🛒
Summer's Eve Herbal Freshness Disposable Douche ✓ 6				🛒	🛒
Summer's Eve Hint of Musk Disposable Douche ✓ 6				🛒	🛒
Vagisil Creme Medication 6, 9, 18				🛒	🛒
Vagisil Feminine Powder ✓ 6				🛒	🛒
Yeast-Gard Medicated Cream 6, 9, 18				🛒	🛒

FEMININE CARE AND BODY POWDERS (TALC AND CORNSTARCH)

Product Type

Powder.

Health Advisory

Carcinogens

Frequent and prolonged use of talcum powder applied directly to the genital area is associated with increased risk for ovarian cancer. In 1982, Daniel Cramer, M.D., an obstetrician and gynecologist, reported in *Cancer* the results of a study of 215 Boston-area women with ovarian cancer that found that 32 had used talcum powder on their genitals and sanitary napkins. When compared to a group of women without cancer, women who used talc had a three-fold risk of ovarian cancer. These results were further confirmed with a recent report from the National Toxicology Program, which also found that talc is carcinogenic.

Safe Shopping Tips

- Always prefer cornstarch-based powders.
- Parents of newborns, be sure that your baby's powder does not contain talc.

Feminine Care and Body Powders (Talc and Cornstarch)

Product					Health Advisory	
Little to No Risk	Minimal Risk	Caution	Recommended		Contact Dermatitis	Carcinogens
Cornstarch-based powders (generic)					Little to No Risk	Little to No Risk
Talcum-based powders (generic) 40					Little to No Risk	Caution

TAMPONS AND OTHER MENSTRUAL PRODUCTS

Product Types

Tampon; pad; cup; sponge.

Health Advisory

Contact Dermatitis

Tampons alter the vaginal flora by allowing air into the vagina, which is normally oxygen free. As a result, women can become more vulnerable to tampon-associated vaginal ulcers and vaginitis.

Carcinogens

Because of the chlorine bleaching processes used in manufacturing tampons, some are contaminated with dioxin, which is carcinogenic.

Safe Use Tips

Toxic shock syndrome (TSS), which is caused by the high absorbency of tampons that are unchanged for too long, strikes some 1 in 100,000 menstruating women per year. That is down from the 6 to 12 cases per 100,000 in the early 1980s. But it can still be deadly. Beware of the warning signs of TSS: fever, nausea, vomiting, diarrhea, dizziness, and a sunburn-like rash.

- Choose low-absorbency tampons; high-absorbency tampons are more likely to cause TSS.
- Alternate tampons with pads.
- Do not leave tampons in overnight.
- To avoid exposure to dioxin, which is carcinogenic, as well as other pesticides that may contaminate bleached cotton pads, seek pads made with organically grown cotton, available at health food stores.

CHAPTER 12

Nail Products

NAIL POLISHES, HARDENERS, AND PROTECTORS

Product Types

Liquid.

Health Advisory

Contact Dermatitis

The use of "sculptured" artificial nails can cause a burning sensation, tingling, and slight numbness of the fingertips—a condition known as *paresthesia*. The condition may persist for weeks after the acute dermatitis has subsided. The bonding materials used are powerful solvents that readily penetrate damaged skin and produce an inflammation of the nerve endings. Use such products with caution.

Facial irritation often occurs because women do their nails immediately before they make up their face, and they end up contaminating their facial skin with the strong irritants in nail products.

Safe Use Tips

Nail products pose an extreme poisoning hazard to children. This is true for all nail products containing solvents such as toluene, and amyl, butyl, and ethyl acetate, which are all neurotoxins. Furthermore, nail remover contains acetonitrile,

263

a chemical that breaks down into lethal cyanide when swallowed. In 1990, some twenty-nine hundred children up to age four were admitted to hospital emergency rooms because of nail preparation–related poisonings. Be sure to store all nail products as safely as you would any household poison, completely out of reach of children.

- Nail products frequently contain neurotoxins such as toluene. They should be applied in very well ventilated areas, and users should avoid inhaling the vapors.
- Many products are extremely flammable. Keep from heat and flame.
- Do not do makeup immediately until after nail polish has completely dried.

Nail Polishes, Hardeners, and Protectors

Product				Contact Dermatitis	Carcinogens
(cart) Little to No Risk	(cart) Minimal Risk	(cart) Caution	✓ Recommended		
Clarion Nails 20, 27, 33, 34				(Caution)	(Minimal)
Cutex Color Quick Nail Enamel with Conditioners 20, 33				(Caution)	(Minimal)
De Lore Chip Proof ✓				(Caution)	(Caution)
De Lore Nail Fix ✓				(Caution)	(Caution)
De Lore Nail Hardener ✓ 19				(Caution)	(Caution)
De Lore Nail Protector ✓				(Caution)	(Caution)
L'Oréal Nail Enamel 20, 33				(Caution)	(Little to No Risk)
Sally Hansen Hard as Nails 20, 33				(Caution)	(Minimal)
Sally Hansen Hard as Nails with Nylon 20, 33				(Caution)	(Little to No Risk)

CHAPTER 13

Skin Products

ANTIPERSPIRANTS AND DEODORANTS

Product Types

Aerosol; cream; roll-on; solid stick. Antiperspirants stop perspiration. Deodorants mask odor.

Health Advisory

Because aluminum could be involved in the onset of Alzheimer's disease, the burning question consumers have about antiperspirants is whether or not their aluminum content could be associated with increased risk. The best answer so far comes from a study, published in the *Journal of Clinical Epidemiology* that, in fact, found that the risk for Alzheimer's disease increased along with the use of antiperspirants. The researchers noted that "a statistically significant trend emerged between increasing lifetime use of aluminum-containing antiperspirants and the estimated relative risk of [Alzheimer's disease]." While this is the only known study of its kind, its results certainly suggest that concerned consumers would do just as well to avoid antiperspirants containing aluminum compounds.

Contact Dermatitis

Aluminum-based compounds are one of the leading causes of skin irritation among users of antiperspirants. Inflammation may spread beyond armpits to other areas of the body.

Triclosan, contained in many deodorants, can be absorbed through the skin and has caused liver damage in tests with experimental animals. The FDA has determined that the use of triclosan in deodorants is probably safe—although it also has warned of potential hazards that may be associated with chronic, long-term use.

Zirconium-based compounds can cause some people to develop underarm granulomas (small nodules of chronically inflamed tissue) after prolonged use of antiperspirants.

Irritants commonly found in antiperspirants include the following:

Ingredient	*Potential for Skin Irritation*
Aluminum chloride	High
Aluminum chlorohydrate	Fairly Low
Aluminum phenolsulfate	Moderate
Aluminum sulfate	Moderate
Zinc phenolsulfonate	Moderate
Zirconium chlorohydrate	Moderate
Zirconyl chloride	Moderate

Avoid the use of products containing quaternium 18, which can act as a sensitizer, causing rashes beyond the area of application.

Carcinogens

Avoid use of products containing BHT, DEA, TEA, D&C Red 33, D&C Green 5, FD&C Green 3, FD&C Blue 1, FD&C Red 4, FD&C Yellow 5, and FD&C Yellow 6. These ingredients are wholly unnecessary for the product's effectiveness and will be absorbed through the skin.

Many products contain talc. Its use in roll-on and solid products does not pose a health risk.

Safe Use Tips

- The gentleness of products will vary depending on the skill of the formulator and individual skin sensitivities. Generally, however, stick antiperspirants and deodorants are gentlest—while aerosols, creams, and roll-ons are more irritating.
- Be sure that the antiperspirant brand you choose contains one or more of the following ingredients, which buffer and reduce the irritation of aluminum- and zirconium-based compounds:

Magnesium oxide
Zinc oxide

• Do not use aerosols.

Antiperspirants and Deodorants

Product				Health Advisory	
Little to No Risk	Minimal Risk	Caution	Recommended	Contact Dermatitis	Carcinogens
Almay Anti-Perspirant Solid Deodorant Unscented ✓ 16				Caution	Caution
Ban Antiperspirant Basic Neutral Scent Nonaerosol Spray 6, 22				Minimal Risk	Caution
Ban Clear Solid Deodorant (Cool Breeze, Fresh & Clean, Lightly Scented, Powder Fresh, Spring Bouquet) 6, 16, 29				Minimal Risk	Caution
Ban Roll-On Antiperspirant & Deodorant (Body Fresh Scent) 6, 31				Minimal Risk	Caution
Ban Roll-On Antiperspirant & Deodorant (Ocean Breeze & Unscented) ✓ 6				Minimal Risk	Little to No Risk
Ban Roll-On Antiperspirant & Deodorant (Powder Fresh) 6, 22				Minimal Risk	Caution
Ban Roll-On Antiperspirant & Deodorant (Regular Scent) 6, 22, 31				Minimal Risk	Caution
Barth Roll-On Deodorant 6, 8, 14, 16, 21				Caution	Caution
Barth Stick Deodorant ✓ 6, 14, 16, 19				Minimal Risk	Little to No Risk
Bellmira Deodorant ✓ 16				Caution	Little to No Risk
Brut Deodorant Stick 6, 34				Minimal Risk	Caution
CamoCare Deodorant ✓ 6, 19				Caution	Little to No Risk
Canoe Deodorant Stick ✓ 6, 14				Caution	Little to No Risk
Chaps Deodorant Stick 6, 16, 27, 29, 33, 34				Minimal Risk	Caution
Degree Antiperspirant & Deodorant Aerosol (Powder Fresh & Shower Clean) 6				Caution	Little to No Risk
Degree Roll-On Antiperspirant & Deodorant (Powder Fresh, Regular & Shower Clean) ✓ 6				Minimal Risk	Little to No Risk
Degree Solid Antiperspirant & Deodorant (Powder Fresh, Regular, Shower Clean, Sport, & Unscented) ✓ 6				Minimal Risk	Little to No Risk

Product				Health Advisory	
				Contact Dermatitis	Carcinogens
Desert Essence Tea Tree Deodorant ✔				🛒	🛒
Earth Science Liken Deodorant ✔				🛒	🛒
Earth Science Liken Deodorant (Unscented) ✔				🛒	🛒
English Leather A Man's Deodorant Stick 6, 14, 16, 27, 30, 34				🛒	🛒
English Leather Stick Longer Lasting Deodorant (Musk & Regular) 6, 16				🛒	🛒
Fabergé Deodorant (Cool Scent) 6, 28				🛒	🛒
Fabergé Deodorant (Fresh) 6, 28, 29				🛒	🛒
Fabergé Deodorant (Musk) 6, 24, 31, 33				🛒	🛒
Fabergé Power Stick Antiperspirant & Deodorant (Active Sport, Cool Scent, Musk, & Regular) ✔ 6				🛒	🛒
Fabergé Power Stick Antiperspirant & Deodorant (Unscented) ✔				🛒	🛒
Fabergé Power Stick Deodorant (Active Sport) 6, 24				🛒	🛒
Five-Day Antiperspirant & Deodorant (Pads) ✔ 6				🛒	🛒
Head Green Tea Roll-On Deodorant ✔ 6, 14				🛒	🛒
Head Green Tea Stick Deodorant 6, 14, 16, 28				🛒	🛒
Head Unscented Stick Deodorant 14, 16, 28				🛒	🛒
Hi & Dri Antiperspirant & Deodorant Roll-On (Powder Fresh) 6				🛒	🛒
Home Health Roll-On Deodorant (Scented) ✔ 6				🛒	🛒
Home Health Roll-On Deodorant (Unscented) ✔				🛒	🛒
Irish Spring Solid Antiperspirant & Deodorant (Classic) 1, 6, 29, 33				🛒	🛒
Irish Spring Solid Antiperspirant & Deodorant (Morning Breeze, Sport Fresh) ✔ 1, 6				🛒	🛒
Irish Spring Solid Deodorant (Classic) 6, 16, 33				🛒	🛒
Irish Spring Solid Deodorant (Sport Fresh) 6, 16, 29				🛒	🛒
Jason Apricot & E Roll-On Deodorant ✔ 7, 14, 16, 19				🛒	🛒

Legend: 🛒 *Little to No Risk* · 🛒 *Minimal Risk* · 🛒 *Caution* · ✔ *Recommended*

Product				Health Advisory	
Little to No Risk	Minimal Risk	Caution	Recommended ✓	Contact Dermatitis	Carcinogens
Jason Apricot & E Stick Deodorant ✓				🛒	🛒
Jason Herbs & Spice Roll-on Deodorant ✓ 7, 14, 16, 19				🛒	🛒
Jason Tea Tree Roll-on Deodorant ✓ 14, 16, 19				🛒	🛒
Jason Tea Tree Stick Deodorant ✓ 16, 19				🛒	🛒
Jean Naté Spray Deodorant 6, 16				🛒	🛒
Jövan Musk for Men Stick Deodorant 6, 16, 34				🛒	🛒
Lady Speed Stick Antiperspirant & Deodorant (No Dyes or Fragrance) ✓				🛒	🛒
Lady Speed Stick Antiperspirant & Deodorant (Aloe Fresh) 1, 6, 33				🛒	🛒
Lady Speed Stick Antiperspirant & Deodorant (Soft Lilac) 1, 6, 27, 29				🛒	🛒
Lady Speed Stick Antiperspirant & Deodorant (Scented) 1, 6, 31				🛒	🛒
Lady Speed Stick Crystal Clear Deodorant (Caribbean Cool) 6, 16, 29, 33				🛒	🛒
Lady Speed Stick Crystal Clear Deodorant (Light Musk) 6, 16, 31				🛒	🛒
Lady Speed Stick Crystal Clear Deodorant (Powder Soft) 6, 16, 29				🛒	🛒
Lavilin Foot Deodorant ✓				🛒	🛒
Lavilin Underarm Deodorant ✓				🛒	🛒
Le Crystal Naturel Deodorant ✓				🛒	🛒
Logona Deodorant ✓				🛒	🛒
Logona Roll-On Deodorant ✓				🛒	🛒
Mitchum Super Dry Roll-On Antiperspirant & Deodorant (Unscented) ✓				🛒	🛒
Mum Gentle Formula Antiperspirant & Deodorant 6, 16, 17				🛒	🛒
Nature De France Gardenia Scent Deodorant Stick ✓ 16				🛒	🛒
Nature De France Unscented Stick Deodorant ✓ 16				🛒	🛒
Nature De France Herbal Scent Stick Deodorant ✓ 16				🛒	🛒

Product	Contact Dermatitis	Carcinogens
Little to No Risk — *Minimal Risk* — *Caution* — ✔ *Recommended*		
Nature De France Floral Scent Stick Deodorant ✔ *16*	Little to No Risk	Little to No Risk
Nature's Gate Roll-On Deodorant (all) 16, 28	Little to No Risk	Minimal Risk
Nature's Gate Stick Deodorant 16, 28	Little to No Risk	Minimal Risk
Old Spice Aerosol Deodorant 6, 16	Caution	Little to No Risk
Old Spice Antiperspirant & Deodorant Stick (Musk) 6, 22	Minimal Risk	Minimal Risk
Old Spice Antiperspirant & Deodorant Stick (Original) ✔ *6*	Minimal Risk	Little to No Risk
Old Spice Pump Deodorant (Classic Sport, Fresh, Musk & Original) ✔ *6*	Minimal Risk	Little to No Risk
Old Spice Stick Deodorant (Fresh) 6, 30, 33	Minimal Risk	Minimal Risk
Pierre Cardin Man's Stick Deodorant 6, 32, 33	Minimal Risk	Minimal Risk
Queen Helene Aloe Deodorant Stick ✔ *6, 16*	Minimal Risk	Little to No Risk
Queen Helene Herbal Deodorant Stick 6, 28	Minimal Risk	Minimal Risk
Queen Helene Mint Julep Deodorant ✔ *6, 16*	Minimal Risk	Little to No Risk
Queen Helene Aloe Deodorant Stick ✔ *6, 16*	Minimal Risk	Little to No Risk
Queen Helene Spice Deodorant Stick 16, 28	Little to No Risk	Minimal Risk
Queen Helene Vitamin E Deodorant Stick ✔ *16, 19*	Little to No Risk	Little to No Risk
Right Guard Sport Stick Antiperspirant & Deodorant (Alpine Air, Fresh, Musk, & Surf Spray) ✔ *6, 14*	Minimal Risk	Little to No Risk
Right Guard Sport Stick Deodorant (Fresh) ✔ *6, 16*	Minimal Risk	Little to No Risk
Right Guard Sport Stick Deodorant (Musk) 6, 16, 30, 31	Little to No Risk	Minimal Risk
Right Guard Sport Stick Deodorant (Original Scent) 6, 16, 29	Minimal Risk	Minimal Risk
Secret Antiperspirant & Deodorant Aerosol (Regular, Powder Fresh, & Spring Breeze) 6	Caution	Little to No Risk
Secret Antiperspirant & Deodorant Cream 6, 29	Minimal Risk	Minimal Risk
Secret Roll-On Antiperspirant & Deodorant (Fresh, Regular, Sporty Clean, & Spring Breeze) ✔ *6*	Minimal Risk	Little to No Risk

Product	Health Advisory	
Little to No Risk / **Minimal Risk** / **Caution** / ✓ **Recommended**	Contact Dermatitis	Carcinogens
Secret Roll-On Antiperspirant & Deodorant (Unscented) ✓	Little to No Risk	Little to No Risk
Speed Stick Antiperspirant & Deodorant Super Dry (Classic Scent, Fresh Scent, Musk, & Spice Scent) ✓ *6*	Minimal Risk	Little to No Risk
Speed Stick Antiperspirant & Deodorant Super Dry (Unscented) ✓	Little to No Risk	Little to No Risk
Speed Stick Deodorant Solid (Cool Spice) 6, 16, 24, 31	Caution	Caution
Speed Stick Deodorant Solid (Lime) 6, 16, 29	Caution	Caution
Speed Stick Deodorant Solid (Spice) 6, 16, 24, 31	Caution	Caution
Speed Stick Deodorant Solid (Sport Talc) 6, 16, 29, 31	Caution	Caution
Speed Stick Deodorant Solid (Fresh Scent) 6, 16, 29	Little to No Risk	Caution
Speed Stick Deodorant Solid (Mountain Herbal) 6, 16, 24, 33	Little to No Risk	Caution
Stetson Easy to Wear Deodorant Stick 6, 16, 29, 31, 33	Little to No Risk	Caution
Suave Aerosol Antiperspirant & Deodorant (Regular Scent) 6	Caution	Little to No Risk
Suave Deodorant Super Stick (Fresh) 6, 16, 29	Caution	Caution
Suave Deodorant Super Stick (Musk) 6, 16, 31	Caution	Caution
Suave Stick Antiperspirant & Deodorant (Aloe Fresh, Baby Powder, Regular, Unscented, & Sport) ✓ *6*	Caution	Little to No Risk
Suave Stick Antiperspirant & Deodorant (Unscented) ✓	Little to No Risk	Little to No Risk
Sure Pro Stick Deodorant (Classic, Fresh, Musk, & Spice) 6, 16, 40	Caution	Caution
Sure Solid Antiperspirant & Deodorant (Desert Spice, Outdoor Fresh, Powder Dry, & Regular) ✓ *6*	Little to No Risk	Little to No Risk
Teen Spirit Roll-On Antiperspirant & Deodorant (Baby Powder Soft & California Breeze) ✓ *1, 6*	Little to No Risk	Little to No Risk
Teen Spirit Wide Solid Antiperspirant & Deodorant (Caribbean Cool, Ocean Surf & Romantic Rose) ✓ *1, 6*	Caution	Little to No Risk
Thursday Plantation Roll-On Deodorant ✓	Little to No Risk	Little to No Risk
Tom's of Maine Stick Deodorant (All Scents) ✓ *16*	Little to No Risk	Little to No Risk

Product					Health Advisory	
(Little to No Risk)	(Minimal Risk)	(Caution)	✓ Recommended		Contact Dermatitis	Carcinogens
Tom's of Maine Roll-On Deodorant (Aloe & Buffered Alum) ✓ 16					🛒	🛒
Tom's of Maine Roll-On Deodorant (Aloe & Coriander) ✓ 16					🛒	🛒
Tussy Cream Deodorant (Powder Fresh) ✓ 6, 8					🛒	🛒
Tussy Roll-On Antiperspirant & Deodorant ✓ 6, 14					🛒	🛒
Tussy Stick Deodorant 6, 16, 29					🛒	🛒
Weleda Citrus Deodorant ✓					🛒	🛒
Weleda Sage Deodorant ✓					🛒	🛒

BUBBLE BATHS, MINERAL BATHS, AND BATH OILS

Product Types

Liquid; powder.

Health Advisory

Contact Dermatitis

Fragrances can be a significant problem with bubble baths, where they are often found in very high concentrations. The potential for allergic reactions is greatest with highly fragranced, carbonated bubble baths.

Irritation-related health problems associated with bubble baths were serious enough for the FDA to publish a regulation in 1980 requiring products intended for children to bear adequate directions for safe use, including a warning that the product should be used only moderately and that excessive use can result in rashes, redness, and irritation. Physicians have found that bubble baths strip away the mucous lining of the genito-urinary tract and make the area vulnerable to infection, especially in young girls.

Carcinogens

People taking bubble baths not only have an extended duration of skin contact, but also the hot water increases skin permeability, and the entire body is exposed. For children the exposure is even more concentrated. Products containing cocamide

DEA or TEA, PEG compounds, ethoxylated alcohols, or polysorbate 60 or 80 should not be used—unless the manufacturer provides label certification that states the product is free from nitrosamines or 1,4-dioxane.

Safe Use Tips

- Fragrance-sensitive people should take bubble baths in well-ventilated areas—especially when using carbonated-type products.
- If your baby or child develops any irritation or rashes in the genital area, discontinue bubble baths.

Bubble Baths, Mineral Baths, and Bath Oils

Product	Contact Dermatitis	Carcinogens
Little to No Risk / Minimal Risk / Caution / Recommended		
Abracadabra California Bath ✓	🛒 Little to No Risk	🛒 Little to No Risk
Abracadabra Foaming Aloe Vera Bath ✓	🛒 Little to No Risk	🛒 Little to No Risk
Abracadabra Kid's Bubble Bath ✓ 6	🛒 Minimal Risk	🛒 Little to No Risk
Abracadabra Luxury Bubble Bath ✓	🛒 Little to No Risk	🛒 Little to No Risk
Abracadabra Mineral Bath ✓	🛒 Little to No Risk	🛒 Little to No Risk
Abracadabra Sport Therapy ✓	🛒 Little to No Risk	🛒 Little to No Risk
Actibath (Light & Fresh, Moisture Treatment, & Spring Floral) 6, 19, 29	🛒 Minimal Risk	🛒 Caution
Actibath Moisture Treatment 6, 19, 29	🛒 Minimal Risk	🛒 Caution
Aubrey Chamomile Bubbles Bath Oil ✓ 13, 19	🛒 Little to No Risk	🛒 Little to No Risk
Aubrey Eucalyptus Spa Bath ✓	🛒 Little to No Risk	🛒 Little to No Risk
Aura Cacia Massage and Bath Oils (all) ✓	🛒 Little to No Risk	🛒 Little to No Risk
Aubrey Rosa Mosqueta Bath Jaléa ✓ 19	🛒 Little to No Risk	🛒 Little to No Risk
Aubrey Relax-R-Bath ✓ 19	🛒 Little to No Risk	🛒 Little to No Risk
Aura Cacia Mineral Bath (Deep Heat, Energize, Heart Song, Inspiration, & Tranquility) ✓	🛒 Little to No Risk	🛒 Little to No Risk
Bellmira Fruit Baths ✓	🛒 Little to No Risk	🛒 Little to No Risk

Product	Health Advisory	
Little to No Risk *Minimal Risk* *Caution* ✓ *Recommended*	Contact Dermatitis	Carcinogens
Bellmira Herbal Baths (Chamomile, Eucalyptus, Hayflowers, Melissa Balm, Peppermint & Rosemary) 28	🛒	🛒
Bellmira ✓ *19*	🛒	🛒
Bellmira White Magnolia Cream Bath 28	🛒	🛒
Calgon Bath Oil Beads (Light Floral with Aloe Vera) 6, 29	🛒	🛒
Calgon Bouquet Bath (Country Lilac) 6, 29	🛒	🛒
Calgon Bubbling Milk Bath (Powder Fresh with Baby Oil) ✓ *6*	🛒	🛒
Calgon Moisturizing Foam Bath (Powder Fresh with Foaming Milk & Baby Oil) ✓ *6, 7, 14*	🛒	🛒
Calgon Moisturizing Foam Bath (Soft Musk with Lanolin & Vitamin E) 6, 8, 14, 19, 27, 29	🛒	🛒
Calgon Moisturizing Foam Bath (Spring Rain with Aloe Vera) 6, 14, 30, 33	🛒	🛒
Earth Preserv Bath Crystals (all scents; JCPenney) ✓	🛒	🛒
Earth Preserv Nourishing Body Bath (all scents; JCPenney) ✓ *14*	🛒	🛒
Ecco Bella Detox Foaming Body Soak ✓	🛒	🛒
Ecco Bella Dieters Body Soak ✓	🛒	🛒
Ecco Bella Love Foaming Body Soak ✓	🛒	🛒
Ecco Bella Sleep Foaming Body Soak ✓	🛒	🛒
Faith in Nature Essential Bath Foam ✓	🛒	🛒
Jean Naté Energizing Bubble Bath 2, 6, 14, 16, 28, 29, 31, 34	🛒	🛒
Jean Naté Sheersilk Bath and Body Oil ✓ *6, 19*	🛒	🛒
Kermit's Krazi Berri Bubbles Bubble Bath 6, 27, 28, 34	🛒	🛒
Kid Care The Little Mermaid Mild Formula Bubble Bath 6, 17, 28, 34	🛒	🛒
Kid Care Teenage Mutant Ninja Turtles Bubble Bath 6, 17, 28, 34	🛒	🛒
Kiss My Face Active Athletic Muscle Relaxant Bath 14, 19, 28	🛒	🛒
Kiss My Face Anti-Stress Bath 14, 19, 28	🛒	🛒

Product	Contact Dermatitis	Carcinogens

Little to No Risk   Minimal Risk   Caution   ✓ Recommended

Product	Contact Dermatitis	Carcinogens
Kiss My Face Romance Bath 14, 19, 28	Little to No Risk	Minimal Risk
Logona Herbal Bubble Bath Refresh ✓	Little to No Risk	Little to No Risk
Logona Bubble Bath Relax with Hops-Chamomile ✓	Little to No Risk	Little to No Risk
Miss Piggy's Pink Bananas Bubble Bath 6, 27, 28	Minimal Risk	Minimal Risk
Mr. Bubble Bubble Bath Powder ✓ 6	Minimal Risk	Little to No Risk
Mr. Bubble Bubbleberry with Aloe Liquid 6, 17, 27, 28, 29	Caution	Minimal Risk
Mr. Bubble Original Fragrance Liquid 6, 17, 27, 28	Caution	Minimal Risk
Naturade Aloe Bubble Bath 6, 14, 19, 28	Minimal Risk	Minimal Risk
Nature's Gate Invigorating Bath Oil 6, 14, 16, 28	Minimal Risk	Minimal Risk
Nature's Gate Moisturizing Bath Oil 6, 14, 16, 28	Minimal Risk	Minimal Risk
Nature's Gate Relaxing Bath Oil 6, 14, 16, 28	Minimal Risk	Minimal Risk
Olbas Bath ✓	Little to No Risk	Little to No Risk
O'Naturel Bath & Shower Foam (Cinnamon & Orange, Lavender, Rosemary & Tangerine) 14, 16, 28	Minimal Risk	Minimal Risk
Paul Penders Calming Flower Bath Oil ✓ 14	Little to No Risk	Minimal Risk
Pure Approach Seaweed Bubble Bath ✓ 16	Little to No Risk	Little to No Risk
Pure Approach Seaweed Non-Foaming Bath ✓ 16	Little to No Risk	Little to No Risk
Queen Helene Batherapy ✓ 6	Minimal Risk	Little to No Risk
Rainbow Research Bubble Bath 14, 19, 28	Little to No Risk	Minimal Risk
Sesame Street Bubble Bath Liquid 6, 17, 27	Caution	Minimal Risk
Sesame Street Bubble Bath Powder ✓ 6	Minimal Risk	Little to No Risk
Sofies's Botanical Bath Creations (All) ✓	Little to No Risk	Little to No Risk
Spanish Bath Bath & Shower Gel 6, 14, 19, 28	Minimal Risk	Minimal Risk
Vaseline Intensive Care Moisturizing Bath Beads with Aloe Vera 6, 14, 17, 29, 33	Caution	Minimal Risk

Product				Health Advisory	
Little to No Risk	Minimal Risk	Caution	Recommended	Contact Dermatitis	Carcinogens
Vaseline Intensive Care Moisturizing Bath Beads with Musk 6, 14, 17, 29				Minimal Risk	Minimal Risk
Vaseline Intensive Care Moisturizing Bath Beads with Vitamin E 6, 14, 17, 19, 29				Caution	Minimal Risk
Vaseline Intensive Care Moisturizing Foam Bath (Aloe Vera) 6, 14, 33				Minimal Risk	Minimal Risk
Vaseline Intensive Care Moisturizing Foam Bath (Floral Scent) 6, 14, 19, 29				Minimal Risk	Minimal Risk
Vaseline Intensive Care Moisturizing Foam Bath (Lanolin) 6, 9, 14, 22, 27				Minimal Risk	Minimal Risk
The Village Bath Private Moments Moisturizing Foam Bath Enriched with Vitamin E and Collagen 6, 19, 27, 28				Minimal Risk	Minimal Risk
The Village Bath Aromatic Bath Tablets (Floral Lavender) 6, 14, 17, 27, 29				Minimal Risk	Minimal Risk
The Village Bath Aromatic Bath Tablets (Fresh Green) 6, 14, 17, 30				Minimal Risk	Minimal Risk
Weleda Bath Oils (all) ✓				Little to No Risk	Little to No Risk

SHAVING CREAMS

Product Types

Brushless shave cream (aerosol); shaving soap; emulsions.

Health Advisory

Carcinogens

We recommend against the use of products with BHA, FD&C Blue 1, FD&C Red 4, FD&C Red 40, DEA, and TEA.

Shaving Creams

Product				Health Advisory	
Little to No Risk	Minimal Risk	Caution	Recommended	Contact Dermatitis	Carcinogens
Alba Botanica Cream Shave 14, 19, 21				Minimal Risk	Minimal Risk
Aubrey Mint & Ginseng Shaving Cream ✓ 19				Little to No Risk	Little to No Risk

Product				Health Advisory	
![Little to No Risk]	![Minimal Risk]	![Caution]	✓	Contact Dermatitis	Carcinogens
Little to No Risk	*Minimal Risk*	*Caution*	*Recommended*		
Barbasol Original 6, 21					
Barbasol Sensitive Skin 6, 10, 21					
Barbasol Skin Conditioner 6, 8, 21					
Colgate Aloe 6, 14, 16, 21					
Colgate Regular Shave 6, 21					
Colgate Sensitive Skin 6, 21					
Earth Science Azulene Shaving Cream 1, 19, 21					
Edge Extra Rich Gel Aloe Formula 6, 21, 29					
Edge Extra Rich Gel Lanolin Formula 6, 8, 21, 29					
Edge Extra Rich Gel Lime Formula 6, 21, 29					
Edge Extra Rich Gel Tough Beards 6, 21, 29					
Gillette Foamy Lemon-Lime 4, 6, 21, 22					
Gillette Foamy Regular 6, 21, 22					
Gillette Foamy Sensitive Skin 6, 17, 21, 22					
Gillette Foamy Skin Conditioning 4, 6, 17, 21, 22					
Hers Shave Cream For Women 6, 16, 19, 21, 32, 34					
Kiss My Face Moisture Shave 6, 14, 19, 28					
Logona Men's Shaving Cream ✓ 8, 19					
Noxzema Aloe & Lanolin 6, 8, 16, 21, 29					
Noxzema Cocoa Butter & Vitamin E Skin Softening Formula 6, 19, 21, 31					
Noxzema Extra Sensitive Skin Emollient Rich 6, 16, 21, 28, 29					
Noxzema Medicated Regular 6, 21					
Paul Penders Lemon Balm Shave Cream ✓					
Soft Sense Shave Gel For Women Dry Skin Formula 6, 9, 19, 21, 22, 28, 32					

Product				Health Advisory	
🛒 *Little to No Risk*	🛒 *Minimal Risk*	🛒 *Caution*	✓ *Recommended*	Contact Dermatitis	Carcinogens
Soft Sense Shave Gel For Women Lanolin & Vitamin E 6, 9, 19, 22, 28, 32				🛒	🛒
Soft Sense Shave Gel Dry Skin Formula 6, 9, 19, 22, 28, 32				🛒	🛒
Soft Sense Shave Gel For Women Sensitive Skin Formula With Aloe & Vitamin E 6, 19, 21, 22, 29, 32				🛒	🛒
Soft Sense Shave Gel For Women Ultra Protection Formula 6, 19, 21, 22, 32				🛒	🛒
Soft Shave Moisturizing Shave Lotion for Women 6, 9, 17				🛒	🛒
Tom's of Maine Shave Cream ✓ 6				🛒	🛒

SKIN LOTIONS

Product Types

Cream; lotion; moisturizer; oil.

Health Advisory

Contact Dermatitis

People who are chemically sensitive should avoid using products containing fragrance and quaternium 15. Some people are sensitive to lanolin compounds.

DMDM hydantoin is another formaldehyde releaser that may cause problems.

Carcinogens

Avoid products containing 2-bromo-2-nitropropane-1,3-diol, DEA, and TEA, as these may expose you to formaldehyde or nitrosamines. Furthermore, stay away from products with artificial colors.

Safe Use Tip

If you develop irritation after using skin lotion, it may be fragranced; your first step should be to find one without fragrance. After eliminating fragrance, eliminate the major allergens such as parabens, propylene glycol, and quaternium 15.

Skin Lotions

Product	Health Advisory	
Little to No Risk Minimal Risk Caution Recommended	Contact Dermatitis	Carcinogens
Alba Botanica Emollient Body Lotion ✓ *1, 14, 19*	Minimal Risk	Minimal Risk
Alba Botanica Unscented Very Emollient Body Lotion ✓	Minimal Risk	Minimal Risk
Almay Stress Body Moisturizer *1, 7, 14, 19, 32, 34*	Minimal Risk	Little to No Risk
Aloe Vera—Real Aloe Company Hand & Body Lotion *6, 13, 14, 21*	Little to No Risk	Little to No Risk
Aubrey Cell Therapy ✓ *19*	Minimal Risk	Minimal Risk
Aubrey Collagen & Almond Oil ✓ *19*	Minimal Risk	Minimal Risk
Aubrey Collagen TCM Therapeutic Cream Moisturizer ✓ *19*	Minimal Risk	Minimal Risk
Aubrey Elastin NMF ✓ *19*	Minimal Risk	Minimal Risk
Aubrey Evening Primrose Complexion & Body Lotion ✓ *19*	Minimal Risk	Minimal Risk
Aubrey Evening Primrose Oil ✓ *19*	Minimal Risk	Minimal Risk
Aubrey Ginseng Face Cream Men's Stock ✓ *19*	Minimal Risk	Minimal Risk
Aubrey Vegacell Herbal Cellular Complex ✓ *19*	Minimal Risk	Minimal Risk
Aubrey Maintenance for Young Skin ✓ *19*	Minimal Risk	Minimal Risk
Aubrey Mandarin Magic Moisturizer ✓ *19*	Minimal Risk	Minimal Risk
Aubrey Rejeunesse Moisturizing Cream ✓ *19*	Minimal Risk	Minimal Risk
Aubrey Rosa Mosqueta Hand & Body Lotion ✓ *19*	Minimal Risk	Minimal Risk
Aubrey Rosa Mosqueta Rose Hip Moisturizing Cream ✓ *19*	Minimal Risk	Minimal Risk
Aubrey Rosa Mosqueta Rose Hip Seed Oil ✓ *19*	Minimal Risk	Minimal Risk
Aubrey Vegetal Collagen Moisturizer ✓ *19*	Minimal Risk	Minimal Risk
Aubrey Seaherbal Massage Lotion ✓ *19*	Minimal Risk	Minimal Risk
Aubrey Swimmers Moisturizer ✓ *19*	Minimal Risk	Minimal Risk
Autumn Harp Body Lotion ✓	Minimal Risk	Minimal Risk
Beauty Without Cruelty Aloe and E Moisture Creme ✓ *14, 19, 21*	Minimal Risk	Little to No Risk

Product		Health Advisory	
		Contact Dermatitis	Carcinogens
🛒 *Little to No Risk* 🛒 *Minimal Risk* 🛒 *Caution* ✓ *Recommended*			
Beauty Without Cruelty Oil Free Moisture Creme ✓ 14, 16, 19		🛒	🛒
Beehive Botanicals Honey and Almond Hand & Body Lotion ✓ 6, 14, 21		🛒	🛒
Beehive Botanicals Home and Bee Pollen Body Moisturizer ✓ 6, 7, 14		🛒	🛒
Beehive Botanicals Therapeutic Derma Cream ✓ 14, 19		🛒	🛒
Body Love Aroma Lotion ✓		🛒	🛒
Camo Care Hand & Body Lotion 1, 14, 16, 19, 21		🛒	🛒
Chanel Emulsion Pour Le Corps Body Lotion 1, 3, 6, 9, 14, 16, 19, 21, 31, 33		🛒	🛒
Chanel Hydra-Système Moisture Lotion 3, 6, 14		🛒	🛒
Chica Bella Cloud Forest Avocado ✓		🛒	🛒
Clarins Revitalizing Body Lotion with Cell Extracts 6, 14, 16, 21, 33, 34		🛒	🛒
Clinique Dramatically Different Moisturizing Lotion 9, 14, 16, 21, 27, 33, 34		🛒	🛒
Corn Huskers Lotion Heavy Duty Hand Treatment 6, 14, 21		🛒	🛒
Curê Moisturizing Cream/Lotion (Fragrance-Free) ✓ 14		🛒	🛒
Curê Moisturizing Cream/Lotion ✓ 6, 14		🛒	🛒
Deep Magic Moisturizing Lotion 6, 8, 14, 21		🛒	🛒
Desert Essence Jojoba Rosemary Lotion ✓ 14, 19		🛒	🛒
Dry Skin Pacquin Plus 6, 14, 28		🛒	🛒
Earth & Body Care Aloe Vera Family Lotion ✓ 6, 7, 19		🛒	🛒
Earth Preserv Skin Moisturizer (all scents; JCPenney) ✓ 1, 14, 19		🛒	🛒
Earth Science Hand and Body Lotion ✓ 19		🛒	🛒
Ecco Bella After Workout Skin Nourisher ✓ 19		🛒	🛒
Ecco Bella Calm Spirit Skin Nourisher ✓ 19		🛒	🛒
Ecco Bella Dry-Mature Skin Facial Nourisher ✓ 19		🛒	🛒

Product	Health Advisory	
	Contact Dermatitis	Carcinogens
Ecco Bella Energy Boost Skin Nourisher ✔ 19	🛒	🛒
Ecco Bella Erotic Skin Nourisher ✔ 19	🛒	🛒
Ecco Bella Farewell Cellulite Skin Nourisher ✔ 19	🛒	🛒
Ecco Bella Natural Moisture Day Cream ✔ 19	🛒	🛒
Ecco Bella Normal-Sensitive Skin Facial Nourisher ✔ 19	🛒	🛒
Ecco Bella Oily-Problem Skin Facial Nourisher ✔ 19	🛒	🛒
Ecco Bella Tocca Mi Skin Nourisher ✔ 19	🛒	🛒
Ecco Bella Vanilla Body Lotion ✔ 14, 19	🛒	🛒
Estée Lauder Maximum Care Body Lotion 6, 7, 14, 19, 28	🛒	🛒
Faith in Nature Jojoba Moisturizing Lotion 14, 21	🛒	🛒
Home Health Skin Lotion (Almond, Coconut, Jasmine, & Unscented) ✔ 10, 19	🛒	🛒
Home Health Liquid Lanolin ✔ 10	🛒	🛒
Jacki's Magic Lotion (Almond) ✔ 8	🛒	🛒
Jacki's Magic Lotion (Coconut, Jasmine, & Rose) ✔ 6, 8	🛒	🛒
Jacki's Magic Lotion Lavender ✔ 8	🛒	🛒
Jacki's Magic Lotion Orange-Vanilla ✔ 8	🛒	🛒
Jacki's Magic Lotion Rose-Mint ✔ 8	🛒	🛒
Jason Aloe Vera Gel Hand & Body Lotion 1, 16, 19, 21	🛒	🛒
Jason Apricot Hand & Body Lotion 13, 14, 16, 19, 21	🛒	🛒
Jason Cocoa Butter Hand & Body Lotion 1, 7, 14, 19, 21	🛒	🛒
Jason E.F.A. Hand and Body Lotion 1, 7, 14, 19, 21	🛒	🛒
Jason Herbal Hand & Body Lotion 7, 14, 16, 19, 21	🛒	🛒
Jason Vitamin E Hand & Body Lotion ✔ 7, 14, 19	🛒	🛒

Legend: Little to No Risk | Minimal Risk | Caution | ✔ Recommended

Product				Health Advisory	
(cart) Little to No Risk	(cart) Minimal Risk	(cart) Caution	✓ Recommended	Contact Dermatitis	Carcinogens
Jergens Advanced Therapy Lotion Aloe & Lanolin 6, 8, 14, 17				Caution	Minimal Risk
Jergens Advanced Therapy Lotion (Extra Dry Skin Treatment) 1, 6, 10, 14, 17				Minimal Risk	Minimal Risk
Jergens Advanced Therapy Lotion (Original Scent) 6, 10, 14, 16, 17				Caution	Minimal Risk
Jergens Ever Soft Dry Skin Lotion (Scented) 2, 6, 14, 16, 17				Caution	Minimal Risk
Jergens Ever Soft Dry Skin Lotion (Unscented) 2, 14, 16, 17				Little to No Risk	Minimal Risk
Jergens Vitamin E & Lanolin ✓ 6, 8, 14, 19				Little to No Risk	Minimal Risk
Keri Lotion Silky Smooth Formula For Soft Skin Everyday (Fragrance-Free) ✓ 2, 17				Caution	Minimal Risk
Keri Lotion Silky Smooth Formula For Soft Dry Skin Everyday 2, 6, 17				Caution	Minimal Risk
Kiss My Face Fragrance-Free Olive & Aloe Moisturizer ✓ 6, 13, 14, 19				Little to No Risk	Minimal Risk
Kiss My Face Honey & Calendula Moisturizer ✓ 6, 13, 14, 19				Little to No Risk	Minimal Risk
Kiss My Face Oil-Free Moisturizer ✓ 14, 16				Minimal Risk	Minimal Risk
Kiss My Face Vitamin A & E Moisturizer ✓ 6, 14, 19				Little to No Risk	Minimal Risk
Logona Almond Body Lotion ✓ 19				Minimal Risk	Minimal Risk
Logona Almond Extra Care Cream ✓ 19				Minimal Risk	Minimal Risk
Logona Aloe & Hypericum Cream ✓ 9, 19				Minimal Risk	Minimal Risk
Logona Avocado Extra Care Cream ✓ 8, 19				Minimal Risk	Minimal Risk
Logona Carrot Extra Care Cream ✓ 9, 19				Minimal Risk	Minimal Risk
Logona Chamomile Bodycare Oil ✓ 19				Minimal Risk	Minimal Risk
Logona Cistacea Intensive Moisturizing Cream ✓				Minimal Risk	Minimal Risk
Logona Free Body Lotion ✓ 19				Minimal Risk	Minimal Risk
Logona Free Facial Moisturizing Cream ✓ 19				Minimal Risk	Minimal Risk
Logona Hand Cream ✓ 19				Minimal Risk	Minimal Risk
Logona Herbal Blossom Body Lotion ✓ 19				Minimal Risk	Minimal Risk

Product				Health Advisory	
(cart) *Little to No Risk*	(cart) *Minimal Risk*	(cart) *Caution*	✓ *Recommended*	Contact Dermatitis	Carcinogens
Logona Hypericum Bodycare Oil ✓ *19*				Caution	Caution
Logona Linden Blossom Extra Care Cream with Vitamin E ✓ *19*				Caution	Caution
Logona Mallow & Jojoba Cream ✓ *9, 19*				Caution	Caution
Logona Marigold Bodycare Oil ✓ *19*				Caution	Caution
Logona Massage Oil ✓ *19*				Caution	Caution
Logona Rose & Wheat Germ Cream ✓ *19*				Caution	Caution
Logona Rosemary & Chamomile Cream ✓ *19*				Caution	Caution
L'Oréal Plénitude Active Daily Moisture Lotion Fluide Hydratant *3, 6, 14*				Minimal Risk	Little to No Risk
Lubriderm Lotion (Fragrance-Free) *8, 9, 14, 21*				Caution	Little to No Risk
Lubriderm Lotion (Regular) *6, 8, 14, 21*				Minimal Risk	Little to No Risk
Moisturel Lotion ✓ *2, 18*				Caution	Caution
Nature's Gate Moisturizing Lotion ✓ *1, 8, 13, 14*				Caution	Caution
Nature's Gate Fragrance-Free Moisturizing Lotion ✓ *1, 10, 14, 19*				Caution	Caution
Nature's Gate Papaya Moisturizing Lotion *14, 19, 21*				Caution	Little to No Risk
Nature's Gate Skin Therapy Lotion ✓ *1, 14, 19*				Caution	Caution
Nivea Creme Ultra Moisturizing ✓ *6, 9*				Minimal Risk	Caution
Nivea Moisturizing Lotion Extra Enriched Formula ✓ *6, 9*				Minimal Risk	Caution
Nivea Moisturizing Lotion Original European Formula *6, 14, 21*				Minimal Risk	Little to No Risk
Oil of Olay Moisture Replenishing Cream *6, 31*				Minimal Risk	Little to No Risk
Oil of Olay Daily UV Protectant Moisture Replenishing Cream *6, 14, 21, 28, 31, 33*				Minimal Risk	Little to No Risk
Oil of Olay Daily UV Protectant Beauty Fluid Moisture Replenishment *6, 14, 21, 28, 31, 33*				Caution	Little to No Risk
Paul Penders Oriental Flower Body Lotion ✓				Caution	Caution
Pond's Dry Skin Cream Extra Rich Formula *6, 7, 14, 21*				Minimal Risk	Little to No Risk

Product	Contact Dermatitis	Carcinogens
Legend: Little to No Risk / Minimal Risk / Caution / ✓ Recommended		
Rain Tree Aloe Dry Skin Lotion 6, 7, 9, 14, 21, 29, 33	Minimal Risk	Little to No Risk
Reviva Elastin Body Lotion ✓ *6, 14*	Minimal Risk	Caution
Shi Kai Apricot/Rose Hand & Body Lotion ✓ *6, 7, 19*	Minimal Risk	Caution
Shi Kai Cucumber/Melon Hand & Body Lotion ✓ *6, 7, 19*	Minimal Risk	Caution
Shi Kai Fragrance-Free Hand & Body Lotion ✓ *7, 19*	Caution	Caution
Soft Sense Skin Essentials Skin Lotion (Extra Moisturizing for Dry Skin with Vitamin E) ✓	Caution	Caution
Stony Brook Oil-Free Body Lotion (Scented) ✓ *6, 14, 19*	Caution	Caution
Stony Brook Oil-Free Body Lotion (Unscented) ✓ *14, 19*	Caution	Caution
Suave Skin Lotion (Aloe Vera) 6, 14, 21	Minimal Risk	Little to No Risk
Suave Skin Lotion (Baby Care Skin Lotion) 6, 14, 21	Minimal Risk	Little to No Risk
Suave Skin Lotion (Extra Relief) 6, 14, 21	Minimal Risk	Little to No Risk
Suave Skin Lotion (Vitamin E & Lanolin) 6, 10, 14, 21	Minimal Risk	Little to No Risk
Sunshine Products Aromassage Lotion/Refreshing Herbal Magic ✓ *14, 19*	Caution	Caution
Sunshine Products Aromassage Lotion/Sensual Bouquet ✓ *14, 19*	Caution	Caution
Swiss Formula Aloe Vera Moisturizing Hand & Body Lotion 6, 14, 16, 17, 21, 29	Caution	Little to No Risk
Swiss Formula Collagen Elastin Dry Skin/Sensitive Skin Lotion 14, 16, 17, 21	Minimal Risk	Little to No Risk
Swiss Formula Collagen Elastin Dry Skin Lotion/Extra Relief 6, 14, 17, 19, 21, 27, 29, 33	Minimal Risk	Little to No Risk
Swiss Formula Vitamin E Nutrient Rich Hand & Body Lotion with Vitamin A 1, 6, 14, 16, 17, 19, 21, 33	Caution	Little to No Risk
Ten-O-Six Oil-Free Moisturizer for Normal to Oily Skin 1, 14, 21	Caution	Little to No Risk
Therapeutic Keri Lotion Original Formula for Dry Skin Care 6, 10, 14, 16, 17, 21	Caution	Little to No Risk
Trader Joe's Moisturizing Skin Lotion ✓	Caution	Caution
Tropical Botanicals Babacu Nut Body Lotion ✓ *6, 14, 19*	Minimal Risk	Caution

Product				Health Advisory	
Little to No Risk	Minimal Risk	Caution	✓ Recommended	Contact Dermatitis	Carcinogens
Vaseline Intensive Care Lotion Aloe & Lanolin 6, 8, 14, 21, 28, 29, 33				🛒	🛒
Vaseline Intensive Care Lotion Extra Strength 6, 8, 14, 21, 28				🛒	🛒
Vaseline Intensive Care Lotion Relieves Over-Dry Skin 6, 8, 14, 21, 28				🛒	🛒
Vaseline Intensive Care Lotion Sensitive Skin Formula with Vitamin E 6, 8, 14, 19, 21, 28				🛒	🛒
Vaseline Intensive Care Lotion UV Daily Defense Lotion 6, 8, 14, 21, 28				🛒	🛒

SOAPS

Product Types

Bar; liquid. Generally, soaps are made of either animal or vegetable fats or synthetic detergent cleansers.

Health Advisory

Contact Dermatitis

Soaps can cause skin irritation that is commonly called housewife eczema, soap dermatitis, or winter itch. Researchers say that there are tremendous differences in the degree of skin irritation that different soap brands cause. Glycerin soaps are among the mildest. Tallow soaps containing sodium tallowate may be less irritating than coconut soaps containing sodium cocoate.

Of the eighteen most popular major brands of soaps today, the gentlest include the following, listed in order of most gentle to least gentle:

- Dove (mildest)
- Aveenobar
- Purpose
- Dial
- Alpha Keri
- Fels Naphtha
- Neutrogena
- Ivory
- Oilatum

- Lowila
- Jergens
- Lubriderm
- Cuticura
- Basis
- Irish Spring
- Zest
- Camay
- Lava (harshest)

Soaps

Product				Health Advisory	
Little to No Risk	Minimal Risk	Caution	✔ Recommended	Contact Dermatitis	Carcinogens
Alexandra Avery Wild Mountain Herbs Soap ✔ 19				🛒	🛒
Alexandra Avery Jungle Blossoms Soap ✔ 19				🛒	🛒
Aloe Vera—Real Aloe Company Aloe Vera Soap ✔ 6				🛒	🛒
Aubrey Rose Mosqueta Moisturizing Cleansing Bar ✔				🛒	🛒
Aura Cacia Deep Heat Bath Soap ✔				🛒	🛒
Aura Cacia Energize Bath Soap ✔				🛒	🛒
Aura Cacia Euphoria Aromatherapy Bath Soap ✔				🛒	🛒
Aura Cacida Heart Song Bath Soap ✔				🛒	🛒
Aura Cacia Inspiration Bath Soap ✔				🛒	🛒
Aura Cacia Tranquility Bath Soap ✔				🛒	🛒
Barth Aloe Vera Soap ✔				🛒	🛒
Barth Cocoa Butter Soap ✔ 6				🛒	🛒
Barth Lecithin Soap ✔ 6				🛒	🛒
Bindi Herbal Cleanser ✔				🛒	🛒
Boraxo Powdered Hand Soap ✔				🛒	🛒
Brookside Soap Oatmeal/Almond ✔				🛒	🛒

Product	Health Advisory	
Little to No Risk Minimal Risk Caution ✓ Recommended	Contact Dermatitis	Carcinogens
Brookside Soap Spearmint ✓		
Brookside Soap Rosemary/Lavender ✓		
Brookside Soap Cinnamon ✓		
Brookside Soap Extra Mild Herbal ✓		
Brookside Soap Extra Mild Unscented ✓		
Brookside Soap Lemongrass/Lime ✓		
Brookside Soap Lime ✓		
Calben Pure Soap ✓		
Chandrika Soap ✓		
Camay 6, 31		
Caress Body Bar ✓ 6, 22		
Caress Light Body Bar with Bath Oil 6, 22		
Cashmere Bouquet Soap ✓ 6		
Clearly Natural Glycerine Bar ✓		
Clean & Smooth Antibacterial Soap 6, 27, 28, 33		
Chica Bella Bird of Paradise ✓		
Chica Bella Costa Rican Honey ✓		
Chica Bella Deep Earth Clay ✓		
Chica Bella Deep Sea Algae ✓		
Chica Bella Honey Jasmine ✓		
Chica Bella Monteverde Aloe Vera ✓		
Chica Bella Organic Orange Peel ✓		
Chica Bella Rare Orchid ✓		
Dial 6, 22		

Product				Health Advisory	
				Contact Dermatitis	Carcinogens

Little to No Risk Minimal Risk Caution ✓ Recommended

Product	Contact Dermatitis	Carcinogens
Dial Liquid Antibacterial Soap 6, 28, 31, 33	🛒	🛒
Dove Beauty Wash 6, 14, 16, 17, 22	🛒	🛒
Dove Pink Beauty Bar ✓ 6, 22	🛒	🛒
Dove Unscented ✓ 6, 22	🛒	🛒
Dove White ✓ 6, 22	🛒	🛒
Dr. Bronner's Soaps (all) ✓	🛒	🛒
Earth Preserv Cream Soaps (all; JCPenney) ✓	🛒	🛒
Earth Preserv Glycerine Soaps (all; JCPenney) ✓	🛒	🛒
Eastern Star Soap ✓ 6	🛒	🛒
Faith in Nature Lavender Bar Soap ✓	🛒	🛒
Faith in Nature Orange Bar Soap ✓	🛒	🛒
Faith in Nature Pine Bar Soap ✓	🛒	🛒
Faith in Nature Rosemary Bar Soap ✓	🛒	🛒
Fight 6	🛒	🛒
Head Green Tea Deodorant Soap ✓ 6	🛒	🛒
Head Green Tea Liquid Body Soap 6, 14, 21, 28	🛒	🛒
Head Lotus Body Scrub Bar ✓ 6	🛒	🛒
Home Health Palma Christi Cleansing Bar ✓ 8, 19	🛒	🛒
Ivory 6, 22	🛒	🛒
Jason Aloe Vera Satin Body Wash 1, 14, 16, 19, 28	🛒	🛒
Jason Apricot Satin Soap 1, 6, 14, 16, 19, 28	🛒	🛒
Jason Apricot Satin Body Wash 14, 16, 19, 28	🛒	🛒
Jason Herbal Satin Body Wash 1, 6, 14, 16, 19, 28	🛒	🛒
Jergens Lotion Enriched Liquid Soap 6, 10, 14, 17, 28	🛒	🛒

Product				Health Advisory	
🛒 *Little to No Risk*	🛒 *Minimal Risk*	🛒 *Caution*	✓ *Recommended*	Contact Dermatitis	Carcinogens
Kappus Body Shampoo 2, 6, 16, 28				🛒	🛒
Kappus Cream Soaps ✓ 6				🛒	🛒
Kappus Glycerine Soaps ✓ 6				🛒	🛒
Kiss My Face Liquid Moisture Soap 1, 6, 14, 19, 28				🛒	🛒
Kiss My Face Soap ✓				🛒	🛒
Kiss My Face Olive & Aloe Soap ✓				🛒	🛒
Kiss My Face Olive & Herbal Soap ✓				🛒	🛒
Lever 2000 6, 22				🛒	🛒
Lifebuoy 6, 22				🛒	🛒
Logona Body Soaps (Chamomile, Herbal, Honey & Marigold) ✓				🛒	🛒
Logona Cistacea Intensive Cleansing Lotion ✓				🛒	🛒
Logona Facial Scrub Cream ✓ 19				🛒	🛒
Logona Free Soap ✓				🛒	🛒
Mountain Fresh 6, 22				🛒	🛒
Naturade Cactus Edition Hand & Body Gel 6, 14, 21				🛒	🛒
Nature De France Algoli Soap ✓				🛒	🛒
Nature De France Argile Blanche Soap ✓				🛒	🛒
Nature De France Argile Rose Soap ✓				🛒	🛒
Nature De France Argile Soap ✓				🛒	🛒
Nature De France Argimiel Soap ✓				🛒	🛒
Nature's Gate Antiseptic Liquid Soap 14, 28				🛒	🛒
Nature's Gate Deep Cleansing Liquid Soap 14, 28				🛒	🛒
Nature's Gate Moisturizing Liquid Soap 6, 14, 28				🛒	🛒
Nature Works Herbal Balm Soap ✓				🛒	🛒

Product	Health Advisory	
	Contact Dermatitis	Carcinogens
Little to No Risk / Minimal Risk / Caution / Recommended		
Nature Works Herbal Camomile Soap ✓	🛒	🛒
Nature Works Herbal Lavender Soap ✓	🛒	🛒
Nature Works Herbal Marigold Soap ✓	🛒	🛒
Nature Works Herbal Rosemary Soap ✓	🛒	🛒
NutriBiotic Nonsoap Skin Cleanser ✓ *1, 14*	🛒	🛒
Palmolive Gentle Skin Care Bar *6, 8, 22, 24*	🛒	🛒
Pond's Cold Creme ✓ *6*	🛒	🛒
Pond's Dry Skin Cream *6, 7, 14, 21*	🛒	🛒
Pond's Moisturizing Cleansing Bar *6, 22*	🛒	🛒
Pure Approach Clay Soaps ✓	🛒	🛒
Pure Approach Combination Skin Soap ✓	🛒	🛒
Pure Approach Dry Skin Soap ✓	🛒	🛒
Pure Approach Emile Soaps (Honey, Olive/Lavender, Passion Fruit, Vanilla) ✓	🛒	🛒
Pure Approach Emile's Honey Shower Gel ✓ *14*	🛒	🛒
Pure Approach Loofa Soap ✓	🛒	🛒
Pure Approach Sea Mud Soap ✓	🛒	🛒
Pure Approach Sensitive Skin Soap ✓	🛒	🛒
Pure Approach Shea Butter Soap ✓	🛒	🛒
Rainbow Research Aloe/Oatmeal Bar ✓ *19*	🛒	🛒
Rainbow Research Clay Cleansing Bar ✓ *19*	🛒	🛒
Revivia Aloe Chamomile Soap ✓	🛒	🛒
Reviva Honey and Almond Scrub ✓ *6, 16*	🛒	🛒
Reviva Oatmeal Soap ✓ *6*	🛒	🛒

Product				Health Advisory	
Little to No Risk	*Minimal Risk*	*Caution*	*Recommended*	Contact Dermatitis	Carcinogens
Reviva Silica Scrub 6, 14, 21				⊞	⊞
San Francisco Soap Co. Soaps (all) ✓ 6, 19				⊞	⊞
Sappo Hill Glycerine Creme Soap ✓ 6				⊞	⊞
Shield 6, 22, 30				⊞	⊞
Sirena Coconut Soap ✓				⊞	⊞
Sirena Vitamin E Soap ✓ 19				⊞	⊞
Softsoap Moisturizing Soap 6, 28, 30				⊞	⊞
Softsoap Aloe Vera Formula 6, 28, 30				⊞	⊞
Softsoap Sensitive Skin Cleansing Liquid ✓ 6				⊞	⊞
Tone The Skin Care Bar with Cocoa Butter 6, 22, 33, 34				⊞	⊞
Weleda Calendula Baby Soap ✓				⊞	⊞
Weleda Iris Soap ✓				⊞	⊞
Weleda Rose Soap ✓				⊞	⊞
Weleda Rosemary Soap ✓				⊞	⊞
Zest ✓ 6				⊞	⊞

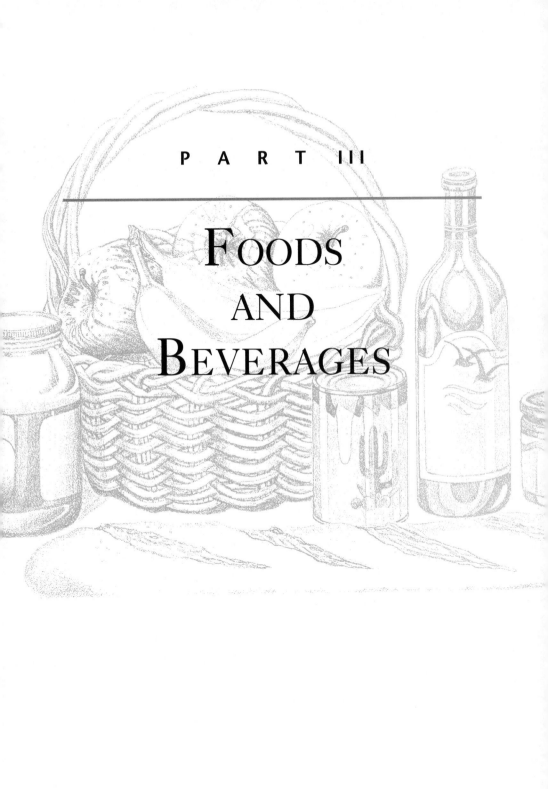

PART III

FOODS
AND
BEVERAGES

Danger of Carcinogens in the Food Supply

Foods and beverages may be contaminated with a variety of chemicals that have been intentionally or unintentionally added during their production, handling, storage, and processing. Fruits, vegetables, nuts, seeds, and grains are contaminated primarily with pesticides and sometimes molds. Dairy, meat, seafood, and processed foods are also contaminated with industrial chemicals, additives, hormones, growth stimulants, antibiotics, and other animal drugs as well as occasionally molds and bacteria. Many of these chemicals have carcinogenic, neurotoxic, reproductive, or immunotoxic (i.e., immune-damaging) effects. In addition to threatening the health of workers involved in growing and processing agricultural crops and livestock, they are a threat to your health and your children's health.

Of primary concern to consumers, and rightfully so, is the wide range of animal drug, industrial, chemical, and pesticide residues that show up in the foods that are placed on the dining tables of families across America each day. In 1993, two important studies provided overwhelming evidence that the pesticides used in food production are a public health menace, especially to the nation's children. *Pesticides in the Diets of Infants and Children,* issued by the National Academy of Sciences, and *Pesticides in Children's Food,* prepared by the Environmental Working Group, a Washington-based nonprofit research organization, both concluded that infants and children are at high risk for future cancers because of their exposure to carcinogenic pesticides, quite apart from neurotoxic, teratogenic, and other toxic effects. These reports are merely the latest in a long line of such findings, dating from the 1960s and earlier, detailing the health hazards of our nation's farmers' reliance on pesticides. The tragedy is that these reports, like those produced earlier, have been largely ignored by U.S. policymakers. In fact, pesticide use on American farms has increased 125 percent over the past twenty-five years.

The push for change is coming, not from Washington, but from citizens who have decided to boycott foods and beverages contaminated with carcinogens that pose health risks. But it is going to take a lot more consumer outrage and anger and the willingness of shoppers to vote with their consumer dollars.

"We've got a lot of pesticides out there and we ought to be doing something to reduce them," said FDA Commissioner Dr. David A. Kessler in 1993. However, Dr. Kessler's agency has not yet taken any action requiring labeling of foods for carcinogenic pesticides and other contaminants. Meanwhile, although Congress has passed consumer disclosure legislation forcing the food industry to list fat, cholesterol, and additional nutritional information on labels, consumers have no legal right to know of the carcinogenic and other toxic chemicals whose residues are found in the food supply. The bottom line is that consumers have a legal right to know about cholesterol and fat in the food supply; but when it comes to pesticides in the food supply, consumers have no such right.

Recent reports have focused on the risk to children posed by chemicals in the food supply. But adults are also at risk, from both their childhood and current exposures to chemical contaminants, and if you care about your health, then it is time to get these poisons out of your diet. A 1993 study found that women with the highest blood levels of DDT had four times the breast cancer risk of women with the least exposure. This study is only one of many since the 1970s—all largely unpublicized—to associate DDT and other related pesticides and industrial chemicals with breast cancer risk. In fact, there is growing evidence that the nation's present breast cancer epidemic is related to exposure to a wide range of environmental contaminants, including DDT, other carcinogenic pesticides, and estrogenic stimulants.

Many other cancers related to toxic exposures, including brain cancer, non-Hodgkin's lymphoma, bladder cancer, prostate cancer, testicular cancer, and leukemia, have also shown major (age-adjusted) increases in incidence since 1950. Consumers, anxious about the presence of carcinogenic residues in the food supply, have been told that there is no cause for concern and that these amounts are trivial. But when one in three Americans is now stricken with cancer, up from one in four in 1950, reducing exposure to carcinogenic substances is prudent.

The regulatory system in place today can trace its origin to the enactment of the Federal Insecticide, Fungicide, and Rodenticide Act (FIFRA) in 1947. Congress intended FIFRA to "balance" the alleged economic benefits from pesticides with their established environmental and human health harm. In other words, rather than prevent cancer by preventing exposure to carcinogens in the food supply, the government attempts only to "manage" cancer, knowing that some people will be stricken and others will not.

The term used by scientists and government regulators to describe this system of cancer roulette is "quantitative cancer risk assessment (QCRA)." The scientific validity of QCRA has been seriously challenged, despite the government's reliance on the system to ensure your health and freedom from cancer. These are "rubber" numbers that can vary by a factor of up to ten million. Furthermore, most independent and informed scientists agree that there is simply no such thing as a "safe" level of exposure to a carcinogen.

Although it is well established that chemicals in the food supply cause many human health problems beyond cancer, *The Safe Shopper's Bible* focuses primarily on carcinogens. This decision should not be construed as trivializing the effects of neurotoxicity, teratogenicity, immunotoxicity, and other damaging health effects; it simply reflects the limited scope of research in this area. Cancer is the only major chronic adverse effect for which there is enough epidemiological information on incidence and mortality, together with quantifiable animal data, to give scientists enough tools to work with to make even remotely accurate assessments of human risk. Furthermore, most carcinogens are also neurotoxins. By eliminating carcinogens from the food supply, we can make a great deal of progress in eliminating neurotoxins, and even some reproductive toxins.

There are two ways to prevent cancer. The first is to mount a strong national grassroots movement that will force government to label foods for carcinogenic residues and to phase out the use of carcinogenic pesticides within the next few years. The second is to protect yourself in the meantime by buying organic foods and pressuring supermarkets, by boycott if necessary, to stock them.

To this end, *The Safe Shopper's Bible* provides alphabetical lists of hundreds of individual foods and beverages that are coded to show their degree of contamination with carcinogens.

We have tried to provide quick, solid information that shows which foods are most and which are least contaminated with carcinogens. By following the guidelines in this book, readers can reduce their exposure to carcinogenic chemicals.

THE ADVANTAGES OF ORGANIC FOODS

How can you be sure that foods are truly organic? Are organic foods really purer and better than conventionally grown foods? These are important questions.

Unlike conventional crops, which may have fifteen or more separate applications of pesticides before they reach supermarkets, organic produce is supposed to be grown without the use of pesticides that persist in the environment or on the food crop. The chemicals and other growing practices used by the organic farmer (such as the use of sulfur, beneficial insects, and natural pyrethrins) are safe for you and the environment.

Some organic produce may occasionally have residues of a pesticide, either from contaminated soil that was sprayed many years earlier, or from the drift of a neighboring farm.

A recent analysis of samples of organic produce tested by the California Department of Food and Agriculture found clear evidence that organic foods are purer than conventional crops. In 1989, a total of 170 samples were taken of California-grown organic produce. Of these, 55 were from farms certified as organic by the California Certified Organic Farmers (CCOF) and 49 from CCOF-pending farms. There were also 66 samples taken from farms not in the CCOF program. Out of the total samples, 7 showed detected levels of pesticides. Only one of these was from a CCOF-certified grower; drift was the suspected source of contamination. In 1990, 108 samples were taken from CCOF-certified farms and 11 from CCOF-pending farms. Three samples had pesticide residues. Researchers concluded that "the amount and concentration of pesticides detected in organic produce is significantly lower than for conventional produce."

In the state of Washington, as of 1990, the state's organic agriculture department had found no samples with detectable pesticide residues.

These results speak to the purity of organic foods and should stimulate consumer confidence. Organic foods are also free from artificial colors, preservatives such as BHA, and nitrites, which are precursors of nitrosamines.

Organic meats make up another important part of the organic foods movement. Organic meat and poultry contain none of the antibiotics, hormones, growth stimulants, veterinary drugs, and other substances that go along with the factory farm and that threaten the health of consumers. Furthermore, organic meat is free from freshly applied pesticides and herbicides that may contaminate the feed given animals raised nonorganically.

However, you should know that simply buying produce and meat from a health food store is not a guarantee that it is organically grown. You can verify that produce is organically grown by looking for certifying groups' logos. Certification ensures crops are grown according to strict organic standards. Make sure that a label statement on the food, its packaging, or its food bin states the food is "certified" organic by any one of several internationally recognized certifying groups. Look for labels from these certification groups:

Biodynamic
California Certified Organic Farmers (CCOF)
Colorado Department of Agriculture
Demeter Association
Farm Verified Organic (FVO)
Florida Organic Growers and Consumers
Georgia Organic Growers Association

Maine Organic Farmers' & Gardeners' Association (MOFGA)

Natural Organic Farmers Association (NOFA)

Ohio Ecological Food and Farm Association

Oregon Tilth

Organic Certification Association of Montana

Organic Crop Improvement Association (OCIA)

Organic Foods Production Association of North America (OFPANA)

Organic Growers and Buyers Association

Organic Growers of Michigan

Ozark Organic Growers Association

Texas Department of Agriculture

Virginia Association of Biological Farmers

Washington State Department of Agriculture

Washington Tilth

Wisconsin Natural Food Associates

If food isn't certified, it may still be organic; when you are at a farmer's market or speaking with a knowledgeable produce manager in a health food store or at a roadside produce stand, ask lots of questions. Who was the farmer? What does the farmer use for pest control? (If questioning whether or not meat or poultry is organic, ask if the farmer uses any medications for stimulating growth or treatment of disease. In California, organic livestock farmers may use specific medications for a specific illness but not within ninety days of slaughter.)

Organic Foods—Probably More Nutritious

For years, people have been buying organic foods for what they do not get, namely dangerous residues of pesticides, industrial chemicals, hormonal contaminants and other animal drugs, and dangerous preservatives. Now consumers are beginning to realize that they should also be buying organically grown foods for what they *do* get: added nutritional value.

There is growing evidence that organically grown foods are more nutritious than commercially grown foods. A 1993 study published in the *Journal of Applied Nutrition* reports that organically grown foods contain significantly higher amounts of trace elements than foods grown conventionally with pesticides. In this study, the average elemental concentration in organic foods was found to be about twice that of commercial foods. Organically grown foods had nearly two to four times more nutritional trace elements, including boron, calcium, chromium, copper, iodine, magnesium, manganese, molybdenum, phosphorus, selenium, silicon, strontium, and zinc than commercially grown foods. Organic foods also had lesser amounts of toxic trace elements such as aluminum, lead, and mercury.

Among the study's highlights:

- Organically grown wheat had twice the calcium, four times more magnesium, five times more manganese, and thirteen times more selenium.
- Organically grown pears had two to nearly three times greater amounts of chromium, iodine, manganese, molybdenum, silicon, and zinc.
- Organically grown corn had nearly twenty times more calcium and manganese, and two to five times more copper, magnesium, molybdenum, selenium, and zinc.
- Organically grown potatoes had two or more times the boron, selenium, silicon, strontium, and sulfur, and 60 percent more zinc.
- Overall, of the twenty-two beneficial trace elements measured in the study, organically grown foods significantly exceeded conventionally grown crops for twenty.

Other studies have also found organic foods to contain superior nutritional value. Organically grown foods have been shown to have higher amounts of vitamin C and higher protein content.

Do these results have a practical impact on your health? Yes.

A three-year study with rabbits compared the effect of a "common diet" that was a commercial preparation with one of similar, organically grown components. The number of animals born alive was significantly higher, and the number of animals alive after ninety days was highest when the rabbits were fed with the organic diets. The percentage of animals born dead was highest in the common diet group.

In 1994, Danish researchers reported in the British medical journal *The Lancet* that organic food consumers enjoy health benefits in the area of sexual reproduction. Organic farmers and other people who frequently consume foods grown without pesticides have "an unexpectedly high sperm density . . . *despite a lower period of sexual continence.*" The organic food consumers had *twice* the sperm count of the control group of men in blue-collar jobs who do not consume organic foods.

Although the researchers say they "have no plausible hypotheses to explain this finding," the differences—if they are indeed real—may be accounted for by either improved nutritional content of the organic farmers' foods or their reduced exposure as consumers and workers to reproductive toxins used in agricultural crop production—or a combination of both.

This area of research, of course, deserves much greater study with public funds and independent researchers. But the results so far suggest that choosing organically grown foods leads to greater nutrient intake.

Organic Foods' Increasing Popularity

The Wall Street Journal reported in 1994 that one in three shoppers seeks out organically grown fruits and vegetables and that more shoppers would be purchasing organic foods except for those twin bugaboos of cost and appearance. It is true that organic foods can sometimes be up to 50 percent more expensive than their chemically grown counterparts—although their cost is decreasing as the nation's number of organic farmers and their production increase. As for appearance, organic produce is also becoming better looking all the time as farmers improve their agricultural skills.

Some two-thirds of all shoppers in the United States have now tried organic produce and nearly 90 percent reported they would purchase organic foods if their cost were the same as nonorganic products; yet, 41 percent were willing to buy organically grown foods even if they cost more, the paper reported.

Furthermore, major produce companies are getting into the organic foods market in a big way; Dole, for example, has purchased organic fruit packing and produce distribution companies. Welch's, the grape jelly company, now owns a substantial interest in Cascadian Farm, one of the nation's leading producers of organic jams and jellies. Indeed, the largest organic farmer in California is now the Gallo wine company. Even clothing manufacturers are beginning to use organically grown cotton. Get used to it: Americans are going organic.

How to Obtain Organic Foods

If your neighborhood supermarket does not supply organic foods or your area is without a health food store that sells organically produced foods, see Appendix A beginning on page 381 for addresses and telephone numbers of organic food mail-order outlets.

HOW WE EVALUATED FOODS AND BEVERAGES

To know which foods and beverages pose the greatest potential for cancer because of their contaminants, it is essential to know the following information: what carcinogens are present; their potency; and average concentration.

The formula we generally used to evaluate various foods was to multipy the average concentration of each carcinogenic pesticide in each food by the potency of each individual carcinogenic pesticide. The result provided a relative ranking for each food.

Foods and beverages were evaluated for their carcinogenic risks, based on a review of thousands of pages of reports from the federal government, private industry, international agencies, research institutions, and public interest groups. These various reports list concentrations of carcinogenic pesticides in a wide range of foods and beverages, along with the country or state where the food was grown or imported from and the year that the food was sampled and analyzed.

Much of this information was obtained through requests made via the federal Freedom of Information Act (FOIA) or through requests to individual groups and institutions. In general, approximately ten or more samples up to one hundred of each food item were used for each evaluation. When data were more limited, results were evaluated in relation to information from other sources.

Potency of Each Individual Carcinogenic Pesticide

Once you know which pesticides are in a food and their average concentration, it is important to know the carcinogenic potency of each. Carcinogenic chemicals vary in potency.

The EPA has assigned "cancer potency numbers" called Q* values to many carcinogenic pesticides found in foods and beverages. The EPA derives a chemical's cancer potency number from experimental studies in which laboratory animals are dosed with a carcinogenic pesticide at various levels and the incidence of cancers at each of these levels is determined. This cancer potency number represents the calculated incidence of cancers in animals that would be expected at the lower concentrations of the carcinogen found in the human diet. High and low cancer potency values indicate strong and weak carcinogenic responses, respectively. For example, the Q* values are 16 for dieldrin, .019 for 2,4-D, and .0035 for the folpet. Thus, dieldrin is roughly 840 times more potent than 2,4-D, and roughly 4,000 times more potent than folpet.

However, these cancer potency estimates can actually *underestimate* a carcinogen's potency. The main problem is in calculating risks associated with carcinogens at concentrations in the human diet from the higher concentrations used in carcinogenicity testing. When you are dealing with the very high concentrations of carcinogenic chemicals to which experimental animals are exposed, a "flattening" of the dose-response curve occurs. Even as the dosage is increased, virtually no change in response will occur. This ultimately leads to an underestimate of chemical potencies at the lower concentrations found in the human diet.

For most foods we were able to compile data on the average concentration of each carcinogen the food contains and its potency in order to arrive at the food's overall carcinogen advisory value. Table 6, for instance, shows data on apples and oranges.

As you can see from looking at the data for apples, the average concentration of benomyl is .138 ppm. Multiplying the average concentration of benomyl (.138 ppm) by the potency number (.0042) yields a cancer advisory value of .0006. Similarly, the concentration of captan is .0799 ppm, its potency number .0036.

Table 6: How We Rated Foods for Their Cancer Risk

Food Item	Residue Concentration in Parts per Million (ppm)	Cancer Potency Number	Carcinogen Advisory Value
Apples			
Azinphos-methyl	.044	.00000015	0
Benomyl	.138	.0042	.0006
Captan	.0799	.0036	.0003
Dicofol	.0053	.31	.0016
Dimethoate	.0035	—	—
Mancozeb/Maneb (Ethylene bisdithiocarbamate)	.0937	.11	.01
Propargite	.217	.031	.0067
Total ×100			1.9
Oranges			
Dacthal	.05	—	—
Lead	.04	—	—
Parathion	1.05	.0018	.002
o-Phenylphenol	.7463	.0022	.002
Total ×100			.4

Multiplying the average concentration of captan (.0799 ppm) by the potency number (.0036), yields .0003. We did this for each carcinogenic pesticide residue. In some cases, such as azinphos-methyl, the carcinogen advisory value was so low we listed it as "0."

The sum total of carcinogenic advisory values for all seven contaminants, multiplied by 100, is the overall "Carcinogen Advisory" value for that food. It is 1.9 for apples.

The same procedure for oranges results in an overall Carcinogen Advisory value of .4. That means that, relatively, apples present the consumer with roughly five times more carcinogenic risk than oranges.

In the charts in this section, those foods with a carcinogenic advisory value of less than 1 are rated for "little to no risk." Foods with a value of 1 to 5 are rated for "minimal risk." Foods with a value of 6 or more are rated for "caution." Of course, factors other than contamination with pesticide or industrial chemical residues also may have influenced our evaluations. These factors include presence of carcinogenic animal drugs or a wide range of pesticide residues with possible synergistic interactions. We have also rated for minimal risk some foods for which better—often organic—choices are readily available (as in the case of some produce and meat items with identical organic counterparts), and some unhealthy foods that are not part of an optimum diet (e.g., various hydrogenated oils, corn syrup, and white sugar), except in the case of desserts and snacks.

Although we have tried to be as accurate as possible, several factors may skew the results: We have probably underestimated Carcinogen Advisory values for several reasons.

- Some foods are contaminated with carcinogens without assigned potency factors or found in "trace" amounts.
- The government's routine monitoring programs detect chemicals at only about .05 parts per million and above.
- Specialized government monitoring programs, such as the Total Diet Study, measure contaminants at much lower levels, but they do not look for all the possible contaminants on a food item.
- Government laboratories routinely miss about half the chemicals known to contaminate foods and beverages, resulting in a gross underestimate of food contamination.
- Government sampling programs do not routinely test for most carcinogenic feed additives and animal drugs, including hormones.

This information will not tell you how many cancers might be caused in the population because of exposures to these carcinogenic residues. Nor will it tell you about the synergistic interactions of chemicals that may produce greater toxicological dangers when they are grouped together than they would if they were in isolation. These answers are impossible to determine. *The Safe Shopper's Bible* is simply estimating which foods and beverages present the greatest cancer risk from man-made contaminants and ingredients in the food supply.

HOW TO USE THE SHOPPING CHARTS

It is important to keep your diet as free as possible from carcinogens. But organically grown foods are not always easy to find and often cost more than ordinary supermarket food.

You can still find the safest foods for you and your family no matter where you shop. The charts in this section of *The Safe Shopper's Bible* will point up your safest choices in every food and beverage category. As with the earlier charts on household products, cosmetics, and personal care items, a black circle indicates foods posing the highest risk; shaded circle, intermediate risk; and white circle, least risk.

The information in the following charts represents generic foods and beverages, such as hot dogs, hamburgers, milk shakes, apples, sweet potatoes, wheat bread, swordfish, and apple pie. Do not worry about brand names; there is not that much of a difference in their food safety—unless they are organic.

Table 6 on page 306 lists carcinogens commonly detected in foods and beverages, together with their identifying number. You will find their corresponding numbers listed in the charts. For example, in the fruit chart, you will see the first column lists "Food and Carcinogenic Contaminants," and the "apple" entry contains seven numbers (2, 3, 6, 12, 14, 26, 35). These represent the seven carcinogenic pesticide residues most often found in apples. As you can see by referring to table 6, these carcinogens are azinphos-methyl (2), benomyl (3), captan (6), dicofol (12), dimethoate (14), Mancozeb/Maneb (ethylene bisdithiocarbamate) (26), and propargite (35).

Similarly, under "oranges," you will see four numbers (10, 23, 29, 31), representing the four carcinogenic residues found most often in this fruit: dacthal (DCPA) (10), lead (23), ortho phenylphenol (29), and parathion (31).

Fruits

Column One				Two
Food and Carcinogenic Contaminants				Health Advisory
Little to No Risk	Minimal Risk	Caution	Recommended	Carcinogen Advisory
Apples 2, 3, 6, 12, 14, 26, 35				◉
Oranges 10, 23, 29, 31				🛒

Under the second column, "Carcinogen Advisory," you will see a shaded circle for apples, which pose a minimal risk, and a clear circle for oranges, which pose little to no risk. Oranges would make a better shopping choice. In fact, as you go through the charts, you will see a lot of fruits that make safer shopping choices.

By applying this formula to hundreds of the most commonly eaten foods, consumers are able to determine which present the greatest risk from carcinogenic contaminants. This information will help you to make informed shopping decisions for all foods and beverages.

While these ratings reflect primarily pesticide and industrial chemical contaminants, the text accompanying the tables will also provide more limited available information on additional risks from other carcinogens such as additives, preservatives, food dyes and colors, packaging and wrapping materials, growth stimulants, hormones, industrial chemicals, irradiation, and naturally occurring carcinogens.

Our recommendations are indicated in the charts by the symbol ✓ following the food. These are your best choices.

Finally, the cancer risk of individual foods is due to its carcinogenic ingredients and contaminants, not to the food itself. Foods *can* be grown and processed practically and economically without contamination by pesticides and other carcinogens.

Table 7: Carcinogenic Contaminants Commonly Found in Foods and Beverages

1. Acephate	14. Dimethoate
2. Azinphos-methyl	15. Dioxin
3. Benomyl	16. Endrin
4. Benzene hexachloride (BHC)	17. Ethylenethiourea (ETU)
	18. Folpet
5. Captafol	19. Heptachlor
6. Captan	20. Hexachlorobenzene (HCB)
7. Chlordane	21. Hormone additives
8. Chlorobenzilate	22. Imidan/Phosmet
9. Chlorothalonil	23. Lead
10. Dacthal (DCPA)	24. Lindane
11. DDT, DDE, DDD	25. Linuron
12. Dicofol/Kelthane	26. Mancozeb/Maneb (ethylene
13. Dieldrin	bisdithiocarbamate)

27. Nonachlor *

28. Octachlor †

29. o-Phenylphenol and Na salt

30. Oxadiazon

31. Parathion

32. Pentachlorophenol ("Penta")

33. Permethrin

34. Polychlorinated biphenyls (PCBs)

35. Propargite

36. Radiation (Chernobyl-related)

37. Toxaphene

---

* *Nonachlor is contained in the pesticide chlordane, which is carcinogenic. It concentrates in body tissues and is an indicator of chlordane, exposure. No data are available on its carcinogenicity.*

† Octachlor is one of the trade names of a chlordane formulation.

CHAPTER 14

Foods

FRUITS

Health Advisory

Prefer fruits and vegetables over meat and dairy foods, even if you do not have organically grown produce available. While nonorganic fruits and vegetables are contaminated with pesticides, so are animal foods—even more so. Plant foods, however, also provide vital nutritional content, including beta-carotene (the plant form of vitamin A), vitamin C, and fiber; all are extremely important for the prevention of a wide range of diseases, including heart attack and cancer. Meat, poultry, and dairy simply cannot duplicate the nutritional benefits of fresh produce, and they also bring a lot of saturated fat into the diet, which is not only bad for your heart and your arteries, but also is where many of the most potent and toxic pesticides and industrial chemicals that permeate the food supply concentrate. Best to favor organic produce!

Carcinogens

Artificial colors: Citrus Red No. 2 is used to dye the skins of Florida oranges to conceal color variations in the fruit so that they can compete with California oranges, which are not dyed. Citrus Red No. 2 is carcinogenic.

Pesticides: Fruits are contaminated with a wide range of carcinogenic pesticides. While you can always find safer fruits at any supermarket by using the accompanying shopping charts, your best bet is to buy organically grown produce whenever possible.

Radiation: Apple juice made from concentrate sometimes contains radioactive contaminants because of the Chernobyl nuclear explosion in 1986, reports the FDA's Radionuclides in Foods program. Most consumers do not know that some U.S. suppliers of apple juice made from concentrate import their raw materials from Austria, Germany, Hungary, and Yugoslavia. Government records indicate that cesium 137 isotopes, traced to the Chernobyl disaster, have been found in samples of apple juice concentrate from these nations. In the years since Chernobyl, levels have diminished dramatically, but Chernobyl-related contamination still is occasionally present. Since the concentration of radiation falls within what U.S. guidelines term *acceptable exposures*, such apple juice products are allowed to be sold legally.

Waxes: Waxes contain fungicides such as benomyl and sodium ortho-phenyl phenate; both are carcinogenic. Fruits most likely to be waxed include apples, avocados, cantaloupes, grapefruits, lemons, limes, melons, oranges, passion fruit, peaches, and pineapples.

Safe Shopping and Cooking Tips

- Peeling may remove some of the contaminants on a fruit, as well as some nutrients. On the other hand, some contaminants are systemic, meaning they permeate the entire fruit, and peeling will not do much good. It is a better solution to simply buy organic varieties.
- Washing fruit with soap or detergent may reduce pesticide residues, but it will not eliminate them altogether. Since waxes containing pesticides cannot be removed with water, you will need a mild liquid dish soap and bristled scrub brush. (To find a safe dish soap see our recommendations under dishwashing detergents.) A report in the April 1988 issue of *Food Science and Technology Abstracts* noted that apples sprayed with pesticides retained 50 percent to 100 percent of the chemical contaminants' residues—even after several months in cold storage and a detergent wash. However, other studies have shown that washing and peeling can reduce pesticides' residues, sometimes quite significantly. The bottom line is that washing should not take the place of buying organically grown fruits. But it is a good idea to wash your fruits anyway, whether or not they are organic.
- If you enjoy marmalade, make sure only peels from organically grown oranges are used to avoid contamination from artificial colors and pesticides.
- Buy organically grown apple juice from U.S. apples.
- See Appendix A for a listing of mail-order sources of organically grown fruits.

Fruits

Food and Carcinogenic Contaminants	Health Advisory
	Carcinogen Advisory

Icons legend: 🛒 *Little to No Risk* 🛒 *Minimal Risk* 🛒 *Caution* ✓ *Recommended*

Food and Carcinogenic Contaminants	Carcinogen Advisory
Acerola ✓	Little to No Risk
Apple 2, 3, 6, 12, 14, 26, 35	Minimal Risk
Apple, Dried ✓	Little to No Risk
Apple (organic) ✓	Little to No Risk
Applesauce ✓ 14, 17, 23, 31	Little to No Risk
Apricot ✓ 2, 6	Little to No Risk
Apricot, Canned ✓	Little to No Risk
Avocado ✓ 10	Little to No Risk
Banana ✓ 3, 26	Little to No Risk
Banana Chips ✓	Little to No Risk
Blackberry 2, 5, 6	Minimal Risk
Black Currant ✓	Little to No Risk
Blueberry 5, 6	Minimal Risk
Boysenberry 6, 10, 12, 18, 31	Caution
Breadfruit ✓	Little to No Risk
Cantaloupe 1, 9, 10, 11, 12, 13, 17, 23, 29, 31, 37	Minimal Risk
Cassava ✓	Little to No Risk
Cherry 2, 3, 6, 14, 31	Minimal Risk
Cherry (organic) ✓	Little to No Risk
Coconut Meat ✓	Little to No Risk
Clementine ✓	Little to No Risk
Cranberry 5, 9, 11, 18, 22, 31	Minimal Risk
Crenshaw Melon ✓	Little to No Risk

Food and Carcinogenic Contaminants	Health Advisory
	Carcinogen Advisory
Little to No Risk — Minimal Risk — Caution — ✓ Recommended	
Currants ✓ 6	(Little to No Risk)
Dates ✓	(Little to No Risk)
Figs ✓	(Little to No Risk)
Fruit Cocktail, Canned ✓ 12, 23, 35	(Little to No Risk)
Gooseberry ✓ 6	(Little to No Risk)
Grapes 1, 2, 6, 11, 12, 14, 17, 18, 35	(Caution)
Grapes (organic) ✓	(Little to No Risk)
Grapefruit ✓ 2, 6, 12, 29	(Little to No Risk)
Guava ✓	(Little to No Risk)
Honeydew ✓ 9	(Little to No Risk)
Kiwifruit ✓ 22, 33	(Little to No Risk)
Lemon ✓ 6, 31	(Little to No Risk)
Lime ✓	(Little to No Risk)
Loganberry ✓ 6	(Little to No Risk)
Mandarin Orange ✓	(Little to No Risk)
Mandarin Orange, Canned ✓	(Little to No Risk)
Mango ✓	(Little to No Risk)
Nectarine ✓ 2, 3, 5, 12, 22	(Little to No Risk)
Orange ✓ 10, 23, 29, 31	(Little to No Risk)
Papaya ✓	(Little to No Risk)
Passion Fruit ✓	(Little to No Risk)
Peaches (fresh) 2, 3, 11, 12, 14, 17, 22, 31, 35	(Caution)

Food and Carcinogenic Contaminants	Health Advisory

	Carcinogen Advisory
🛒 *Little to No Risk* 🛒 *Minimal Risk* 🛒 *Caution* ✓ *Recommended*	
Peaches, Canned ✓ *1, 23*	🛒
Peaches, Dried ✓	🛒
Pears *2, 6, 12, 14, 17, 22, 31*	🛒
Pears, Asian ✓ *2, 31*	🛒
Pears, Canned ✓	🛒
Pears, Dried ✓	🛒
Pears (organic) ✓	🛒
Persimmons ✓	🛒
Pineapple (fresh or canned) ✓ *3, 4, 23, 24*	🛒
Plantains ✓	🛒
Plums *12, 14, 18, 22, 23, 35*	🛒
Plums (organic) ✓	🛒
Pomegranates ✓	🛒
Prickly Pear Cactus ✓	🛒
Prunes ✓ *31*	🛒
Raisins *11, 12, 14, 23, 34, 35*	🛒
Raisins (organic) ✓	🛒
Raspberries *2, 6, 31*	🛒
Strawberries *3, 6, 11, 12, 17, 18, 31*	🛒
Strawberries (organic) ✓	🛒
Sweet Carambola ✓	🛒
Tamarinds ✓	🛒

Food and Carcinogenic Contaminants	Health Advisory
🛒 Little to No Risk 🛒 Minimal Risk 🛒 Caution ✓ Recommended	Carcinogen Advisory
Tangelos ✓	🛒
Tangerines ✓	🛒
Watermelon ✓ 20, 23	🛒

Jams, Jellies, and Spreads

Food and Carcinogenic Contaminants	Health Advisory
🛒 Little to No Risk 🛒 Minimal Risk 🛒 Caution ✓ Recommended	Carcinogen Advisory
Apple Spread ✓	🛒
Apricot Jam ✓	🛒
Banana Puree ✓	🛒
Cherry Jam ✓	🛒
Cranberry Topping/Syrup ✓ 31	🛒
Gooseberry Jam ✓	🛒
Grape Jelly ✓	🛒
Guava Jam/Jelly ✓	🛒
Mango Chutney ✓	🛒
Orange Marmelade (organic) ✓	🛒
Orange Marmelade (nonorganic)	🛒
Peach Jam ✓	🛒
Plum Preserve ✓	🛒
Pear Jelly ✓	🛒
Raspberry Jam ✓	🛒
Raspberry Preserve ✓	🛒

Food and Carcinogenic Contaminants	Health Advisory
Little to No Risk • Minimal Risk • Caution • Recommended	Carcinogen Advisory
Red Currant Jam ✓	🛒
Strawberry Jam ✓	🛒
Strawberry Marmelade ✓	🛒

Fruit Juices

Food and Carcinogenic Contaminants	Health Advisory
Little to No Risk • Minimal Risk • Caution • Recommended	Carcinogen Advisory
Apple Juice (imported from Europe) 36	🛒
Apple Juice (nonorganic) 1, 14, 23	🛒
Apple Juice (organic, U.S) ✓	🛒
Cranberry Juice ✓	🛒
Grape Juice ✓ 14, 23	🛒
Grapefruit Juice ✓ 8	🛒
Guava Juice/Nectar ✓	🛒
Lemonade ✓ 8, 12	🛒
Mango Drink/Nectar ✓	🛒
Orange Drink ✓	🛒
Orange Juice ✓ 12, 14	🛒
Pear Juice ✓	🛒
Pineapple Juice, Canned ✓ 23	🛒
Prune Juice, Bottled ✓ 23	🛒
Strawberry Juice ✓	🛒

NUTS AND SEEDS

Health Advisory

Most nuts and seeds are safe and make nutritious snacks. But shoppers should be aware of a few notable exceptions.

Carcinogens

Aflatoxins: A naturally occurring carcinogenic toxin produced by a fungal mold, aflatoxin contaminates some peanut products. The FDA has established so-called safe tolerances, and even now a high percentage of peanut-based foods contain legally allowable residues of this mold.

Pesticides: The American peanut crop—protestations from the Southern peanut growers notwithstanding—is heavily contaminated with carcinogenic pesticide residues, a trend that has been apparent since at least 1982.

Sesame seeds and cashews from India are extremely contaminated with highly toxic pesticides.

Sesame seeds from Mexico also are relatively contaminated with carcinogenic pesticide residues.

Tahini spreads, which are made from sesame seeds, will be similarly contaminated depending on where the sesame seeds originate.

Safe Shopping Tips

- Prefer organically grown peanuts and peanut butter from companies that provide certification on their labels that their products are free from aflatoxin. If a company refuses your request for evidence of certification that their products are free from aflatoxin, you should avoid these products. A number of organic brands of peanut butter do offer such assurances.
- Buy organic sesame seed products.
- If buying a nonorganic nut spread, prefer almond butter or safflower butter over peanut butter.
- Choose brands that avoid the use of hydrogenated oils or salt; both hydrogenated oils and salt are either direct or indirect risk factors for cardiovascular or kidney disease.

Nuts and Seeds

Food and Carcinogenic Contaminants				Health Advisory
🛒 Little to No Risk	🛒 Minimal Risk	🛒 Caution	✓ Recommended	Carcinogen Advisory
Almonds ✓				🛒
Brazil Nuts ✓				🛒
Cashews ✓				🛒

Food and Carcinogenic Contaminants	Health Advisory
	Carcinogen Advisory

🛒 *Little to No Risk*   🛒 *Minimal Risk*   🛒 *Caution*   ✓ *Recommended*

Food	Carcinogen Advisory
Cashews (from India) 4, 24	🛒
Chestnuts ✓	🛒
Filberts ✓	🛒
Macadamia Nuts ✓	🛒
Peanuts, dry roasted 11, 13, 19, 20, 32, 37	🛒
Peanuts (organic) ✓	🛒
Pecans ✓ 23	🛒
Pine Nuts ✓	🛒
Pistachio Nuts ✓	🛒
Pumpkin Seeds ✓	🛒
Sesame Seeds (from India) 4, 11, 24	🛒
Sesame Seeds (from Mexico) 4, 11, 24	🛒
Sunflower Seeds ✓	🛒
Walnuts ✓	🛒
Watermelon Seeds ✓	🛒

VEGETABLES

Health Advisory

Carcinogens

Pickling Vegetables: Traditional pickled vegetables from Asia have shown evidence of posing a cancer risk, based on epidemiological studies that have found a high rate of stomach and nasopharyngeal cancer among people consuming them.

Pesticides: As with fruits, vegetables are contaminated with a wide range of carcinogenic pesticides. The accompanying safe shopping charts will detail your safest choices in any supermarket, but it is always best to buy organically grown vegetables whenever possible.

Radiation: Some wild European mushrooms still have excess radiation because of the 1986 Chernobyl nuclear disaster. These include boletes and chanterelles, which are often found in gourmet shops and sections of stores.

Waxing: Waxes on vegetables may contain carcinogenic fungicides. Vegetables most likely to be waxed include cucumbers, eggplants, parsnips, peppers, pumpkins, rutabagas, squashes, and sweet potatoes.

Shopping and Cooking Tips

- If you are unable to find organic vegetables in your area, see Appendix A for a list of mail-order sources.
- Discard the outer leaves of lettuce and other leafy vegetables; these may be most contaminated with pesticides.
- Peeling vegetables reduces exposure to pesticide residues but may result in some loss of nutrients.
- Washing can reduce pesticide residues in some cases. See *Fruits*.

Vegetables

Food and Carcinogenic Contaminants	Health Advisory
🛒 Little to No Risk 🛒 Minimal Risk 🛒 Caution ✓ Recommended	Carcinogen Advisory
Artichoke ✓	🛒
Asparagus 13, 23	🛒
Bean Sprouts ✓	🛒
Bean Curd ✓ 1, 31	🛒
Beets 1	🛒
Bell Pepper (organic) ✓	🛒
Bell Pepper, Sweet, Green 10, 11, 14, 31, 33	🛒
Black Beans ✓	🛒
Black-eyed Peas ✓ 1	🛒
Bok Choy 10, 11, 14	🛒
Broccoflower ✓	🛒
Broccoli 1, 9, 10, 11, 13, 33	🛒
Broccoli (organic) ✓	🛒
Brussels Sprouts (U.S.) ✓	🛒

Food and Carcinogenic Contaminants	Health Advisory

	Carcinogen Advisory
🛒 *Little to No Risk* 🛒 *Minimal Risk* 🛒 *Caution* ✔ *Recommended*	
Cabbage 1, 10, 31, 33	🛒
Cabbage (organic) ✔	🛒
Carrot, raw 11, 17, 25	🛒
Carrot, raw (organic) ✔	🛒
Cauliflower 10, 13, 23	🛒
Cauliflower (organic) ✔	🛒
Celery 1, 3, 9, 10, 11, 33	🛒
Celery (organic) ✔	🛒
Cherry Tomato ✔ 5, 9	🛒
Chin Choy ✔	🛒
Chinese Broccoli ✔	🛒
Collard Greens 1, 2, 9, 10, 11, 13, 14, 17, 23, 33, 37	🛒
Collard Greens (organic) ✔	🛒
Corn, Canned ✔	🛒
Corn, Cream Style ✔	🛒
Corn, Fresh, Sweet ✔ 23, 24	🛒
Cucumber, Pickling 7, 9, 11, 13	🛒
Cucumber 1, 9, 13, 19, 23, 37	🛒
Daikon ✔	🛒
Eggplant ✔ 9	🛒
Endive ✔ 14, 33	🛒
Escarole ✔ 9	🛒
Garbanzo Beans ✔	🛒
Green Beans ✔ 5, 14, 26	🛒

Food and Carcinogenic Contaminants	Health Advisory
	Carcinogen Advisory
Little to No Risk 🛒 *Minimal Risk* 🛒 *Caution* 🛒 ✓ *Recommended*	
Kale 1, 2, 10, 11, 33	🛒
Kale (organic) ✓	🛒
Kidney Beans ✓	🛒
Kohlrabi ✓	🛒
Leeks 11	🛒
Lentils 24, 31	🛒
Lettuce (Iceberg) 1, 9, 10 11, 14, 17, 33	🛒
Lettuce (Iceberg, organic) ✓	🛒
Lima Beans, Immature 1, 10, 12, 14, 24	🛒
Lima Beans, Mature ✓ 10, 24	🛒
Lo Bok ✓	🛒
Mixed Vegetables, Canned ✓ 1, 23	🛒
Mung Beans ✓	🛒
Mushrooms ✓ 1, 17, 23	🛒
Mushrooms (European Boletes and Chanterelles) 36	🛒
Mustard Greens 17	🛒
Navy Beans ✓ 13	🛒
Okra ✓	🛒
Onions, Green (Scallions) ✓ 10, 11	🛒
Onions, Raw ✓	🛒
Onions, Yellow ✓	🛒
Parsley (fresh) 4, 13, 19, 20, 24, 31	🛒
Parsnips 11	🛒
Peas, Garden 6, 9, 14, 17	🛒

Food and Carcinogenic Contaminants	Health Advisory
	Carcinogen Advisory

Little to No Risk   Minimal Risk   Caution   Recommended ✓

Food	Carcinogen Advisory
Peas, Dried ✓	Little to No Risk
Pepper, Hot 1, 17	Minimal Risk
Pepper, Jalapeño 1	Minimal Risk
Pinto Beans ✓ 24	Little to No Risk
Potato, Baked 7, 11, 13, 17, 19, 23	Caution
Potatoes, Boiled (potato skin removed) ✓ 11, 19	Little to No Risk
Potatoes, Mashed (potato skin removed) ✓ 11	Little to No Risk
Potatoes, organic ✓	Little to No Risk
Radicchio ✓	Little to No Risk
Radishes 10, 13, 19, 24, 37	Minimal Risk
Rapini ✓	Little to No Risk
Red Beans ✓ 24	Little to No Risk
Rhubarb ✓	Little to No Risk
Snow Peas ✓	Little to No Risk
Soy Beans (nonorganic) 4, 13, 19	Minimal Risk
Soy Beans (organic) ✓	Little to No Risk
Spinach 4, 7, 10, 11, 13, 14, 17, 23, 33, 37	Minimal Risk
Spinach (organic) ✓	Little to No Risk
Squash, Summer 7, 11, 13, 19, 23, 27, 31, 37	Caution
Squash, Winter 1, 7, 13, 19, 23, 27, 37	Minimal Risk
Sugar Beets ✓	Little to No Risk
Sweet Potatoes, Baked 11, 13, 23	Minimal Risk
Swiss Chard ✓ 10	Little to No Risk
Tomatillo 9	Minimal Risk

Food and Carcinogenic Contaminants	Health Advisory
🛒 Little to No Risk 🛒 Minimal Risk 🛒 Caution ✓ Recommended	Carcinogen Advisory
Tomatoes 1, 9, 12, 17, 31, 33	🛒
Tomatoes (organic) ✓	🛒
Tong-Ho ✓	🛒
Turnips ✓ 10	🛒
Turnip Greens 9, 10, 11, 33	🛒
Watercress ✓	🛒
Yams ✓	🛒

Vegetable Juices

Food and Carcinogenic Contaminants	Health Advisory
🛒 Little to No Risk 🛒 Minimal Risk 🛒 Caution ✓ Recommended	Carcinogen Advisory
Carrot Juice ✓	🛒
Mixed Vegetable Juice ✓	🛒
Tomato Juice ✓ 1	🛒

GRAINS

Health Advisory

Carcinogens

Conventionally grown grain products are generally free from residues of carcinogenic pesticides (except for products from India); yet carcinogenic pesticides are used extensively in the production of grain products, and they pose a threat to the health of farmers and farm workers. Researchers have noted high rates of non-Hodgkin's lymphoma among farmers. The probable explanation is agricultural exposure to herbicides. Researchers from Sweden and the United States have found a five- to six-fold increase in the risk of non-Hodgkin's lymphoma and also excesses of brain cancer, multiple myeloma, and leukemia among persons frequently exposed to herbicides. You can do a lot for the health of farmers and farm workers by insisting on buying only organically grown grains.

Colors: Cereals should be avoided if they contain the following colors that have been shown to be carcinogenic or to contain carcinogenic impurities:

- FD&C Blue 1
- FD&C Green 3
- FD&C Red 4
- FD&C Red 40
- FD&C Yellow 5
- FD&C Yellow 6

Safe Shopping Tips

- Prefer organically grown whole grain products; they are readily available either at health food stores or in the gourmet/health food sections of supermarkets. Buying organically grown grains will not only reduce your exposure to pesticides and additives, but also ensure that you receive all of grains' nutritional value; many valuable nutrients, antioxidant minerals, and fiber are lost when grains are refined. Fortunately, most organic products are made with whole grains. You can also find organic tortillas, bread, muffins, hamburger and hot dog buns, rolls, cold and hot cereals, and many other items, all priced competitively with conventional brands.
- Products with labels that state they are made from "enriched" flours or simply "wheat flour" are refined and have no place in your shopping cart.
- Buy cereals free from artificial colors.

Grains

Food and Carcinogenic Contaminants	Health Advisory
🛒 Little to No Risk 🛒 Minimal Risk 🛒 Caution ✓ Recommended	Carcinogen Advisory
Barley ✓	🛒
Bread Crumbs ✓	🛒
Bread Mix ✓	🛒
Bread, Rye ✓	🛒
Bread, White, Enriched ✓	🛒
Bread, Whole Wheat ✓ 23	🛒
Breadsticks ✓	🛒

Food and Carcinogenic Contaminants	Health Advisory
Little to No Risk Minimal Risk Caution ✓ Recommended	Carcinogen Advisory
Bulgar Wheat ✓	
Buckwheat ✓	
Cereal, 40% Bran Flakes ✓	
Cereal, Cornflakes ✓	
Cereal, Fruit Flavored (with artificial colors) 12, 23	
Cereal, Crisped Rice ✓	
Cereal, Oat Ring ✓	
Cereal, Puffed Wheat ✓	
Cereal, Raisin Bran 12, 14, 35	
Cereal, Raisin Bran (organic) ✓	
Cereal, Shredded Wheat ✓	
Cornbread, Southern Style ✓ 11	
Crackers, Saltine ✓	
Egg Noodles ✓ 40	
Farina, Cooked ✓	
Flour, Amaranth ✓	
Flour, Oat ✓	
Flour, Wheat, Enriched ✓	
Flour, Whole Wheat ✓	
Granola, Plain ✓ 23	
Hominy Grits, Cooked ✓	
Linguini, Enriched ✓	
Macaroni, Enriched ✓	
Muffins ✓ 23	

Food and Carcinogenic Contaminants	Health Advisory

				Carcinogen Advisory
🛒 Little to No Risk	🛒 Minimal Risk	🛒 Caution	✓ Recommended	
Oats ✓ 17				🛒
Pancakes ✓ 11				🛒
Pasta ✓				🛒
Psyllium Husk (from India) 4, 24				🛒
Rice, Basmati (except India) ✓				🛒
Rice, Basmati (from India) 4, 24				🛒
Rice, Brown, Whole Grain ✓				🛒
Rice Flour (from Mexico) 4, 24				🛒
Rice, Jasmine ✓				🛒
Rice, Polished ✓				🛒
Rice Sticks ✓				🛒
Rice, White ✓				🛒
Rolls, Soft, White ✓				🛒
Spaghetti ✓				🛒
Spaghetti, Vegetable ✓				🛒
Tortilla, Corn ✓				🛒
Tortilla, Flour ✓				🛒
Wild Rice ✓ 11, 13				🛒

MEAT, POULTRY, AND MEAT SUBSTITUTES

Health Advisory

Bacterial Contamination

Because of continual outbreaks of bacterial disease among consumers of meat and poultry products, in September 1993 the federal government required meat packers to carry a warning on labels of meat and poultry products that they are contaminated with dangerous bacteria such as salmonella and *E. coli*. Illness resulting from such bacteria can be deadly to babies of less than two years and the elderly, as well as to those people whose immune systems have been compromised by AIDS, cancer, cirrhosis, or other conditions. For the healthy mature adult, salmonellosis usually means a distressing bout of fever, diarrhea, and stomach cramps.

Following guidelines for safe handling and cooking of meat and poultry products will reduce your risk of contracting a bacterial illness such as salmonellosis.

Carcinogens

Meat and poultry contain a wide range of carcinogens, including pesticides, animals drugs, hormones, and radiation.

Pesticides: Pesticides remaining as residues in animal feed crops may be ingested by livestock and concentrate in their tissues. Pesticides may be applied directly on feed crops or come from general environmental contaminants in the soil, barns, or elsewhere. These include past use of chlordane, DDT, and dieldrin, which are among the potent pesticides commonly found in the food supply. A study by Dr. Mary S. Wolff, associate professor of community medicine at the Mount Sinai School of Medicine in New York City, found that women with blood levels of DDT in the top 10 percent had four times the breast cancer risk as women in the bottom 10 percent. In addition, several other pesticide contaminants found in meat and poultry have been implicated as causing breast cancer. Yet, quite apart from those substances that induce breast cancer, many other carcinogens are found in meat and poultry products.

Animal drugs: Animal drugs are widely used nationwide. Drugs administered to livestock, which include antibiotics such as sulfas, are often misused, leaving illegal residues in animal tissues and subsequently in meat and poultry. Forty of the animal drugs and pesticides known to occur as residues in meat and poultry are carcinogens. Furthermore, another eighteen cause birth defects. There is virtually no monitoring of these substances—even though at least 143 pesticides and drugs are known to leave chemical residues in meat and poultry. Only 46 of the 143 drugs and pesticides found in edible animal tissues are monitored by the USDA, and they are poorly and rarely monitored. A 1985 congressional subcommittee concluded that FDA officials believe that as many as 90 percent or more of the twenty thousand to thirty thousand new animal drugs estimated to be on the market have not been approved by FDA as safe and effective and, therefore, are being marketed in violation of the Food, Drug, and Cosmetic Act. The committee went on to estimate that as many as four thousand of these new animal drugs could have potentially significant adverse health effects on animals or humans.

Simply choosing poultry instead of beef will not protect you from exposure to animal drugs. Unless raised organically, poultry is also contaminated. Says one former poultry industry executive who worked for one of the nation's major producers, "At Perdue we allocated three-quarters of a square foot for each animal.

They are very crowded, and walking and pecking in their own excrement. That is why disease passes so rapidly through a flock of chickens. You go into a chicken house every week and do a post mortem and if there is a sick bird you treat the whole flock uniformly. They are medicated in the feed or in the water. Or you go into a [chicken] house with something that looks like a leaf blower and spray an atomized mixture of antibiotics in solution. It is like a fog."

One group of animal drugs that pose serious health risks is sulfa drugs. Sulfamethazine and other sulfa drugs have been used since the 1940s to prevent respiratory disease among market hogs and veal calves. Sulfamethazine is carcinogenic. Although in the past sulfamethazine residues have been found frequently in market pork as well as milk-fed veal, the USDA claims that the incidence is presently minimal. Certainly, there has been improvement among ranchers; however, the continued use of sulfamethazine remains a significant food safety issue, primarily because ranchers have replaced sulfamethazine, not necessarily with better animal husbandry and improved conditions, but with other structurally similar sulfa drugs. A report from the federal General Accounting Office (GAO) recognizes that if a structural feature in one compound is found to cause cancer, the presence of that same structural feature in other compounds greatly increases the probability that they too can cause cancer.

Growth stimulating hormones: Sex hormones, both natural and synthetic, which are given to up to 90 percent or more of the cattle raised for slaughter in the United States, also leave residues in edible portions of meats. Industry experts claim there is no danger to humans from these hormones when they are used properly. But, like antibiotics, growth hormones are sold to ranchers over the counter without a veterinary prescription, and the federal system of inspection for hormone levels in meat and poultry is notoriously inadequate—despite the fact that hormones are listed as known human carcinogens by the International Agency for Research on Cancer. Only 1 in 8,000 livestock and 1 in 700,000 poultry are tested in USDA laboratories for chemical residue content and rarely ever for hormones. That means that a consumer who carefully checks the meat and poultry she buys to determine that it has a USDA-inspected stamp on it is merely getting a product that has been inspected for cleanliness and general health—but in no way does that imply that there has been only testing to determine whether or not it has high residues of carcinogenic hormones. Most meat and poultry products containing illegal levels of chemical residues are sold to the public. Most of this meat bears the USDA inspection stamp.

While the body produces hormones and hormones are naturally present in foods, the use of natural and synthetic hormones should be banned.

Federal regulators and the beef industry claim that the hormones implanted in cattle are not harmful. The facts tell a different story. Although the government banned the synthetic hormone DES (diethylstilbestrol) in 1979, its illegal use by American meat producers continued until at least 1983 when nearly fifteen hundred veal calves from five different farms in upstate New York were found to be contaminated with residues of this illegal growth stimulator. Furthermore, rather than finding safe alternatives following the DES ban, the meat industry promptly switched to other carcinogenic additives, particularly forms of the natural sex hormones estradiol, progesterone, and testosterone, which are legally implanted in the ears of commercially raised feedlot cattle. These substances are carcinogenic. And unlike the synthetic DES, whose residues can be monitored and whose use was conditional on a seven-day preslaughter withdrawal period, residues of natural hormones are not detectable, and they cannot be practically differentiated from the same hormones produced by the body, except by their higher levels. Since 1983, however, the FDA has allowed virtually unregulated use of these additives up to the time of slaughter, subject only to the theoretical and nonenforceable requirement that residue levels in meat must be less than 1 percent of the daily hormonal production of young children. The result is that virtually the entire U.S. population consumes, without any warning, labeling, or information, unknown and unpredictable amounts of hormonal residues in meat products over a lifetime.

In 1986, as many as half of all cattle sampled in feedlots as large as six hundred animals were found to have hormones illegally implanted in muscle, rather than the ear skin, to induce further increased growth. This practice results in very high residues in meat, which even the FDA has admitted could produce "adverse effects." Left unanswered is whether or not such chronic and uncontrolled estrogen dosages are involved in increasing cancer rates (now striking one in three Americans), particularly the alarming 50 percent increase in the incidence of breast cancer since 1965. These questions are of further concern in light of long-standing evidence confirming the association between breast cancer and oral contraceptives, whose estrogen dosage over a fraction of a lifetime is known and controlled, in contrast with that from residues of hormones in meat products. More than a decade ago, Roy Hertz, then director of endocrinology of the NCI and a world authority on hormonal cancer, warned of the carcinogenic risks from life-long exposure to estrogenic feed additives, particularly for hormonally sensitive tissues such as breast tissue, because they could increase normal body hormonal levels and disturb delicately poised hormonal balances. Hertz pointed to evidence from innumerable animal tests and human clinical experience that such imbalances can be carcinogenic. Hertz also warned of the essentially uncontrolled and unregulated use of these extremely potent biological agents, no dietary levels of which can be regarded as safe. Even a dime-sized piece of meat contains billions or trillions of molecules of these carcinogens. Such exposures are particularly critical for young children.

A dramatic warning of the dangers of growth-promoting additives was triggered by an epidemic of premature sexual development and ovarian cysts involving about three thousand Puerto Rican infants and children from 1979 to 1981. These toxic effects were traced to hormonal contamination of fresh meat products, and were usually reversed by simple dietary changes. The meat products were found to be contaminated with estrogen residues more than ten times above the normal ranges. The epidemic also was associated with increased rates of uterine and ovarian cancers in adult women.

Nitrites: Cured meats such as bacon, ham, beef jerky, salami, and luncheon meats contain nitrites. These substances inhibit the growth of dangerous botulism-causing bacteria, and maintain the meat's red color. Although nitrite itself is not carcinogenic, it combines with naturally occurring chemicals called secondary or tertiary amines to form carcinogenic nitrosamines. This reaction will occur in the food itself while it is sitting on the shelf or in the refrigerator or when being fried, but it also occurs within the stomach once the food is ingested. Nitrite-contaminated food is thought to be a cause of stomach cancer in the United States, Japan, and other nations. Recently, researchers reported that children who eat hot dogs cured with nitrite a dozen or more times monthly have a risk of leukemia ten times higher than normal. Furthermore, children born to mothers who consume hot dogs once or more weekly during their pregnancy are twice as likely to have childhood brain tumors. Stay away from nitrites! You can find safer choices that use far less toxic preservatives such as ascorbic acid (vitamin C). See *Safe Shopping and Cooking Tips* for methods of self-protection.

Charcoal broiling, grilling, oven cooking, and pan frying: In the 1700s, soot containing polycyclic aromatic hydrocarbons (PAHs) was linked to scrotal cancer in chimney sweeps. Today, grilled meat is the major source of PAHs in food.

Heavy charring of meats produces high concentrations of carcinogenic PAHs such as benzopyrene.

Some eighteen different PAHs have thus far been found in food. Although the data are not entirely conclusive, researchers believe that at least five and perhaps as many as twelve of these eighteen PAHs cause cancer. PAHs form when fat from grilled meats falls down on flames or hot coals. The PAHs that are formed in this reaction rise with the smoke and permeate the meat.

Although the formation of PAHs appears limited primarily to barbecuing and grilling, you must be careful when broiling and pan frying meats to prevent formation of another group of cancer-causing chemicals known as heterocyclic amines (HAs), which are created when amino acids and other substances in meats are burned. The National Cancer Institute estimates that HAs may increase the number of human cancers in the United States by about two thousand cases annually. (It is of interest to note that NCI has made no such estimates for excess cancers related to exposure to pesticides, hormones, and industrial contaminants in meats.)

Occasionally eating grilled meat or meats cooked at high temperatures, as in broiling or frying, is not a problem. But if you like to grill your meats regularly, then you should learn a few cooking techniques that can help make consuming grilled foods safer and healthier.

Radiation: Some meat products are contaminated by environmental radiation from nuclear accidents such as Chernobyl. Radiation is carcinogenic. The meat products of four countries that export significant amounts to the United States have been shown to have trace levels of radioactivity because of the 1986 Chernobyl explosion. Such products include canned ham from Poland, Hungary, Yugoslavia, and Brazil (which processes European meats), as well as other meat and poultry products from Finland and Switzerland. Countries whose meat products were least affected include France, Germany, Italy, and the Netherlands.

Safe Shopping and Cooking Tips

Shopping

- Buy "organically raised" meat and poultry. See Appendix A for sources of organic meat and poultry.
- Consider the use of meat substitutes such as tempeh or tofu burgers, hot dogs, and bacon, available at health food stores.
- Avoid products containing nitrites. Healthy Choice, a mainstream brand of cold cuts available in most supermarkets, is free from nitrites, as are Coleman Beef and Shelton products, which are sold in health food stores.
- Look for pork bacon without nitrites in the freezer section of your health food store.
- The only meat and poultry that is safe is organically raised. However, these are your best choices when shopping in a market that does not sell organic meat and poultry:

Bologna, Chicken (low-fat/nonfat)	Tofu Bacon
Bologna, Turkey (low-fat/nonfat)	Tofu Burgers
Buffalo	Tofu Hot Dogs
Pheasant	Turkey Breast, Roasted
Quail	(no nitrite)
Rabbit	

Safe Handling

To prevent bacterial illness follow these guidelines:

- Harmful bacteria are most likely to multiply if meat and poultry are stored at temperatures between 40°F and 140°F.
- Defrost frozen ground meats in the cooler—never at room temperature.
- For rapid defrosting, seal meat in a watertight plastic bag and place it in a sink of cold running water. Check food temperature every twenty minutes. Be sure it does not exceed 40°F.

- Always wash hands thoroughly in hot soapy water before preparing foods and after handling raw meat.
- Do not let raw meat or poultry juices touch ready-to-eat foods either in the cooler or during preparation. Store properly wrapped raw meats below ready-to-eat foods in the cooler. Always store raw poultry on the lowest shelf.
- Do not put cooked foods on the same plate that held raw meat. Wash, rinse, and sanitize utensils that have touched raw meat before using them for cooked meats.
- Thoroughly clean and sanitize pots, pans, and utensils.
- Use hot water and the proper detergent to clean counters, cutting boards, and other surfaces raw meats have touched.

Safe Cooking

Follow these guidelines to prevent bacterial illness:

- Cook meat patties and meat loaf long enough so that it is not pink and the juices run clear.
- Cook crumbled ground meats until no pink color remains.
- Eat ground meat patties and loaves when they have reached 155°F in the center, ground poultry patties and loaves, 165°F.
- When broiling, grilling, or cooking on the stove, turn meats over at least once.
- To reheat precooked foods, cover and heat to 165°F or until hot and steaming throughout.
- Verify all final internal product cooking temperatures with a clean and sanitized thermometer.
- Instead of pan frying, cook bacon in a microwave oven to significantly lower levels of nitrosamines.

Grilling Meats

There are several ways to minimize formation of carcinogenic PAHs in grilled meats:

- Avoid charcoal-broiling meats until they are black. That goes for steaks, hamburgers, roasts, poultry, pork, and seafood. Slight grill marks are fine.
- Buy the leanest foods for grilling. The leanest choices for grilling include chicken breast, lobster, scallops, yellowfin tuna, flounder, sole, grouper, monkfish, halibut, and shrimp.
- Broil meat in the oven, where heat comes from above; because the fat does not drip onto the flame, you can eliminate cancer-causing PAHs.

- When buying fuel for your barbecue, prefer regular hardwood charcoal to mesquite. Researchers have discovered that cooking with mesquite produces far higher concentrations of PAHs than cooking with regular hardwood charcoal.
- When grilling, raise the grill higher than usual from the charcoal and place the charcoal on one side of the barbecue and the meat on the other side.
- If you like smoked flavoring, instead of burning in that smoky wood flavoring on your home grill, try liquid smoke products. Such products are filtered; tars, resins, and most PAHs are removed. Supermarkets carry liquid smoke in the condiment section.
- Try a Swedish innovation called the Vertikal Grill, which lets you barbecue meat without allowing its fat to drip into the flames. See Appendix A, page 392, to find out where it can be bought.

Broiling and Oven Cooking

The following guidelines will help reduce the formation of carcinogenic HAs in broiled and oven-cooked meats and poultry:

- Use lower temperatures. Of course, because of bacterial contamination, you should not eat meat, poultry, or seafood raw. But do not overcook. The key is to cook long enough at high enough temperatures to kill bacteria and parasites—without overcooking.
- Before broiling or frying, precook meat in the microwave on high for thirty to ninety seconds and toss out the juice.

Safe Storage

To prevent bacterial illness follow these guidelines:

- Do not let foods stand at room temperature. After cooking, keep them hot at 140°F or higher.
- After eating, refrigerate unused portions immediately in shallow counter pans. Ground meat and ground poultry products should be no deeper than two inches.
- Set your cooler at 36°F or colder; set your freezer at 0°F or below.
- Keep uncooked ground meat and poultry in the refrigerator only one or two days before cooking or freezing. And practice "First in, first out."
- Chill cooked foods to 40°F within four hours.
- Use or freeze cooked meat and poultry stored in the refrigerator within one to two days.

Meat, Poultry, and Meat Substitutes

Food and Carcinogenic Contaminants	Health Advisory
Little to No Risk *Minimal Risk* *Caution* ✓ *Recommended*	Carcinogen Advisory
Alligator 11, 13, 27	🛒
Bacon (with nitrites) 11, 13, 19	🛒
Beef, All Cuts (organic) ✓	🛒
Beef, Chuck Roast, Roasted 11, 13, 20, 21, 23, 34	🛒
Beef, Ground, Fried 11, 13, 19, 20, 21, 23	🛒
Beef, Liver/Calf 11, 13, 21, 23, 32	🛒
Beef, Loin/Sirloin 11, 13, 19, 20, 21	🛒
Beef, Meatloaf 11, 13, 19, 20, 21, 23	🛒
Beef, Round Steak, Stewed 13, 20, 21, 23, 34	🛒
Bologna, Chicken (low-fat/nonfat; nitrite-free) ✓	🛒
Bologna, Pork/Beef (with nitrites) 4, 11, 13, 19, 20, 21, 24	🛒
Bologna, Turkey (low-fat/nonfat; nitrite-free) ✓	🛒
Buffalo ✓	🛒
Chicken, All Cuts (organic) ✓	🛒
Chicken, Drum & Breast, Fried ✓ *11*	🛒
Chicken, Whole, Roasted 11, 23, 32	🛒
Frankfurter, Beef/Pork (with nitrites) 4, 11, 13, 19, 20, 21, 24	🛒
Lamb, All Cuts (organic) ✓	🛒
Lamb Chop 11, 13, 19, 21, 28	🛒
Pheasant ✓	🛒
Pork, All Cuts (organic) ✓	🛒
Pork Chop (raised with sulfa drugs) 24	🛒
Pork, Ham, Cured (with nitrites) 11	🛒

Food and Carcinogenic Contaminants	Health Advisory
🛒 *Little to No Risk* 🛒 *Minimal Risk* 🛒 *Caution* ✓ *Recommended*	Carcinogen Advisory
Pork Roast, Loin (raised with sulfa drugs) 11	🛒 (Caution)
Pork Sausage, Cooked (with nitrites) 11, 19, 24, 28	🛒 (Caution)
Quail ✓	🛒 (Little to No Risk)
Rabbit ✓	🛒 (Little to No Risk)
Salami (with nitrites) 4, 11, 13, 19, 20, 21, 24	🛒 (Caution)
Tempeh Burgers ✓	🛒 (Little to No Risk)
Tofu Bacon ✓	🛒 (Little to No Risk)
Tofu Hot Dogs ✓	🛒 (Little to No Risk)
Turkey Breast, Roasted 11	🛒 (Little to No Risk)
Veal (conventionally raised) 11, 23	🛒 (Caution)
Veal (organic) ✓	🛒 (Little to No Risk)

SEAFOOD

Health Advisory

Natural Toxins

Ciguatera: Food poisoning caused by ciguatera, naturally occurring organisms belonging to the dinoflagellate family, is associated with consuming fish in tropical areas such as Australia, Hawaii, and the Caribbean, including the Bahamas, Cuba, Puerto Rico, and the U.S. Virgin Islands. In the continental United States, the greatest threat of ciguatera occurs along the southern Florida coast. Symptoms of ciguatera include abdominal pain, diarrhea, vomiting, a metallic taste in the mouth, and severe tooth pain. Reversals in nerve sensation may occur in which hot coffee may feel cold and ice cream may feel hot. Cold water can burn the skin. The onset of symptoms is roughly one to six hours after a meal of toxic fish.

Ciguatera can be fatal. The naturally occurring toxins, ciguatoxins, are severe neurotoxins, and their effects may linger for many years after the acute illness has passed. Restaurants in prime tourist spots such as Hawaii do an excellent job of protecting their patrons. But sport fishermen are at risk. Fish most likely to harbor the ciguatoxin include barracuda, forktailed snapper, grouper, mahimahi, royal sea bass, and snapper. Larger fish are more likely to cause illness than smaller fish. These fish from Hawaiian waters may harbor ciguatoxin: amberjack (kahala), barracuda (kaku), black snapper (wahanui), blue-spotted grouper (roi), eel (puhialo), goatfish (weke), jack (ulua), milkfish (awa), thread-fin fish (moi), mullet (uouoa), skipjack (aku), snapper (opakapaka), surgeonfish (manini or palani), and wrasse (po'ou).

Scombroid: Scombroid is caused by poor handling of fishery products aboard fishing vessels, which causes a buildup of a histamine toxin, especially when fish remain at high temperatures for several hours. Symptoms include nausea, abdominal cramps, tingling and burning sensations around the mouth, oral blistering or burning, rashes and itching, redness, headaches, dizziness, and vomiting. One sign of scombroid contamination is a peppery taste to the fish. Sport fishermen should be sure to immediately ice and chill their catch. Fish most likely to cause scombroid poisoning are tuna, mackerel, bonito, bluefish, and mahimahi. Also sometimes involved are herring, sardines, amberjack, anchovy, jack mackerel, and skipjack.

Paralytic shellfish poisoning: Shellfish poisoning may result when naturally occurring dinoflagellates build up in shellfish, often during red tides. They concentrate in mussels, oysters, scallops, and clams. Paralytic shellfish poisoning (PSP) was once widespread. But careful monitoring has sharply decreased its incidence, although a freak red tide off the North Carolina coast in 1987 resulted in forty-eight cases of paralytic shellfish poisoning.

Recreational shellfish harvesters should never eat their catch when taken during or immediately after a red tide. Red tides usually occur in the United States between May and October. You should stop harvesting at the first sign of a red tide. As the red tide recedes, shellfish generally quickly excrete the toxin. PSP symptoms occur within thirty minutes of eating the food and include nausea and vomiting; paralysis may set in. This disease is life threatening and can make you feel as though you have had a stroke. Be especially cautious during clambakes and barbecues when shellfish have been gathered from local areas. *Cooking will not destroy the toxin responsible for paralytic shellfish poisoning.* Victims should get help immediately from a doctor or poison control center.

Carcinogens

Antibiotics: The raising of farm-raised fish is quite similar to the factory farmyard methods used for cattle. As with cattle, fish are given a wide range of antibiotics and other drugs.

This massive new industry is virtually unregulated. As a result farm-raised fish are likely to contain residues of a wide variety of animal drugs, some of which are carcinogenic. Prefer wild deep-water ocean fish whenever possible.

Industrial chemicals and pesticides: Seafood can be one of the most dangerously contaminated food sources in the diet today when uninformed shopping choices are made. In fact, the National Academy of Sciences estimated in 1991 that the risk of cancer to the average consumer who eats seafood can be some seventy-five times greater than normally acceptable guidelines. As you can see from the following charts, some seafood items such as bluefish, farm-raised catfish, lake trout, Maine lobster, and striped bass are contaminated with concentrations of industrial chemicals and pesticides hundreds to thousands of times greater than other food groups. Yet when consumers make choices based on adequate information, seafood can be one of the safest, most nutritious foods.

Carcinogenic industrial chemicals and pesticides commonly found in contaminated seafood include benzene hexachloride, chlordane, DDT, dieldrin, dioxin, heptachlor, hexachlorobenzene, lindane, and polychlorinated biphenyls.

No fish from waters near agricultural and industrial areas or from the nation's major inland waterways or harbors are safe to consume due to industrial chemical and pesticide contamination.

Safe Shopping and Cooking Tips

- Avoid freshwater fish—unless it comes from high mountain lakes and streams.
- Prefer wild fish over farm-raised varieties.
- Fish from the waters off Argentina, Chile, Mexico, and New Zealand are as pure as the seven seas can give.
- Tuna is an excellent choice; however, it is a moderate mercury accumulator, so it should be eaten no more than twice a week during pregnancy because of the reproductive effects of methylmercury.
- Be wary of fish that are heavy mercury accumulators, especially if you are a woman of childbearing age. Mercury-accumulating fish include swordfish, many fish from the inland waters of the Midwest and Florida, shark, and tuna.
- Broil fillets on an open rack and let the juices drip out.
- Research shows that by discarding the oil before serving pan-fried fish you can reduce industrial pollution and pesticide concentrations by as much as 65 percent.
- Because pesticides accumulate in fatty tissue, the way you clean fish is important. Trim and discard the skin and fatty portions from the top, side, and belly of pike, walleye, Great Lakes coho salmon and lake trout, and other Great Lakes fish, if you eat fish from those waters.

Seafood

Food and Carcinogenic Contaminants	Health Advisory
Little to No Risk 🛒 **Minimal Risk** 🛒 **Caution** 🛒 **Recommended** ✓	Carcinogen Advisory
Abalone ✓	🛒
Anchovies ✓	🛒
Barracuda (from California)	🛒
Bass (Freshwater, from Canada) 7, 11, 13, 19, 34	🛒
Bluefish 4, 7, 11, 13, 20, 27, 28, 34	🛒
Bonito (California) 11, 34	🛒
Buffalo Fish 11, 37	🛒
Butterfish (from Virginia) 4, 11	🛒
Cabrilla (Mexico) ✓	🛒
Carp 34	🛒
Catfish (Farm-Raised) 7, 11, 13, 24	🛒
Catfish (River) 7, 11, 13, 15, 16, 19, 28, 34	🛒
Clams, Red 30	🛒
Crab Stick (Korea) ✓	🛒
Cod (Denmark, Iceland) ✓ 4	🛒
Cod (U.S.) 11, 34	🛒
Corvina (California) 11, 34	🛒
Crawfish ✓	🛒
Croaker (from Gulf Coast—Arkansas, Louisiana) 11, 20, 34	🛒
Croaker (from California) 11, 34	🛒
Croaker (from Gulf Coast of Texas) 15	🛒
Croaker (from People's Republic of China, Uruguay) ✓ 11, 20, 34	🛒
Dover Sole ✓ 11	🛒

Food and Carcinogenic Contaminants	Health Advisory
	Carcinogen Advisory

Little to No Risk   Minimal Risk   Caution   Recommended ✓

Eels 11, 13	🛒
Flounder (Imported) ✓	🛒
Flounder (U.S.) ✓	🛒
Geoduck (Canada, Washington) ✓	🛒
Goo (Louisiana) 11, 32	🛒
Grouper ✓ *11*	🛒
Haddock (Canada, Iceland, United Kingdom) ✓	🛒
Halibut (California) 11, 34	🛒
Halibut (Iceland, Mexico) ✓ *20*	🛒
Herring (Atlantic) 7, 11, 13, 20, 27, 34	🛒
Herring (Imported) 4, 10, 11, 16, 19, 24, 27, 34	🛒
Hoki ✓	🛒
Jack Mackerel, Canned (Chile) ✓	🛒
Lake Trout (Great Lakes) 4, 7, 11, 13, 20, 27, 28, 34	🛒
Lingcod (California) 11	🛒
Lobster (Australia, California, Mexico, New Zealand, Thailand) ✓	🛒
Lobster (Canada) ✓ *11, 34*	🛒
Lobster (Maine, Massachusetts, New Hampshire, New Jersey, New York, Rhode Island) 34	🛒
Lobster Tomalley 4, 11, 34	🛒
Mackerel, Canned (Chile) ✓	🛒
Mackerel (Import) 4, 11	🛒
Mackerel (U.S.) 4, 11, 20, 27, 28	🛒
Mahimahi (Dolphin Fish) ✓	🛒
Marlin ✓	🛒

Food and Carcinogenic Contaminants	Health Advisory
	Carcinogen Advisory

⊞ Little to No Risk ⊞ Minimal Risk ⊞ Caution ✓ Recommended	
Menpachi (from Hawaii) ✓	⊞
Milkfish 11, 13, 34	⊞
Mullet (Imported) 11	⊞
Mullet (U.S.) 10, 11, 13, 15, 34	⊞
Ocean Perch 4, 11, 34	⊞
Orange Roughy ✓	⊞
Oysters ✓	⊞
Palani (Hawaii) ✓	⊞
Pike/Pickerel (Canada) 13, 34	⊞
Pollock (Canada, Iceland) ✓ 4, 20	⊞
Pompano (Florida) ✓	⊞
Porgy 7, 11, 13, 27, 34	⊞
Rainbow Trout (Farm-Raised)	⊞
Redfish ✓	⊞
Red Snapper ✓ 11	⊞
Rock Bass (Florida) ✓	⊞
Rockfish (California) 11, 34	⊞
Sablefish (California) 11	⊞
Salmon (Pacific Coast) 4, 11, 15, 34	⊞
Salmon (Imported) 4, 11, 24, 34	⊞
Sand Dabs ✓ 11	⊞
Sardines ✓ 11	⊞
Scallops ✓	⊞
Sea Bass ✓ 11, 34	⊞

Food and Carcinogenic Contaminants	Health Advisory
	Carcinogen Advisory

Legend: 🛒 Little to No Risk · 🛒 Minimal Risk · 🛒 Caution · ✓ Recommended

Food and Carcinogenic Contaminants	Carcinogen Advisory
Sea Trout (Atlantic) 4, 7, 11, 13	🛒
Sea Trout (Argentina, Uruguay) ✓ 11, 34	🛒
Shad 4, 7, 13, 19, 34	🛒
Shark (California) 11, 34	🛒
Shark (Import) 38	🛒
Shrimp, Farm-Raised (United States) ✓	🛒
Shrimp, Farm-Raised (Imported)	🛒
Shrimp (Wild) ✓	🛒
Smelt (from Oregon) ✓	🛒
Sole (California) 11	🛒
Speckled Trout (Mexico) ✓	🛒
Spot (Virginia) ✓ 11, 13, 34	🛒
Squid ✓	🛒
Striped Bass (Atlantic) 4, 7, 11, 13, 15, 20, 27, 28, 34	🛒
Sturgeon 11, 13, 20	🛒
Swordfish 11, 34	🛒
Tarpon ✓	🛒
Tilapia (Farm-Raised) ✓ 11	🛒
Trout (from Iceland) ✓	🛒
Trout (U.S.) 11, 34	🛒
Tuna (Imported) ✓	🛒
Tuna (U.S.) ✓ 4, 11	🛒
Wahoo ✓	🛒
Whitefish/Chub 4, 7, 10, 11, 16, 19, 24, 27, 28, 32	🛒

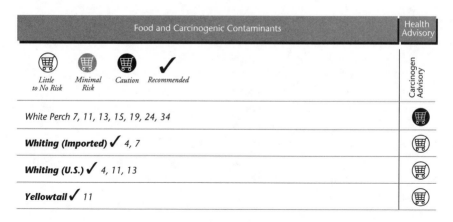

Food and Carcinogenic Contaminants	Health Advisory Carcinogen Advisory
White Perch *7, 11, 13, 15, 19, 24, 34*	🛒
Whiting (Imported) ✓ *4, 7*	🛒
Whiting (U.S.) ✓ *4, 11, 13*	🛒
Yellowtail ✓ *11*	🛒

DAIRY AND DAIRY SUBSTITUTES

Health Advisory

Carcinogens

Pesticides: Many carcinogenic pesticides—including BHC, chlordane, DDT, dieldrin, heptachlor, HCB, and lindane—accumulate in the most fatty dairy products (e.g., butter, ice cream, whole milk, high-fat cheeses).

Animal drugs: The FDA is responsible for assuring the safety of the billions of gallons of milk produced in the United States each year. Concerned about media reports that independent surveys had found a wide range of animal drugs in the milk supply, the FDA conducted three surveys to determine the presence of selected antibiotic drug residues in milk between 1988 and 1990. Although the FDA insists that these surveys confirmed their belief that the nation's milk supply is safe, we cannot support such statements because of flaws in the survey methods. For one thing, the number of samples tested was small; for another, the testing methods were grossly inadequate for detecting the many drugs used by the dairy industry.

One major concern is the use of sulfa drugs in dairy cows. Sulfamethazine is carcinogenic, and its residues are often found in milk. *FDA's own 1990 screening tests indicate that 46 percent of all milk samples tested contained more than one sulfa drug residue.* According to the GAO, other sulfa drugs exhibit toxic effects like those produced by sulfamethazine. In setting alleged safety levels, however, the FDA has allowed residues of up to ten parts per billion (ppb) for each sulfa drug, while ignoring their aggregate or synergistic effect.

The problem is compounded further because sulfamethazine metabolites (i.e., breakdown products) may also be present in milk. They also present carcinogenic risks; however, metabolites of sulfamethazine cannot be detected by the analytic methods FDA has used in past milk surveys.

Quite apart from sulfamethazine, other highly dangerous drugs such as chloramphenicol, which can cause the often fatal blood disease aplastic anemia, have also been found in the milk supply.

Dioxin: The Health Protection Branch of Canada has reported dioxin levels in the parts per trillion range in several samples of milk and cream packaged in bleached milk cartons manufactured in the United States. Dioxin, which is a by-product of the process used to bleach paper products at pulp and paper mills, had migrated from the cartons to the milk. Very likely U.S. milk products are similarly contaminated with dioxin. Dioxin's carcinogenicity is up to 500,000 times more potent than that of DDT. This problem can be easily prevented by using the self-protection methods outlined in *Safe Shopping and Cooking Tips.*

Allergies and Milk Sensitivity

Some 70 percent of the world's population lack the enzyme required to digest lactose, a sugar occurring naturally in milk. Especially vulnerable are people of African and Asian descent. Drinking just one glass can trigger symptoms of milk sensitivity such as diarrhea and cramps. Some companies offer lactose-free dairy products. Allergic responses to penicillin, tetracycline, and sulfa drugs, all of which may leave residues in retail milk supplies, are also of concern. See *Safe Shopping and Cooking Tips.*

Biosynthetic Hormones

In 1993, the FDA began allowing use of bovine growth hormone (BGH), a genetically engineered hormone that can boost milk production by 10 percent to 25 percent. Furthermore, the FDA stipulated that label disclosure will not be required to notify consumers whether or not their milk has been produced with biosynthetic hormones.

Biosynthetic hormones, which in addition to BGH includes bovine somatotropin (BST), are manufactured by giant chemical companies—Monsanto, American Cyanamid, Upjohn, and Eli Lilly together with Dow—who anticipate $1 billion in annual worldwide sales. Industry claims these are natural hormones. In fact, biosynthethic growth hormones are not "natural." The FDA now admits that they are up to "three percent different in molecular structure" from the normal hormone. Increased BGH levels in milk and blood have been found in injected cows. BGH and its digested products could be absorbed from milk into blood, particularly in infants, and produce hormonal and allergic effects.

In December 1994, the Commission of the European Community extended a ban to prohibit the marketing and use of BST/BGH until the year 2000. The decision of the seventeen-member commission was based on research that indicated authorization of BST would cause smaller dairies to go out of business and would be contrary to European agricultural policy, which aims to decrease current milk production. The commission also pointed out that the safety of BST could be ensured only under extremely controlled conditions not commonly found in current dairy management practices. In July 1994, the Canadian government decided to impose a moratorium on the marketing and use of BST/BGH for that nation's dairy industry.

The use of BGH raises fundamental ethical, social, and economic considerations, including the continued viability of the small family dairy farm and adverse veterinary effects. The past and expanding use of BGH poses potential public health hazards that so far have not been investigated.

The biotech industry claims that the hormones are natural, increase milk yields up to 25 percent, do not harm cows, do not alter milk quality, and are safe for humans. (The FDA also agrees that bovine growth hormones are safe and even allowed the sale of unlabeled milk and meat from BGH cows for about five years before formal approval was required. Some twenty thousand cows were treated in the past with BGH/BST in experimental trials, and their milk was allowed to be sold with the general milk supply. The figure now exceeds 5 percent of all cows and is rapidly increasing.) These claims, which are based on industry-contracted research at more than twenty U.S. university dairy science departments, are misleading.

Apart from the national surplus of milk and anticipated loss of thousands of small dairy farms if milk production is increased and milk prices are reduced, the effectiveness of BGH is exaggerated. Furthermore, the nutritional quality of milk and cheese is altered; fat is increased as much as 27 percent, and casein (milk protein) is decreased. Stress effects have been noted in cows hyperstimulated by BGH. These include increased susceptibility to infection, infertility, loss of fat, heat intolerance, and "burnout" or lactational failure. Severe stress diseases, including gastric ulcers, arthritis, and kidney and heart abnormalities, have also been induced in pigs. Additionally, BGH may be misused as a growth promoter in calves, pigs, and sheep, particularly as there are no practical methods for detecting the hormone in meat.

Apart from economic and veterinary concerns, BGH poses grave potential consumer health risks that have not yet been investigated by the industry or the FDA:

- Increased levels of cell-stimulating insulin-like growth factors (IGF), apparently identical to those in humans, have been reported in BGH milk. These could induce premature growth in infants and possibly promote colon cancer and breast cancer in women.
- Increased bacterial infections in BGH cows will require treatment with antibiotics that will pass into milk. This is likely to result in antibiotic-resistant infections in the general population. Also, the stress effects of BGH in cows could suppress immunity and activate latent

viruses, such as bovine leukemia (leukosis) and bovine immunodeficiency viruses, which are related to cancer and the AIDS complex and may be infectious to humans.

- Steroids and adrenaline-type stressor chemicals induced in cows by these hormones are likely to contaminate milk and may be harmful, particularly to infants and young children.
- The fat and milk of cows are already contaminated with a wide range of carcinogenic contaminants, including dioxins and pesticides. Bovine growth hormones reduce body fat and are likely to mobilize these carcinogens into milk, with cancer risks to consumers.

What is to be done? Politically, state legislatures should be pressured to ban BST/BGH. The FDA should be petitioned to ban the manufacture, domestic sale, and export of the hormones until all safety questions can be resolved. Congressional oversight should be focused on industry's misleading and self-interested claims on BGH and the FDA's regulatory abdication. Finally, consumers should be made to recognize that these hormones are industry's latest unsafe contribution to the brave new world of chemicalized food and mechanized farming.

Individually, consumers should demand certification that a company's products are free from BGH/BST and avoid those that do not provide such assurances.

Radiation

Milk is a prime route by which consumers are exposed to radioactive contaminants released by nuclear plants. Milk is especially dangerous because it is quickly marketed, and short-lived radioactive isotopes are still present when it is consumed. Milk is associated with increased risk for breast cancer, and the combination of pesticides and radiation have been proposed as one possible explanation. If your dairy is near a nuclear plant, don't use their products.

Safe Shopping and Cooking Tips

- Unless a dairy company certifies that its products are free from animal drugs and pesticide residues and that BGH/BST is not used in its cows, the company's products should be suspect and boycotted. If you are unable to find a company that provides explicit assurance, you should use dairy substitutes (except for children under around age two who may require dairy products). To find BGH-free milk from a dairy in your area, call the BGH consumer information line at (202) 466-2823.

- If you must have real dairy foods, then make sure they are produced from organically raised cows. Organic dairy products such as milk, butter, and cheese are becoming increasingly available at health food stores, and they make an excellent shopping choice. Organic dairy products are free of many of the problems described earlier, most importantly residues of animal drugs. Natural Horizons, of Colorado, distributes organic milk and yogurt. Find out where its products are available in your area; or write Natural Horizons, P.O. Box 17577, Boulder, CO 80301.

- Adults and older children (past ages two or three) should always prefer non-fat milk, yogurt, desserts, and other dairy products, as these will have the lowest amounts of chemical contamination. Substitute ice milk or non-fat frozen yogurt for ice cream; low-fat or nonfat dessert topping for whipped cream; low-fat or nonfat cheeses over whole milk cheeses; non-fat milk for whole milk; and tofu spreads or nonfat cream cheese for regular cream cheese. Always make the nonfat variety your first choice.

- Prefer cooking with olive oil or low-fat butter, available at health food stores, whenever possible. (However, do not substitute margarines made from partially hydrogenated vegetable oils, as hydrogenated oils have been implicated as a causal factor in heart disease.)

- Avoid any dairy product that lists "artificial color."

- Whenever possible, buy liquid dairy products in glass containers. This will prevent migration of even trace amounts of dioxin from paper cartons, or other plasticizers from plastic containers. Furthermore, glass containers are recycled.

- Soy milk or rice milk, made with organic tofu, is a fine milk substitute for older children and adults and can be substituted for many milk uses. It works well with cereal. Always be sure products are made with organically grown soybeans. Nut and grain milks can also be used in place of cow's milk. They are made with an almond blend or with cultured rice known as amazake, and they are available in the dairy sections of health food stores. *Please note: babies require greater amounts of fat in their diets until around age two. Consult with your physician first if you are considering the removal of whole milk products from your baby's diet.*

- At restaurants or home, try dairy substitutes such as frozen fruit desserts and sherbets.

Dairy and Dairy Substitutes

Food and Carcinogenic Contaminants	Health Advisory
Little to No Risk *Minimal Risk* *Caution* ✓ *Recommended*	Carcinogen Advisory
Butter, Stick 4, 11, 13, 19, 20, 24, 28	
Buttermilk 13, 19, 23	
Cheese, American 4, 11, 13, 19, 20, 24, 28	
Cheese, Blue ✓	
Cheese, Brie ✓	
Cheese, Camembert ✓ *4, 11, 13*	
Cheese, Cheddar 4, 11, 13, 19, 20, 24, 28	
Cheese, Feta ✓ *4, 11*	
Cheese, Goat ✓	
Cheese, Gouda ✓	
Cheese, Gruyère 21	
Cheese, Havarti ✓	
Cheese, Jarlsberg ✓	
Cheese, Gorgonzola (Italy) ✓	
Cheese, Goya ✓	
Cheese, Monterey Jack ✓	
Cheese, Mozzarella ✓ *11, 13*	
Cheese, Muenster ✓	
Cheese, Parmesan ✓ *11*	
Cheese, Provolone ✓	
Cheese, Reggiano 20	

Food and Carcinogenic Contaminants	Health Advisory
Little to No Risk **Minimal Risk** **Caution** ✓ *Recommended*	Carcinogen Advisory
Cheese, Ricotta ✓	🛒
Cheese, Romano ✓	🛒
Cheese, Roquefort ✓ *11*	🛒
Cheese, Sap Sago ✓	🛒
Cheese, Semi-Soft, Part-Skim ✓	🛒
Cheese, Sheep ✓	🛒
Cheese, Swiss ✓	🛒
Cottage Cheese, 4% Fat or Less ✓ *11, 20*	🛒
Cream Cheese ✓	🛒
Cream, Half & Half 1, 11, 13, 19, 20, 24, 28	🛒
Ice Cream 4, 11, 13, 19, 20, 23, 24, 28	🛒
Ice Cream Sandwich 4, 11, 13, 23, 28	🛒
Ice Milk ✓ *11, 20, 23*	🛒
Milk, Chocolate 11, 13, 19	🛒
Milk, Evaporated 4, 11, 13, 19, 20, 28	🛒
Milk, Goat ✓	🛒
Milk, Lowfat, 2% Fat 11, 13, 19, 20	🛒
Milk, Skim ✓ *11*	🛒
Milk, Whole 11, 13, 19, 20	🛒
Milk shake 11, 13, 19, 20	🛒
Popsicles ✓	🛒
Rice-based Drinks ✓	🛒
Sherbet ✓	🛒

Food and Carcinogenic Contaminants	Health Advisory
Little to No Risk Minimal Risk Caution ✓ Recommended	Carcinogen Advisory
Sour Cream, Nonfat ✓	
Soy-based Drinks ✓	
Tofu Cheeses (organic) ✓	
Tofu Cheese Spreads (organic) ✓	
Yogurt, Frozen, Nonfat ✓	
Yogurt, Plain, Lowfat ✓ 11, 20, 23	
Yogurt, Sweetened with Fruit, Lowfat, Nonfat ✓ 11, 20	

EGGS

Health Advisory

Bacterial Contamination

Salmonella: Raw or lightly cooked eggs pose the threat of bacterial contamination. The number of salmonella-poisoning cases associated with Grade A eggs increased six to seven times from 1976 to 1986. High-risk consumers include children under the age of one, pregnant women, the elderly, and those whose immune systems are compromised, including people undergoing cancer treatment and those with AIDS. Many outbreaks have been associated with Grade A eggs that met all state and federal requirements and underwent shell washing with chlorine disinfectants. These outbreaks occurred because the particular strain of salmonella known to cause illnesses is actually *inside* the eggs.

Quite apart from eggs, a wide range of homemade dishes made with raw, unpasteurized eggs could be contaminated with bacteria: homemade mayonnaise, homemade ice cream, milk shakes, Caesar salad, hollandaise sauce, soft omelets, eggs sunny side up, uncooked batter of cakes and cookies, cake filling, pasta with raw-cheese stuffing, stuffing for seafood dishes, rice balls and meatballs made with eggs, eggnog, and potato-egg salad. Many of these foods, when sold commercially, are made with bulk eggs that are pasteurized and sterilized, and they should be free from this particular hazard.

Carcinogens

Pesticides: Eggs are contaminated with carcinogenic pesticide residues. But when contrasted with meat, dairy, seafood, and poultry, the contamination from U.S. chicken eggs is minimal. Duck and quail eggs from China and Thailand are more highly contaminated with pesticides.

Safe Shopping and Cooking Tips

- For protection from salmonellosis, cook eggs well. Do not eat them raw. Microwave cooking will not necessarily destroy salmonella bacteria.
- Seek eggs from companies that certify that their product is free from animal drugs and that the animals were raised humanely, not in cages, but allowed to roam relatively free. The Nest Eggs brand name certifies that eggs are from hens raised humanely without animal drugs. You can now find such brands in many mainstream supermarkets. See also Appendix A, page 392.
- Fertile eggs are less likely to have any antibiotic residues, because roosters and hens cannot be crammed together into cages. Therefore they are less likely to be overcrowded and require animal drugs to prevent the spread of infection.
- Do not buy unrefrigerated eggs. Temperatures between 40°F and 140°F are ideal for salmonella to breed.
- Never leave eggs unrefrigerated for more than two hours.
- Use only uncracked eggs.
- Always wash your hands after working with raw eggs. Do not let raw eggs touch other foods.

Eggs

Food and Carcinogenic Contaminants	Health Advisory
🛒 Little to No Risk 🛒 Minimal Risk 🛒 Caution ✓ Recommended	Carcinogen Advisory
Eggs, Chicken ✓ 11, 13, 20	🛒
Eggs, Duck (U.S.) ✓	🛒
Eggs, Duck (Tawain) 4, 11, 20	🛒
Eggs, Quail (Thailand) 11, 13, 19	🛒

PREPARED AND PROCESSED FOODS

Health Advisory

Carcinogens

Additives: Some additives such as coal tar food colors, potassium bromate, and BHA are carcinogenic or have shown suggestive evidence of carcinogenicity. Products with such ingredients should not be eaten.

Preserved foods: Especially in processed foods containing cured meats such as pepperoni pizza, sausages, and luncheon meats, the presence of nitrite preservatives deserves caution. Nitrites interact with other secondary or tertiary amines in the food, especially following cooking, or in the stomach, to form carcinogenic nitrosamines. While the preservative effect of nitrites is clearly important, safer alternatives are available. Avoid processed or preserved foods, meats, or fish containing nitrites.

Pesticides: In general, carcinogenic pesticides concentrate in processed foods. Brands using organic ingredients are preferable; so are nonfat and low-fat brands.

Safe Shopping Tips

- Prefer nonfat and low-fat processed foods without added coal tar colors and only safe preservatives. Nonfat products are good choices if you are going to eat prepared foods. Their lower fat content is not only healthier for your heart, but it also lowers exposure to carcinogenic pesticide residues.
- Prefer brands with organic ingredients.
- There are certain brands of prepared foods, available in health food stores and more and more frequently in mainstream supermarkets, that offer excellent choices in prepared and processed foods. Look for these labels:

> Amy's Kitchen (vegetable potpies, macaroni and cheese)
> Arrowhead Mills (easy-to-prepare grains)
> Colonel Sanchez (tamales)
> De Bole's (pasta, macaroni and cheese)
> Enrico's (pasta sauces)
> Graindance Pizza
> Health Valley (wide variety of packaged products)
> Heart & Soul (lasagna, spinach quiche, broccoli quiche, potpies)
> Jaclyn's (soups)
> Lima (ratatouille potage, sietan)

Legume (low-calorie microwavable, diet vegetarian meals)
Medallions (salmon patties)
Millina's Finest (organic pasta sauces)
Muir Glen (pasta sauces)
Old Chicago Pizza
Pizsoy
Soy Deli Tofu Burgers
Soy Powder Baked Tofu
Specialty Grain Company (popcorn)
Wildwood Tofu
Yves Veggie Cuisine (vegetarian burgers, deli slices, hot dogs)

Prepared and Processed Foods

These charts are derived from FDA Total Diet Study results. They reflect the limited number of prepared and processed foods analyzed under this program.

Food and Carcinogenic Contaminants	Health Advisory
![Little to No Risk] ![Minimal Risk] ![Caution] ✓ Recommended	Carcinogen Advisory
Beef & Vegetable Stew 11, 13, 24, 25	🛒
Biscuits, Baking Powder ✓	🛒
Chicken Noodle Casserole 11, 13	🛒
Chicken Potpie ✓ 11, 24	🛒
Chili Con Carne, Beef 4, 11, 19, 20	🛒
Coleslaw ✓ 4, 24	🛒
French Fries 11, 13	🛒
Beef, Quarter-Pound Hamburger, Fast Food 4, 11, 13, 19, 20, 24, 28, 31, 32	🛒
Fried Chicken Frozen Dinner ✓	🛒
Lasagna, Homemade 11	🛒
Macaroni & Cheese ✓ 11	🛒

Food and Carcinogenic Contaminants	Health Advisory
	Carcinogen Advisory
Onion Rings 23	🛒
Pizza, Cheese 4, 11, 13, 19, 23, 24	🛒
Pork & Beans ✓	🛒
Pork Chow Mein 11, 23	🛒
Sauerkraut, Canned 13, 23	🛒
Scalloped Potatoes 11, 13	🛒
Soup, Chicken Noodle 11, 23, 24	🛒
Soup, Cream of Tomato 1, 11, 23, 24	🛒
Soup, Vegetable Beef 13	🛒
Spaghetti with Meatsauce, Canned ✓ 11	🛒
Spaghetti with Tomato Sauce, Canned ✓ 23	🛒
Sweet Potatoes, Candied 11, 13, 23	🛒

Legend: 🛒 Little to No Risk · 🛒 Minimal Risk · 🛒 Caution · ✓ Recommended

DESSERTS AND SNACKS

Health Advisory

Carcinogens

Pesticides: Milk chocolate is highly contaminated with residues of BHC and lindane.

Peanut butter is highly contaminated with carcinogenic pesticides, including DDT, dieldrin, and toxaphene. Peanut butter can also be contaminated with the fungus aflatoxin, which is carcinogenic as well.

Pumpkin pie is contaminated with dieldrin; pumpkin pie made with organically grown pumpkins is a better choice.

Safe Shopping and Cooking Tips

- Prefer nonfat desserts and snacks. Substitute nonfat frozen yogurt for ice cream. Prefer low-fat or nonfat milk shakes.

- Substitute carob (without hydrogenated oils) for milk chocolate.
- Substitute organic peanut butter for mainstream brands. Be sure its label certifies it is free from aflatoxins.
- Substitute almond or safflower butter or organic tahini for peanut butter.
- Look for these brands at your health food store or supermarket:

> El Molino (cookies)
> Glenny's Fruit Drops
> Health Valley (a wide variety of nonfat desserts and snack foods)
> Tree of Life (nonfat cookies and snack foods)
> Westbrae (organic cookies)

Desserts and Snacks

Food and Carcinogenic Contaminants	Health Advisory: Carcinogen Advisory
Little to No Risk / Minimal Risk / Caution / ✓ Recommended	
Apple Pie, Frozen ✓ 12, 23	Little to No Risk
Blue Corn Chips (organic) ✓	Little to No Risk
Brownies 11, 13	Minimal Risk
Butter Cookies ✓	Little to No Risk
Cake, Chocolate with Chocolate Icing 4, 23, 24	Minimal Risk
Cake, Yellow ✓ 23	Little to No Risk
Caramel Candy ✓ 13	Little to No Risk
Caramel Custard ✓	Little to No Risk
Carob Brownies (nonfat) ✓	Little to No Risk
Chocolate Eclair 11, 13	Minimal Risk
Chocolate Powder, Sweetened 4, 23, 24	Minimal Risk
Coffee Cake, Frozen 11, 13, 24	Minimal Risk
Cookie, Chocolate Chip 4, 23, 24	Caution
Cookie, Sandwich Type 4, 19, 23, 24	Minimal Risk

Food and Carcinogenic Contaminants	Health Advisory
	Carcinogen Advisory
🛒 Little to No Risk 🛒 Minimal Risk 🛒 Caution ✓ Recommended	
Corn Chips 23	🛒
Danish Pastry/Sweet Roll 4, 23, 24	🛒
Doughnut, Cake Type, Plain 11	🛒
Gelatin, Strawberry ✓	🛒
Key Lime Pie ✓	🛒
Lemon Cake ✓	🛒
Lemon Meringue Pie ✓	🛒
Milk Chocolate 4, 11, 13, 37, 38, 41	🛒
Mince Pie ✓	🛒
Peanut butter 21, 26, 19, 20, 37	🛒
Popcorn ✓ 23	🛒
Potato Chips 11, 13, 20	🛒
Pretzels ✓	🛒
Pudding, Instant, Chocolate 11, 13, 19, 20, 28	🛒
Pumpkin Pie, Frozen 4, 7, 13, 19, 23, 24	🛒
Rice Pudding ✓	🛒
Soda Crackers ✓	🛒
Taffy, Saltwater ✓	🛒

CONDIMENTS, HERBS, AND SPICES

Health Advisory

Carcinogens

Cucumbers (used for pickling) accumulate carcinogenic pesticide residues. Buy pickles made with organically grown cucumbers.

Neurotoxins

Pickles and table salt often contain aluminum additives. Aluminum is neurotoxic, and there is growing evidence of its role in both hyperkinesis (hyperactivity) in children, and Alzheimer's disease. Avoid products containing aluminum.

Safe Shopping Tips

- Prefer nonfat salad dressing and other condiments such as nonfat mayonnaise.
- A wide variety of reasonably priced condiments with organic ingredients can be found at health food stores.
- Choose table salt with nonaluminum anticaking agents.
- Choose baking powder and baking products without sodium aluminum phosphate. Be sure the label specifies that the product contains no aluminum.

Condiments, Herbs, and Spices

Food and Carcinogenic Contaminants	Health Advisory
	Carcinogen Advisory
Little to No Risk · Minimal Risk · Caution · Recommended	
Allspice (nonirradiated) ✓	🛒
Beef Bouillon ✓ 23	🛒
Black Pepper (nonirradiated) ✓	🛒
Brown Gravy ✓	🛒
Catsup (nonorganic) 11	🛒
Catsup (organic) ✓	🛒
Chives (nonirradiated) ✓	🛒
Cilantro ✓	🛒
Cinnamon (nonirradiated) ✓	🛒
Cloves (nonirradiated) ✓	🛒
Dill Pickles 7, 13, 19, 23, 24, 37	🛒

Food and Carcinogenic Contaminants	Health Advisory
	Carcinogen Advisory

Little to No Risk   Minimal Risk   Caution   ✔ Recommended

Dill Pickles (organic) ✔	
Fennel ✔	
Garlic (nonirradiated) ✔	
Ginger, Pickled ✔	
Grape Leaves ✔	
Lemon Juice ✔	
Mayonnaise, Bottled ✔ 23	
Mustard, Dijon ✔	
Mustard, Yellow ✔	
Nutmeg (nonirradiated) ✔	
Parsley (nonirradiated) ✔	
Pepper, Ground (nonirradiated) ✔	
Relish, Pickle 13	
Rosemary (nonirradiated) ✔	
Sage (nonirradiated) ✔	
Salad Dressing, Blue Cheese (nonfat) ✔	
Salad Dressing, Italian ✔	
Salad Dressing, Ranch (nonfat) ✔	
Salt (no aluminum additives) ✔	
Soy Sauce ✔	
Thyme (nonirradiated) ✔	
Tomato Paste ✔	
Tomato Sauce ✔	

Food and Carcinogenic Contaminants	Health Advisory
🛒 *Little to No Risk* 🛒 *Minimal Risk* 🛒 *Caution* ✓ *Recommended*	Carcinogen Advisory
Vanilla Beans ✓	🛒
Vinegar, Apple Cider ✓	🛒
Vinegar ✓	🛒
Vinegar, Raspberry ✓	🛒
Vinegar, Rice Wine ✓	🛒
Vinegar, White Wine ✓	🛒
White Sauce 4, 11, 13, 19, 20, 24, 28	🛒

VEGETABLE OILS

Health Advisory

Carcinogens

Pesticides: Although most oils tend to be fairly free from carcinogenic pesticide residues, soybean oil is contaminated with residues of dieldrin. Safflower oil is contaminated with lindane, which is carcinogenic.

Rancidity: Oils that are improperly stored can become oxidized, leading to formation of oxygen free radicals that are associated with carcinogenic processes.

Safe Shopping and Cooking Tips

- Prefer organic oils. Many brands are available at health food stores.
- Store oils tightly capped and out of the sun. Adding a capsule of vitamin E can help prevent oxidation.
- Look on the label of virtually any brand of margarine, as well as breads, baked goods, and many other items sold in mainstream supermarkets, and you will see an ingredient called "partially hydrogenated" soybean or another oil. This ingredient signals bad news. This unnatural fat could well be a significant contributor to heart disease. Its connection with cancer has been discussed, but the evidence at this time is inconclusive. Furthermore, hydrogenated oils serve no useful nutritional function and make a poor substitute for more nutritious organic oils.

- One of the problems with frying oils is that excessive heat produces oxygen free radicals, which are thought to contribute to damaging bodily processes. This problem is at least partially surmounted through special cooking methods. For example, Chinese chefs put water in their woks first—then oil. The theory behind this cooking method is that water lowers the cooking temperature. Placing vegetables in the frying pan before the oil is added also keeps the oil from overheating.

Vegetable Oils

Food and Carcinogenic Contaminants	Health Advisory
(icons) Little to No Risk	Minimal Risk	Caution	✓ Recommended	Carcinogen Advisory
Almond ✓	🛒
Canola ✓	🛒
Coconut (hydrogenated)	🛒
Cottonseed (hydrogenated)	🛒
Corn (hydrogenated)	🛒
Hydrogenated oils	🛒
Margarine (made with hydrogenated oil)	🛒
Olive ✓	🛒
Palm Kernel (hydrogenated)	🛒
Peanut ✓	🛒
Safflower (nonorganic) 24	🛒
Safflower (high oleic, organic) ✓	🛒
Sesame ✓	🛒
Soybean (nonorganic) 13	🛒
Vegetable Shortening (hydrogenated)	🛒
Walnut ✓	🛒

SWEETENERS, SYRUPS, AND ADDITIVES

Health Advisory

Carcinogens

Aspartame: Aspartame is used in Equal and NutraSweet, as well as in many brands of low-calorie diet foods, desserts, and soft drinks. In 1980, the FDA convened a public board of inquiry (PBOI) to review concerns over aspartame's potential ability to induce brain tumors. Although the PBOI concluded that ingestion of aspartame would not cause brain damage, scientists who had been asked to review scientific findings expressed doubts. The PBOI concluded that experimental data "do not rule out an oncogenic [i.e., giving rise to tumors or tumor formation] effect of aspartame, and that, to the contrary, they appear to suggest the possibility that aspartame, at least when administered in the 'huge' quantities employed in the studies, may contribute to the development of brain tumors." Until these controversial findings on brain cancer in experimental animals have been resolved,use this product sparingly, if at all.

Cyclamates: Used as a sweetener in Canada, cyclamates have shown limited evidence of carcinogenicity. Do not use them.

Saccharin: Used as a sweetener in the United States in soft drinks and table sweeteners such as Sweet'n Low, saccharin is carcinogenic. Do not use it.

Safe Shopping and Cooking Tips

The most nutritious natural sweetener also happens to be lowest in calories. That sweetener is blackstrap molasses, which contains forty-three calories per tablespoon and provides small amounts of thiamin, riboflavin, niacin, calcium, iron, vitamin B-6, phosphorus, and copper. Compare this to white sugar, which has forty-six calories per tablespoon and provides virtually no nutritional value. Dark brown sugar contains fifty-two calories and provides small amounts of calcium, iron, and magnesium. Honey has sixty-four calories, the most of any of the common natural sweeteners, and provides bare traces of vitamin C, thiamin, riboflavin, niacin, calcium, iron, phosphorus, and copper. Corn syrup contains fifty-seven calories and provides small amounts of iron and copper.

For these reasons, the best sweeteners are: molasses (blackstrap), brown sugar, and honey.

Sweeteners, Syrups, and Additives

Food and Carcinogenic Contaminants	Health Advisory
	Carcinogen Advisory
Aspartame	🛒
Brown Sugar ✓	🛒
Corn Syrup	🛒
Cyclamate	🛒
Equal	🛒
Honey ✓	🛒
Maple Syrup ✓	🛒
Molasses (Blackstrap) ✓	🛒
Rose Syrup ✓	🛒
Saccharin	🛒
Sorghum Syrup	🛒
White Sugar	🛒

Legend: 🛒 *Little to No Risk* · 🛒 *Minimal Risk* · 🛒 *Caution* · ✓ *Recommended*

BABY FOODS

Health Advisory

Carcinogens

Pesticides. The embryo, fetus, infant, and young child are much more sensitive and susceptible to carcinogenic pesticide residues than the adult for the following reasons: (1) Because of their smaller size, pound for pound babies receive a greater dose; (2) The baby's liver often lacks certain enzymes required for breaking down pesticides; (3) Babies' and toddlers' immune systems are not as strong as those of adults; (4) The baby's cells undergo rapid growth and may be more susceptible to carcinogens than cells that are more static. In spite of these concerns, the EPA's tolerance-setting procedures have always been calculated for adults.

One recent report notes that "millions of children in the United States receive up to 35 percent of their entire lifetime dose of some carcinogenic pesticides by age 5. . . . By the average child's first birthday, the combined cancer risk from just eight pesticides on 20 foods exceeds the EPA's estimated lifetime level of 'acceptable risk' of one-in-one-million additional cancers throughout the U.S. population." These exposures can result in a high incidence of childhood and subsequent adult cancers. Thus, it is essential that children be protected from carcinogenic chemicals. The best way to do that is to make sure they receive only organically grown foods and purified water.

Shopping and Cooking Tips

- Buy only organically grown baby food. Earth's Best organic baby foods are available at supermarkets throughout the country. The company is located at: P.O. Box 887, Middlebury, VT 05753, (800) 442-4221.

Baby Foods

Food and Carcinogenic Contaminants	Health Advisory Carcinogen Advisory
🛒 Little to No Risk 🛒 Minimal Risk 🛒 Caution ✓ Recommended	
Applesauce 12, 14, 31, 35	🛒
Beef 11, 13, 20, 23	🛒
Beef & Vegetables 6, 11, 20, 23	🛒
Carrots ✓ 11, 20, 23	🛒
Chicken & Noodles	🛒
Chicken/Turkey 11, 13, 20, 23	🛒
Chicken/Turkey & Vegetables 11, 19, 23	🛒
Corn, Creamed ✓	🛒
Dutch Apple/Apple Betty 12, 23, 31	🛒
Fruit Dessert with Tapioca ✓ 14, 23	🛒
Green Beans ✓ 1, 11, 23	🛒
Ham & Vegetables 11, 13, 23	🛒
Infant Formula with Iron ✓ 23	🛒

Food and Carcinogenic Contaminants	Health Advisory

	Carcinogen Advisory
🛒 Little to No Risk 🛒 Minimal Risk 🛒 Caution ✓ Recommended	
Infant Formula without Iron ✓ 23	🛒
Infant Mixed Cereal ✓ 11	🛒
Juice, Apple/Apple Cherry/Apple Grape ✓	🛒
Juice, Orange/Orange Pineapple ✓	🛒
Oatmeal with Applesauce/Banana ✓ 23	🛒
Peaches 11, 23, 31, 35	🛒
Pears/Pears with Pineapple 11, 13, 23, 31, 33	🛒
Peas ✓	🛒
Pork 11, 20, 23	🛒
Pudding/Custard ✓ 23	🛒
Spinach, Creamed 11, 17, 23, 33	🛒
Sweet Potato 1, 13, 23	🛒
Tapioca with Prunes/Plums 11, 13, 31, 35	🛒
Tapioca with Bananas & Pineapple ✓	🛒
Tomato, Beef & Macaroni	🛒
Turkey & Rice 23	🛒
Vegetables, Mixed ✓ 11, 23	🛒
Vegetables with Bacon/Ham (sulfa drugs)	🛒
Vegetables with Beef 11, 13	🛒
Vegetables with Turkey/Chicken 23	🛒

CHAPTER 15

Beverages

TAP WATER

Health Advisory

Water is the universal elixir, used in virtually all beverages, ranging from soft drinks to coffee and tea, as well as in cooking. But the majority of the water on earth is too salty to use, or it is hidden away in inaccessible underground rivers, seas, and lakes. The little usable water remaining is now under intense pressure from population growth, overuse, and industrial and agricultural pollution.

Our bodies are made of two-thirds water; it touches virtually all our tissues and cells, especially those of the bladder and kidneys, which concentrate contaminants contained in drinking water.

The water Americans drink generally comes from either municipal water supplies or private wells. But the safety of both sources has been seriously undermined by the government's failure to enforce clean water regulations and to protect resources from polluting industries, as well as to ensure that the methods of disinfecting are used safely. As one recent report notes, "Many state programs for protecting drinking water are in disarray due to inadequate funding, inability or unwillingness to adopt EPA's mandatory drinking water regulations in a timely fashion, and failure to enforce the Safe Drinking Water Act's rules requiring drinking water protection." The report also noted that the EPA has found that in men, better control of lead alone in drinking water could prevent over 680,000 cases of hypertension, 650 strokes, 880 heart attacks, and 670 premature deaths from heart disease every year. Furthermore, lead in drinking water harms the health of millions of children and has contributed to blood lead levels in excess of the

Centers for Disease Control's defined level of concern for blood lead levels in more than 560,000 children. Finally, the report noted that there were some 250,000 violations of the Safe Drinking Water Act in 1991 and 1992 in 43 percent of the water systems serving 120 million people.

Lead contamination, however, is only a small part of the concern for the safety of our drinking water. The drinking water of an estimated fifty million people in the United States comes from groundwater that is potentially contaminated from agricultural chemicals, including pesticides and nitrates.

Approximately nineteen million of these people get their water from private wells, which are most vulnerable to water contamination.

Today, your tap water may be contaminated with bacteria, viruses, and other pathogens, trihalomethanes (THMs) and other disinfecting by-products, as well as arsenic, lead, and radioactive contaminants. Contamination is also of concern for beverages made from municipal water, ranging from orange juice to beer, and food cooked in contaminated water.

The problem is exacerbated by the presence of VOCs such as THMs and other industrial pollutants. If you have tap water that contains VOCs, such as the carcinogens benzene or trichloroethylene, roughly one-third or less of your exposure to these volatile organic chemicals will come from drinking and cooking. One-third or greater will come from skin absorption, and approximately another one-third or greater from inhalation from sources such as dishwashers, washing machines, toilets, bathing, and showering. In fact, the exposure from inhalation of volatilized contaminants while showering may be greater than the exposure from drinking. And when you do have contaminated water, purifying methods should ideally account for all of these exposures. See also *Water Filters,* page 170.

Bacterial Contamination

One report notes, "Hundreds of water systems that use surface water do not protect their watersheds or filter their water to remove disease-carrying organisms." Nearly one million Americans get sick each year from microbiologically contaminated water. Some nine hundred die from such contamination. In 1993, between 370,000 and 430,000 residents of Milwaukee became ill from the presence of the microbiological organism *Cryptosporidium* that contaminated their drinking water. And in Cabool, Missouri, three deaths were attributed to contamination of drinking water by *E. coli* bacteria. These are not isolated incidences. At greatest risk are infants, the elderly, and persons with compromised immune systems such as AIDS patients, individuals undergoing chemotherapy, and those with liver disease. See *Water Filters,* especially sections on membrane filters for home protection from many kinds of microbiological contaminants.

Carcinogens

Arsenic: A major cancer risk, arsenic contaminates the drinking water of millions of Americans. One report notes that some 350,000 Americans drink water containing levels of arsenic in excess of lenient federal standards, and that 2.5 million people drink water containing more than twenty-five parts per billion (ppb) arsenic, about half the federal standard of fifty ppb. Even very low levels of arsenic in drinking water present a major cancer threat. A California study found that the EPA standard of fifty ppb presents a cancer risk of one cancer in every one hundred people, one thousand to ten thousand times greater than the government's so-called negligible risk guidelines.

Chlorination and trihalomethanes (THMs): The public water supplies of some two hundred million Americans are chlorinated to reduce bacterial levels. Chlorination is a major disinfecting method that successfully prevents bacterially related illnesses. However, chlorination of water already contaminated with organic compounds and other carcinogenic pollutants produces additional carcinogenic compounds called trihalomethanes. Most major municipal water supplies deliver water that has gone through activated carbon filtration, which sharply reduces the levels of THMs; still, the levels can be elevated to the point of posing clear cancer risks. In the case of small municipalities there may be insufficient water treatment, and levels may be elevated as well.

More than one hundred million Americans consume water contaminated with significant levels of THMs. There is growing evidence that chlorinated drinking water causes bladder cancer and rectal cancer. THMs are responsible for 10,700 or more rectal and bladder cancers annually—more people die each year from THMs than from fires and handguns. Because of widespread pollution of drinking water with organic contaminants, many water supplies that are chlorinated probably contain some amount of THM. If above about ten ppb, they should not be used for human consumption, cooking, showering, or other household chores unless they have gone through an effective home filtration system. THMs are highly volatile and exposure in the home results from all possible avenues, including inhalation and skin absorption.

Public water suppliers should be pressured to switch to a disinfecting process called ozonation, which is safer than chlorination and highly effective. Furthermore, industry should be strictly regulated to prevent the discharge of a wide range of industrial pollutants that also act as catalysts for the formation of THMs. Realistically, because such changes in filtration or industrial discharge are unlikely to occur soon, consumers need to take personal responsibility for making sure their tap water is safe. Adequate home filtration with activated carbon can remove THMs.

Fluoride: There is limited evidence that fluoride is carcinogenic.

Industrial pollutants: Many public water supplies are contaminated with carcinogenic industrial chemicals such as perchloroethylene and trichloroethylene.

Lead: Lead is carcinogenic. Older cities may still be using lead pipes in public water systems built before the 1930s. Any city with soft (i.e., corrosive) water—particularly in northeastern states such as Massachusetts and Pennsylvania where acid rain is a problem—could be delivering lead-tainted water. The government will test water only up to the point of delivery to your home. Once water flows through your home's plumbing, you are on your own. *And most lead exposures result from home plumbing.* For example, in April 1994, the EPA reported that brass fittings on submersible well pumps are capable of leaching high levels of lead into well water; the latest study showed that commonly used well pumps can contaminate drinking water with lead levels some five hundred times greater than federal regulations allow. Consumers must perform their own tests. Such tests cost about thirty-five dollars. See *Water Filters* on page 170 for more information on testing and water testing companies.

Pesticides: If you live in a rural agricultural area and you draw water from a private well, your water may be contaminated with a variety of chemicals ranging from carcinogenic, neurotoxic, teratogenic, and immunotoxic pesticides such as alachlor, aldicarb, atrazine, dibromochloropropane (DBCP), and ethylene dibromide (EDB). A recent study by the U.S. Geological Survey found that more than one-quarter of samples of water from the Mississippi River Basin contained atrazine at levels exceeding the EPA's maximum contaminant level. Atrazine, as with several other pesticides found in drinking water such as DBCP and EDB, causes breast cancer. Atrazine also causes human ovarian cancer. Although many people think of pesticide contamination as a problem associated with private wells, some one out of ten public water supply wells contain pesticides, and nearly ten thousand community drinking water wells contain pesticides. A body of evidence incriminates pesticides in drinking water as a cause of human cancer. Do not drink water that is contaminated with pesticides!

Radiation: More than forty-nine million Americans consume water with significant radioactive contamination, because of radon, radium, and alpha particle emitters, and most ominously because of beta particle emitters from man-made fission products such as strontium 90, which damage the immune cells of the bone marrow and are carcinogenic. There is suggestive evidence that radiation-contaminated water supplies are in part responsible for escalating breast cancer mortality in some areas of the country. Recent evidence suggests that increased breast cancer incidence in the Long Island counties of Suffolk and Nassau, as well as Westchester County north of New York City, are related to radiation-contaminated drinking water. This is due to radioactive contamination of the

Croton River watershed reservoirs; the watershed is located only about five miles downwind to the northeast from the Indian Point nuclear plant that has released radioactive fission products since the early 1960s. As for Suffolk and Nassau counties, their drinking water supplies are derived largely from deep aquifer wells that have become contaminated slowly by nuclear fallout contaminated with radioactive strontium 90.

There are also natural sources of radiation contamination of drinking water. For example, areas with granite rock outcroppings often have elevated levels of radium, a breakdown product of uranium, in their drinking water, especially if their supply is derived from groundwater.

Radon, the breakdown product of radium, is also found in drinking water, especially in the northeastern states such as Maine, New Hampshire, Massachusetts, New Jersey, Pennsylvania, and Vermont.

Although the government should clean up radiation-contaminated drinking water supplies, it does not; therefore, it is important to have tap water tested for radiation contamination. Radiation can be removed from drinking supplies by proper filtration, especially reverse osmosis, distillation, and, to some extent, the use of activated carbon. See *Water Filters* for information on water testing and the best methods of removing radiation from drinking water.

Neurotoxins

Aluminum: Sometimes found in drinking water, aluminum is neurotoxic and appears to play a role in Alzheimer's disease. Aluminum can be removed from drinking water through reverse osmosis.

Pesticides: Several pesticides that contaminate water, including parathion and other members of the organophosphate family, are neurotoxic.

Volatile organic chemicals (VOCs): Many VOCs, such as chloroform, perchloroethylene, and trichloroethylene, are neurotoxic. It is important that filtration methods for VOCs eliminate them from all sources of exposures, including inhalation and skin absorption.

Reproductive Toxins

Lead: Exposure to lead during pregnancy can result in a child's diminished cognitive function, low birth weight, and premature birth.

Safe Use Tips

- Request analytical information from your public water supplier. If you have THMs above ten ppb, or other industrial contaminants or pesticides are present at any level, install adequate filtration or use safe bottled water.

- Use a private laboratory to monitor your water supply for contamination. Several companies perform tests for lead, bacteria, minerals, nitrates, industrial solvents, and pesticides. Costs range from around $30 to over $200 for testing for all contaminants. Your health is worth the expense.
- If you intend to filter your water, a point-of-entry system, which filters all the water entering your home, is best. See *Water Filters*, page 170, for information on decontaminating your home's tap water.
- Since common water contaminants such as THMs and industrial chemicals can be inhaled and absorbed through the skin, it is advisable to filter showers and baths. Such filters can be bought for $50 to $100.
- Never drink water from the tap unless you have let it run for one to two minutes. One New York City couple with a baby discovered that their water had eight ppb lead on the first flush. Allowing their water to run for one or two minutes reduced lead contamination to nondetectable levels.
- If you draw water from a household well with a submersible pump that has brass fittings, check it for lead. The most prudent consumer will replace such pumps. The cost of a new, lead-free pump is $200 to $300.
- There are two toll-free telephone numbers to answer questions about lead and drinking water in general: (800) 426-4791; (800) 424-LEAD.

BOTTLED WATER

Bottled water is an important alternative to tap water, and sales are exploding throughout the country as consumers learn that tap water is often unfit for safe human consumption. And there are indeed times when the use of bottled water is warranted for your health. For example, if your water comes from surface sources that are within twenty or thirty miles of a chemical or nuclear plant or downwind of such plants, bottled water from a deep spring source is a better shopping choice. But consumers must also be aware that some bottled water is no better than water from the tap, and the quality varies tremendously. Surveys have found a wide range of organic contaminants in bottled water, as well as radiation. As consumers are spending hundreds of times more money for bottled water than they would for tap water and relying on its quality for health-related reasons, it is imperative that the bottled water industry be strictly regulated to ensure that their products are free from contamination. For example, one causal factor in hypertension in predisposed individuals is excess sodium intake. Sodium levels in any water source should be nondetectable or no more than a few milligrams per liter. Yet surveys conducted throughout the 1980s found that several popular bottled waters contained excess amounts of sodium.

The quality of bottled water is regulated no more strictly than tap water. Currently, without such regulation, full label disclosure should be provided for the product's chemical content. If this information is not provided on the label or when requested by consumers, such products should be avoided.

If you buy bottled water, then ask the company you patronize for laboratory analyses that provide evidence that its product is free from contaminants. Also, pressure your supermarket to demand from their bottled water suppliers that their products be certified free from contamination. And ideally, to be really certain of the quality of bottled water, consumers should have their favorite bottled water tested.

In some circumstances, bottled water is preferable to tap water—for example, if your home has lead pipes or lead-soldered pipes; if your public drinking water supply is contaminated with THMs, radiation, or other industrial chemicals or pesticides, or exceeds EPA standards for other contaminants such as arsenic or sodium; or if you have a family history of cancer and need to limit your exposure to carcinogens.

To be sure your choice of a bottled water is safer than your tap water:

- Request monitoring reports from your bottled water supplier.
- Test your bottled water privately.
- Prefer bottled waters whose sources are from very deep springs. The deeper the spring, the less likely the water is to be affected by nuclear fallout and petrochemicals.

COFFEE, TEA, SOFT DRINKS, AND
OTHER BEVERAGES CONTAINING CAFFEINE

Health Advisory

Carcinogens

Coffee should be consumed in moderation. Heavy coffee consumption has been cited as a possible cause of urinary bladder cancer.

Methylene chloride, used to decaffeinate coffee, is carcinogenic. Use any brands of decaffeinated coffee with caution, unless the label specifically states it was decaffeinated using the Swiss water process or other similar nonsolvent processes.

Soft drinks can be contaminated with chloroform because of the use of chlorinated tap water in their production, carcinogenic artificial sweeteners such as saccharin, and aluminum, which is neurotoxic, and leaches into the drink from aluminum containers.

Avoid diet soft drinks sweetened with cyclamates or saccharin, all of which have shown evidence of carcinogenicity.

Water used for many canned and bottled beverages is chlorinated and contains chloroform and other trihalomethanes that are carcinogenic. Consume soft drinks with caution, unless the label specifically states that the water has been filtered or purified. Avoid beverages containing aspartame. We mentioned earlier long-standing suggestive evidence of its carcinogenicity. Furthermore, when heated, such as when soft drinks are stored at improperly high temperatures in warehouses, aspartame breaks down into methanol, which is highly toxic, and formaldehyde, which is carcinogenic.

Reproductive Toxins

Both men and women of childbearing age should limit consumption of caffeine. High consumption of caffeine by the father can result in increased incidence of spontaneous abortions, stillbirths, and premature births. In one study, women who consumed seven cups of coffee or more daily were found to have an increased incidence of babies born with defects. Heavy consumption was defined as seven cups of coffee or more daily. Caffeine is added to soft drinks and chocolate and found naturally in coffee and tea.

Aspartame "may cause a few cases of mental retardation a year" in children of women who are unaware that they have the disease phenylketonuria (PKU). Individuals with PKU have difficulty metabolizing the amino acid phenylalanine, which aspartame contains. This inherited disorder can cause mental retardation. All women who are of childbearing age should determine whether they have PKU before ingesting foods containing aspartame during pregnancy.

Safe Shopping Tips

Coffee

- Organic coffees are widely available at health food stores and are priced competitively with other gourmet coffees.
- Prefer coffee decaffeinated with the Swiss water or other nonsolvent processes.
- Prefer teas to coffee, as traditional teas have been shown to be free of carcinogenicity. Be sure to consult a physician, however, if you intend to drink herbal teas during pregnancy, as some herbal teas may cause complications.

Soft Drinks and Other Beverages

- Look for canned drinks and juices that use purified or filtered water.
- Avoid beverages containing saccharin and other artificial sweeteners, as well as artificial colors.

- Prefer beverages in glass containers. Aluminum or plastic containers may leach contaminants into drinks. Do not drink from aluminum containers that have been sitting in storage for longer than a few weeks, as dangerously high amounts of aluminum may migrate from the container into the beverage.

ALCOHOLIC BEVERAGES

Health Advisory

Carcinogens

Pure alcohol is not carcinogenic. However, there is substantial evidence that alcoholic beverages do contain carcinogens. Alcoholic beverages have long been associated with cancers of the mouth, esophagus, and liver. More recent evidence, from a wide range of sources, associates excessive consumption with increased risk for breast cancer, which may be due to alcohol's ability to stimulate women's bodies to produce toxic metabolites of estrogenic hormones. Furthermore, consumption of any kind of alcohol in excess may cause cirrhosis of the liver, which in turn can lead to liver cancer. The problem is compounded by the presence of other unwelcome contaminants, including the following:

Asbestos: Asbestos fibers have been found in a wide range of alcoholic beverages worldwide, probably because of the filters used in clarifying beverages, from water used during production processes, and from asbestos-cement water pipes. Asbestos is a known human carcinogen.

Lead: Many fine wines are contaminated with lead from the foil around their corks.

Pesticides: A wide range of pesticides is used in vineyards. Most commonly detected carcinogenic pesticides in U.S. and European wines include dimethoate and procymidone. Other carcinogenic pesticide residues that may be found in wine include arsenic compounds, metalaxyl, carbendazim, vinclozolin, iprodione, trichlorfon and its metabolite dichlorvos, and ethylenethiourea (ETU), which is a degradation product of the family of ethylene bisdithiocarbamate fungicides zineb, maneb, mancozeb, and nabam. Dichlorvos causes breast cancer in rodents.

Urethane: Urethane is present in many kinds of alcoholic beverages. Urethane has caused breast cancers in 100 percent of experimental animals in one study and has caused them to appear almost twice as early. Urethane promotes the effects of X rays in causing these tumors. Urethane has caused cancers in single doses. Although urethane is a known contaminant of alcoholic beverages and has been known to cause mammary tumors in experimental animal studies since 1962, not a single epidemiological study has been performed. Its widespread presence in alcoholic beverages is troubling, especially considering its cancer-promoting and synergistic effects. The alcohol industry has taken no steps to remove this contaminant. Federal regulators allowed the liquor industry to continue to produce beverages with urethane. The urethane problem will persist for years to come. Follow the safe shopping guidelines to make sure the alcoholic beverages you buy are urethane-free.

Safe Shopping Tips

- Many excellent organic wines are available in health food stores, liquor stores, and sometimes mainstream supermarkets. Mail-order sources are included in Appendix A.
- Use a clean towel or cloth to wipe the neck of wine bottles wrapped with foil to reduce the lead levels.
- Alcoholic beverages most likely to be tainted with urethane are American bourbon whiskeys, European fruit brandies (especially cherry, plum, and other stone fruits), cream sherries, port wines, Japanese sakes, Chinese wines, and European liqueurs. Rums have moderately low levels of urethane. Tequila has very low levels. Vodka and gin have virtually none. Champagne and sparkling wine have low levels. Domestic beers and other malt beverages have very low levels; however, imported beers may be contaminated.

CHAPTER   16

Food Safety Issues

PACKAGING

Health Advisory

Carcinogens

Cling film: Cling film contains carcinogens such as di-2-ethylhexyl phthalate (DEHP) and di-2-ethylhexyl adipate (DEHA), which will migrate into foods, especially fatty foods. Such films are used for wrapping cheese and packaging fruit, vegetables, meat, and fish.

Microwave packaging: The FDA has recognized that chemical components of adhesives, polymers, paper, and paperboard products used in microwave packaging migrate into food but has developed virtually no regulations.

Microwaving some packaging may cause it to disintegrate, allowing carcinogens and other uncharacterized chemicals contained in the packaging to enter food. Heat susceptor packages, which help elevate temperatures during microwaving for browning foods, have been shown to contain chemicals that can migrate into foods. These chemicals have been poorly studied, and nobody really knows how much of a hazard they present to the consumer. But what is known is that one such chemical, contained in microwave packaging, that can migrate into foods—dimethyl terephthalate—has shown suggestive evidence of carcinogenicity. Heat susceptor packaging, in particular, is used for microwaving products such as popcorn, pizza, french fries, fish sticks, and Belgian waffles.

"Dual ovenables" are containers that can be used in either conventional or microwave ovens. Some prepared foods packaged in disposable trays, for use in either conventional or microwave ovens, may be contaminated with packaging chemicals at far higher rates when used in a conventional oven. Again, how much these chemicals pose hazards is difficult to determine.

PET bottling and packaging: Polyethylene terephthalate (PET) is used extensively in soft drink containers. PET bottles can release small amounts of dimethyl terephthalate into foods and beverages. Although the National Cancer Institute claims that dimethyl terephthalate is noncarcinogenic, these results have been questioned. Some experts believe this compound to be carcinogenic. Unfortunately PET bottling and packaging is widely used, and it may be difficult to find substitutes at this time. When possible, however, prefer glass containers to those made from PET.

Plastic wrap: Plastic wrap contains residual vinylidene chloride, which is carcinogenic. We advise against its use.

Neurotoxins

Aluminum foil: Foil-wrapping food may be convenient, but it is not necessarily good for you. Foods cooked or stored in aluminum foil wrap or aluminum cookware invariably have some small quantity of the aluminum leached into them.

Safe Shopping and Cooking Tips

- Buy foods such as fruits in bulk without cling wraps. Use paper bags for carrying them or cloth bags made from organic material such as cotton.
- Buy meat and poultry fresh rather than wrapped in packages with cling wrap or styrene. Have meat and poultry wrapped in butcher's paper or waxed paper.
- Transfer microwavable foods that come in disposable trays for use either in a conventional or microwave oven to a stainless-steel baking pan or Pyrex glassware.
- Use wax paper, freezer paper, or glass food containers such as Pyrex glassware for food storage.
- Whenever possible, buy juices, soft drinks, beer, milk, and other beverages in glass containers rather than in aluminum or plastic. This is especially important for bottled water. If buying products in aluminum or plastic, keep out of the heat and use promptly without extended periods of storage.

POTS AND PANS

Health Advisory

Aluminum: Do not use aluminum pans. Alzheimer's disease is clearly a multifactorial disease, and there is growing evidence that aluminum may be one of the causes, or it may exacerbate the disease. Aluminum is neurotoxic. Aluminum pans can be a substantial source of this toxin in the diet. If you boil an acidic-type vegetable or fruit such as rhubarb for thirty minutes in an aluminum saucepan, you can measure between 300 and 400 milligrams (mg) per liter of aluminum escaping from that pan. If you mix a salad in an aluminum utensil and sprinkle in some vinegar to go with the olive oil, you will be getting aluminum as a dressing additive, researchers note.

Cast iron: Safe.

Ceramic: Generally be wary of ceramic cookware from Italy, India, China, Mexico, and Hong Kong; they can leach dangerous amounts of lead into food.

Copper: Use copper pans only if they are lined with tin or stainless steel. Most high-quality copperware is lined. If the lining has worn out, the pan can be relined.

Glass: Safest cooking material.

Stainless steel: Very safe and an excellent choice for all-around cooking. The only problem may be with people who are allergic to nickel and consume highly acidic foods such as rhubarb or stewed tomatoes cooked in stainless steel.

Teflon: Safe when used properly, teflon is inert except at extremely high temperatures when it may give off fumes. It also allows the use of less oil.

MOLD

Is it safe to eat food when it shows the slightest bit of mold? Because some molds produce carcinogenic aflatoxins, it is a good idea to deal safely with these unwelcome guests. These safe kitchen tips deal with mold:

- If a small moldy spot appears on the following foods, you do not need to throw them out: jam and jelly, hard cheese, and firm fruits and vegetables (e.g., cabbage, bell peppers, and carrots). For hard foods, use a clean knife to slice away the mold and a bit more. Place the food in a clean container and consume promptly. For jam or jelly, use a spoon to clean out the mold. Use a second, clean spoon to remove a larger area around the mold. Any kind of off taste means the food has fermented and gone bad.
- Even the slightest appearance of mold means you should toss out any kind of soft cheese including processed cheese slices and cottage cheese. The

same goes for cream, sour cream, yogurt, bread, cake, buns, pastries, corn on the cob, nuts, flour, whole grains, rice, dried peas or beans, and peanut butter.

IRRADIATION

Health Advisory

Irradiation is the process of exposing foods to high-level radiation to kill bacteria, insects, and molds. Massive doses of ionizing radiation (100,000 rads, roughly equivalent to ten million medical X rays) are used.

Food irradiation was the brainchild of the Atomic Energy Commission's efforts during the Eisenhower administration to find practical uses for the flood of radioactive wastes from nuclear weapons.

Atomic Energy of Canada (Nordion Ltd.), with its virtual monopoly on cobalt-60 and with strong backing from the International Atomic Energy Agency, hopes to operate a chain of U.S. plants with U.S. irradiation companies.

Industry and the FDA insist that irradiated food has been thoroughly tested and is absolutely safe. Foods approved for treatment include fruits and vegetables, dry and dehydrated herbs, spices, teas, pork, poultry, white potatoes, wheat, and wheat flour. However, New York, New Jersey, and Maine have prohibited the sale and distribution of irradiated food, as have foreign governments, including Germany, Denmark, Sweden, Australia, and New Zealand.

Claims of safety are unproven at best. High-energy irradiation produces complex chemical changes in food with the formation of poorly characterized radiolytic products, including benzene. Radiolytic products kill bacteria, molds, and larvae, and thus prevent spoilage, a major attraction to the purveyors of produce and poultry contaminated with salmonella and *E. coli*. However, concentrated extracts of irradiated food products have never been tested for cancer and other delayed adverse effects. The need for such studies is overdue, especially in light of numerous reports of chronic toxic effects in studies on test animals that were fed unextracted, whole irradiated food. The studies found reproductive damage in rodents and chromosomal damage in rodents, monkeys, and children.

An Indian study discovered chromosomal abnormalities in malnourished children fed freshly irradiated wheat.

Irradiation also reduces levels of essential nutrients in food, especially vitamins A, C, E, and the B complex. Cooking irradiated food reduces these levels further. A Japanese study found vitamin C content of potatoes reduced nearly 50 percent. The industry admits to this but suggests that the problem could be taken care of by vitamin supplements. But the decrease in these vitamins suggests that other related nutrients and beneficial plant substances, not available through supplements, may also have been decreased.

Another area of possible carcinogenicity deals with workers who will be exposed to cobalt-60 or cesium-137 and communities where such radioactive materials are transported and stored. In 1988, at a Decatur, Georgia, plant that irradiated medical supplies, some steel rods corroded, exposing employees to radiation and contaminating twenty-five thousand gallons of water with radioactive isotopes.

Despite this evidence, the FDA approved food irradiation in 1986. The FDA based its decision on five questionable or allegedly negative tests and on theoretical estimates on cancer risk, which were claimed to be insignificant and "acceptable." This position is consistent with the FDA's revocation of the Delaney law, which banned the deliberate contamination of food with any amount of carcinogenic chemicals, and its substitution by flexible "rubber number" standards based on "acceptable" cancer risk. Furthermore, the now-approved use of irradiation to solve the bacterial contamination problem associated with poultry is ill-advised; such problems would be better solved through the use of more government inspection and tighter and higher standards for animal care and processing.

Safe Shopping Tips

- Herbs and spices are authorized for irradiation; spices that have been imported or are used in processed foods are likely to have undergone irradiation. Be sure you buy spices whose labels specifically state they are not irradiated. One of the nation's leading spice companies, McCormick, does not irradiate its consumer products. McCormick says it will not do it without full public disclosure.

- Irradiated whole foods, such as strawberries, must be displayed with the radura symbol, which resembles a stylized flower, and a statement such as "treated with ionizing radiation." Look for this symbol and avoid foods that carry it.

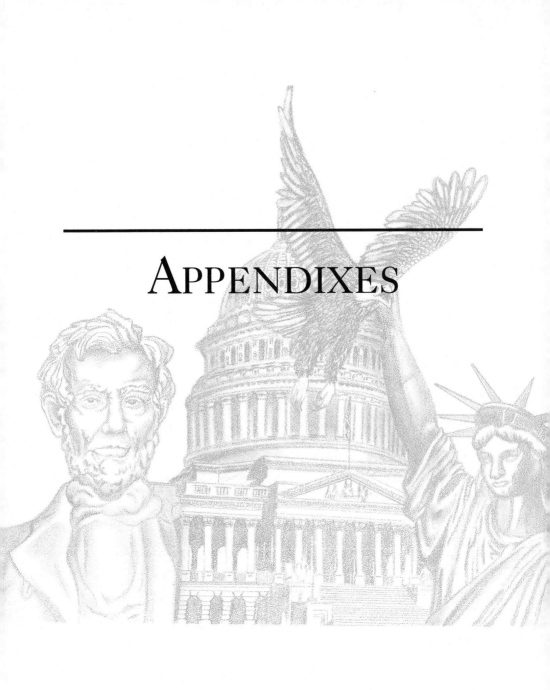

APPENDIXES

Mail-Order Sources for Safer Household Products and Organic Foods

HOUSEHOLD PRODUCTS

Cleaning Products

AFM Enterprises
1960 Chicago Avenue
Suite E-7
Riverside, CA 92507
(909) 781-6860

Auro Organics
Auro/Sinan
P.O. Box 857
Davis, CA 95617-0857
(916) 753-3104

Biofa/Bau, Inc.
P.O. Box 190
Alton, NH 03809
(603) 364-2400

Cal Ben Soap Company
9828 Pearmain Street
Oakland, CA 94603
(510) 638-7091

Chef's Soap
Abbaco Inc.
230 Fifth Avenue
New York, NY 10001

Dasun/Nonscents
P.O. Box M
Escondido, CA 92033
(800) 433-8929

Ecco Bella
6 Provost Square
Suite 602
Caldwell, NJ 07006
(201) 616-0220

Ecover Products
Mercantile Food Company
4 Old Mill Road
P.O. Box 1140
Georgetown, CT 06829
(203) 544-9891

Granny's Old Fashioned
Products
P.O. Box 256
Arcadia, CA 91006
(818) 577-1825

The Greenspan
P.O. Box 4656
Boulder, CO 80306
(303) 444-3440

Infinity Herbal Products
Division of Jedmon
Products Ltd.
Toronto, Canada M3J 3J9

Life Tree Products
A Division of Sierra Dawn
P.O. Box 1203
Sebastopol, CA 95472
(707) 823-3920

Livos Plant Chemistry
1365 Rufina Circle
Santa Fe, NM 87501
(505) 438-3448

Mia Rose Products, Inc.
(714) 662-5465
(800) 292-6339

Natural Chemistry, Inc.
244 Elm Street
New Canaan, CT 06840
(800) 753-1233

Naturally Yours
Ecolo-clean
1405-C North Nias
Springfield, MO 65802
(417) 865-6260

Simmons Pure Soaps
Simmons Handcrafts
42295 Highway 36
Bridgeville, CA 95526
(707) 777-3280

Tropical Soap Company
P.O. Box 31673
Dallas, TX 75231

Wood Finishing Supply
100 Throop Street
Palmyra, NY 14522
(315) 597-3743

Paint Products

AllSafe Paint Company
Albuquerque, NM 87109

Auro/Sinan
P.O. Box 857
Davis, CA 95617-0857
(916) 753-3104

Biofa/Bau, Inc.
P.O. Box 190
Alton, NH 03809

Glidden and the Environment
925 Euclid Avenue
Cleveland, OH 44115
(800) 367-0862

Livos Plant Chemistry
1365 Rufina Circle
Santa Fe, NM 87501
(505) 438-3448

Miller Paint Co., Inc.
12730 NE Whitaker Way
Portland, OR 97230
(503) 255-0190

Pace Chem Industries
779 La Grange Avenue
Newbury Park, CA 91320
(805) 499-2911

Home and Garden Pesticides

Perma Proof Corporation
1927 West Howard Street
Chicago, IL 60626
(312) 764-5559
Boric acid preparations for cockroaches.

Phoenix Farm and Garden
Supply Co.
311 W. 72d Street
Kansas City, MO 64114
Diatomaceous earth.

Natural Gardening Resource
Center
P.O. Box 149
Sunman, IN 47041

Arizona Biological Control
P.O. Box 4247 CRB
Tucson, AZ 85738
(602) 825-9785
Natural enemies.

Beneficial Insectary
14751 Oak Run Road
Oak Run, CA 96069
(916) 472-3715
Natural enemies.

Beneficial Insects, Inc.
P.O. Box 40634
Memphis, TN 38174-0634
(901) 276-6879
Natural enemies.

Biosys
1057 E. Meadow Circle
Palo Alto, CA 94303
Nematodes.

Nematec
P.O. Box 758
San Leandro, CA 94577
Nematodes.

Evans BioControl Inc.
895 Interlocken Parkway,
Unit A
Broomfield, CO 80020
Nematodes.

Biologic
418 Briar Lane
Chambersburg, PA 17201
Nematodes.

Pet Products

The Natural Pet Care
Company
2713 East Madison
Seattle, WA 98112
(800) 962-8266

Wow-Bow Distributors
13B Lucon Drive
Deer Park, NY 11729
(516) 254-6064
(800) 326-0230

Air Filters

AllerMed Corporation
31 Steel Road
Wylie, TX 75098
A wide range of air filters including those for cars.

Cotton Clothing

Eco Sport
28 James Street
South Hackensack, NJ 07606
(201) 489-0389
(800) 486-4326

Earth Care
Ukiah, CA 95482-8507
(800) 347-0070

Jantz Design
PO Box 3071
Santa Rosa, CA 95402
(800) 365-6563

Natural Lifestyle Supplies
16 Lookout Drive
Asheville, NC 28804
(800) 752-2775

Seventh Generation
Colchester, VT 05446-1672
(800) 456-1177

Carpets

Bremworth Carpets
San Francisco, CA
(415) 347-6254
Long Stable New Zealand wools, dye stocks from Europe, organic mothproofing without surface treatments.

Carousel Carpets
1 Carousel Lane
Ukiah, CA 95482
(707) 485-0333
Natural fiber manufacturer and natural latex backings.

Colin Campbell
1717 W. 5th Avenue
Vancouver, B.C., Canada
(604) 734-2758
In Ontario (416) 367-1180
Distributor of Faskell Comet all-natural wool carpet.

Desso Carpets
P.O. Box 1351
Wayne, PA 19087
(800) 368-1515
Wool carpets with jute backs.

Foreign Accent
407 Rio Grande, NW
Albuquerque, NM 87104
(505) 842-6901
Natural woven area rugs.

Gordon T. Sands Ltd.
40 Torbay Road
Markham, Ontario, Canada
L3R 1G6
(416) 475-6380
Fax: (416) 475-1686
Axminster and Wilton loomed carpets and Nova Bond commercial felt carpet pad.

Hendrickson Naturlick
8031 Mill Station Road
Sebastopol, CA 95472
(707) 829-3959
Natural floor coverings and floor products.

Helios Carpet
P.O. Box 1928
Calhoun, GA 30703
(800) 843-5138
Wide variety of wools without surface treatment.

H&I Carpet Corp.
231 Rowntree Dairy Road
Woodbridge, Ontario, Canada
L4L 8B8
(416) 850-1700
Low-emission wool and cotton carpets with jute and cotton backs.

Lilin Products Ltd.
P.O. Box 80988
Burnaby, B.C., Canada
V5H 4K1
(604) 649-8910
Imports genuine rice straw tatami floor mats.

Jack Lenor Larsen
41 East 11th Street
New York, NY 10003-4685
(212) 674-2446
Natural fibers—wool, sisal, coir. No treatments or adhesives used in construction.

Pure Podunk
RR1, Box 69
Thetford Center, VT 05075
Area rugs on linen backing from organic domestic wool.

Toy Safety

The Institute for Injury
Reduction
P.O. Box 1621
Upper Marlboro, MD 20773
(301) 249-0090
(800) 544-3694

Water Filters

Certifiers of Water Filters

National Sanitation
Foundation
3475 Plymouth Road
P.O. Box 130140
Ann Arbor, MI 48105
(313) 769-8010

Water Quality Association
4151 Naperville Road
Lisle, IL 60532
(708) 505-0160
*General information about water
quality problems and point-of-use
technologies that can be used in the
home or office.*

Mail-Order Suppliers and General Catalogs for Household Products

*These mail-order suppliers offer a wide
range of household products.*

Allergy Relief Shop
2932 Middlebrook Pike
Knoxville, TN 37921
(615) 522-2795

Baubiologie
207B 16th Street
Pacific Grove, CA 93950
(408) 372-8626

The Environmental Health
Shopper
P.O. Box 239
Fate, TX 75132
(800) 447-1100

The Living Source
3500 MacArthur Drive
Waco, TX 76708
(817) 756-6341

Nigra Enterprises
5699 Kanan Road
Agoura, CA 91301
(818) 889-6877

Seventh Generation
49 Hercules Drive
Colchester, VT 05446
(802) 655-3116
(800) 456-1177

Foods and Beverages
Vegetables and Fruits

*No matter where you live today it is easy
to find organically grown fresh fruits, vegetables, nuts, and seeds. Many nationwide
distributors have mail-order service and
home delivery.*

Ahler's Organic Date and
Grapefruit Garden
P.O. Box 726
Mecca, CA 92554
(619) 396-2337
Organic dates by mail.

Lee Anderson's Calvalda
Date Company
51-392 Highway 86
P.O. Box 908-N
Coachella, CA 92236
(619) 398-3441
*Organically grown dried apples,
apricots, black mission figs, peaches,
pears, and Thompson seedless raisins by
mail.*

Blooming Prairie
Warehouse, Inc.
2340 Heinze Road
Iowa City, IA 52240
(319) 337-6448
*Organic produce by mail in nine-state
Midwestern region.*

Blue Heron Farm
P.O. Box 68
Rumsey, CA 95679
(916) 796-3799
Organic nuts by mail.

Community Mill and
Bean, Inc.
267 Route 89 South
Savannah, NY 13146
(315) 365-2664
Fax: (315) 365-2690
*Organic beans, wheat, and grain by
mail.*

Dach Ranch
P.O. Box 44
Philo, CA 95466
(707) 895-2635
*Organically grown apples, pears, and
vinegars by mail throughout the
country.*

Dharma Farms
HC 68
Box 140
Green Forest, AR 72638
(501) 553-2550
*Apples and pears mailed throughout the
country.*

Ecology Sound Farm
42126 Road 168
Orosi, CA 93647
(209) 528-3816
*Organically grown navel and Valencia
oranges, plums, Asian pears, Fuyu
persimmons, and kiwifruit available by
mail nationwide.*

Garden Spot Distributors
438 White Oak Road,
Box 729A
New Holland, PA 17557
(717) 354-4936
*Organically grown nuts, dried fruits,
seeds, and beans. In shops, look for their
retail brand name Shiloh Farms.*

Gold Mine Natural Food
Company
1947 30th Street
San Diego, CA 92102-1105
(800) 475-FOOD
Fax: (619) 234-9749
*Organic grains, macrobiotic and
earthwise products for your home.*

Golden Angels Apiary
P.O. Box 2
Singers Glen, VA 22850
(703) 833-5104
Pesticide-free honey by mail.

Great Date in the Morning
P.O. Box 31
Coachella, CA 92236
(619) 398-6171
Organic dates by mail.

Greek Gourmet Ltd.
5 Pond Park Road
Hingham, MA 02043
(617) 749-1866
Organic olives, olive oil by mail.

Green Knoll Farm
P.O. Box 434
Gridley, CA 95948
(916) 846-3431
Organically grown kiwifruit by mail.

Hill and Dale Farms
R.D. 2, Box 1260
Putney, VT 05346
(802) 387-5817
*Northern Vermont mountain apples
(Spy, McIntosh, Red Delicious)
available by mail. Vermont Certified.*

Stanley and Marina
Jacobson Citrus
1505 Doherty
Mission, TX 78572
(210) 585-1712
*Organically grown grapefruit, picked
fresh after you order, shipped throughout
the country.*

Jaffe Brothers
P.O. Box 636
Valley Center, CA 92082
(619) 749-1133
*Organically grown dried fruits, nuts,
and seeds by mail.*

Kennedy's Natural Foods
1051 West Broad Street
Falls Church, VA 22046
(703) 533-8484
*Dried fruits, nuts, and hardy produce by
mail. Mail-order catalog contains many
diverse and useful organic products.*

Mountain Ark Trading
Company
P.O. Box 3170
Fayetteville, AR 72702
(800) 643-8909
Organically grown honey by mail.

Nokomis Farm, Inc.
W2463 Country Road, E.S.
East Troy, WI 53120
(414) 642-9665
Fax: (414) 642-5517
*Organic grains, bakery products, and
organic canned goods such as tomatoes
and sauces.*

Organic Foods Express
11003 Emack Road
Beltsville, MD 20705
(301) 816-4944
*A full line of fresh organically grown
produce, including herbs, shipped
throughout the United States.*

Ozark Organic Growers
Associations/Coop Warehouse
Ozark Mountain Wildflower
Honey
P.O. Box 1211
Fayetteville, AR 72702-1211
Jeff Watson, Managing
Director
(501) 521-0206
*Honey without pesticide or antibiotic
residues.*

Rising Sun Organic Food
P.O. Box 627
PA 150/I-80
Milesburg, PA 16853
(814) 355-9850
Organically grown fruits and vegetables by mail.

Star Organic Produce, Inc.
P.O. Box 561502
Miami, FL 33256-1502
(305) 262-1242
Tropical fruits organically grown in Florida.

Lew Tew Organics
8805 O'Neal Drive
Springdale Estates
Raleigh, NC 27613
(919) 870-0673
(800) 584-4975
Organic sweet potatoes.

Walnut Acres
Penns Creek, PA 17862
(800) 433-3998
(717) 837-0601
A wide variety of fresh produce available by mail. Walnut Acres is the exclusive mail-order distributor of Earth's Best organic baby food.

Water Wheel Sugar House
Route 2
Jefferson, NH 03583
(603) 586-4479
Maple syrup by mail throughout the country.

Grains

Baldwin Hill Bakery
Baldwin Hill Road
Philipston, MA 01331
(508) 249-4691
Organic breads by mail.

Berkshire Mountain Bakery
P.O. Box 785
Housatonic, MA 01236
(413) 274-3412
Organic breads by mail.

Bread Alone
Route 28
Boiceville, NY 12412
(914) 657-3328
Totally organic breads including farm bread (a coarse-grain wheat and rye), six grain bread, miche (yeast-free sourdough), whole wheat walnut, and many others.

Community Mill and Bean
267 Route 89 South
Savannah, NY 13146
(315) 365-2690
Organic whole grain flours, mixes for pancakes, gingerbread, corn bread, organic grains, and organic dried beans.

Diamond K Enterprises
Stockton Roller Mill
P.O. Box 26
Saint Charles, MN 55972
(507) 932-4308 or 932-5433
Organic whole grains in bulk, from alfalfa and barley to oats and soybeans, as well as flours and mixes.

Garden Spot Distributors
438 White Oak Road,
Box 729A
New Holland, PA 17557
(717) 354-4936
A wide variety of organic grains: barley,
buckwheat, millet, rye, rice, sprouted
grain breads, and pesticide-free
granolas.

Mill City Baker
1566 Randolph Avenue
Saint Paul, MN 55105
(612) 699-4784
Some of the best-tasting, purest sour-
dough breads in the nation.

Nokomis Farm Inc.
W2463 Country Road, E.S.
East Troy, WI 53120
(414) 642-9665
Fax: (414) 642-5517
Sourdough bread made with certified
organically grown grains. Nokomis also
sells organically grown flour.

Northern Lake Wild Rice
Company
P.O. Box 28
Cass Lake, MN 56633
Organically grown wild rice.

Pacific Bakery
514 S. Hill Street
Oceanside, CA 92054
(619) 757-6020
or:
P.O. Box 950
Oceanside, CA 92054
Multigrain and oat bread.

Rising Sun Organic Food
P.O. Box 627
PA 150/I-80
Milesburg, PA 16853
(814) 355-9850
Organically grown grain. Rising Sun
also sells organic breads made by the
Baldwin Hill Bakery and by the
Women's Community Bakery, as well as
Sprout's Delight, which uses no yeast;
and organic flours, cereals, and granola.

Sunrise Sourdough Bakery
Bill Hotchkiss
P.O. Box 727
Philomath, OR 97370
(503) 929-3237
Sourdough bread by mail throughout
the western states.

Organic and Hormone-Free Meat and Poultry

Benson Natural, Inc.
Second & State
Osmond, NE 68765
(402) 748-3309
Organic beef and pork. No antibiotics
or hormones are used in
their organic beef.

Brae Beef
45 John Street
Greenwich, CT 06831
(203) 869-0106
Hormone-free beef and poultry by mail
worldwide.

Mike Brodman
6409 East Scipio Top Road 8
Republic, OH 44867
(419) 585-5852
Organic beef.

Dakota Lean Meats
P.O. Box 434
Winner, SD 57580
(800) 727-5326
Hormone-free beef.

Garden Spot Distributors
438 White Oak Road,
Box 729A
New Holland, PA 17557
(717) 354-4936
*A wide variety of organic meat and
poultry products, including whole
chickens and turkeys, chicken and beef
hot dogs, ground beef and bologna. No
nitrites, coloring, fillings or binders in
any products. All organic grains fed to
their animals.*

Green Earth Natural Foods
2545 Prairie Avenue
Evanston, IL 60201
(708) 864-8949
Organic beef, chicken, and pork.

Jordan River Farm
Cory Koral and Miriam Harris
Route 2, Box 103
Huntly, VA 22640
(703) 636-9388
Organic beef and veal.

Lean & Free
R R 3, Box 53
Ackley, IA 50601
(800) 383-BEEF
Hormone-free beef.

Organic Beef, Inc.
P.O. Box 642
Mena, AK 71953
(501) 387-7111
Organic beef and veal.

Organic Cattle Company
Helen Tahmin
P.O. Box 355
White Plains, NY 10605
(914) 684-6529
*Beef without hormones or antibiotics.
Cattle are fed organic grains.*

Rising Sun Organic Food
P.O. Box 627
PA 150/I-80
Milesburg, PA 16853
(814) 355-9850
*Certified organic chicken, turkey, beef,
lamb, and pork.*

Roseland Farms
27427 M-60 West
Cassopolis, MI 49031
(616) 445-8769
Fax: (616) 445-8987
Organic beef.

Summerfield Farm
HCR 4 Box 195A
Brightwood, VA 22715
(703) 948-3100
Veal products available from humanely raised calves. Lamb and game birds are also available. In addition, cruelty-free venison and rabbits.

Walnut Acres
Penns Creek, PA 17862
(800) 433-3998
(717) 837-0601
Organic beef and poultry.

Wolfe's Neck Farm
10 Burnett Road
Freeport, ME 04032
(207) 865-4469
Certified organic beef air-shipped throughout New England.

A Safer Grill

Hermelin, Inc.
130 McCormick Avenue
Suite 109
Costa Mesa, CA 92626
(714) 545-3500
Manufacturers of the "Vertikal Grill," which allows grilling without cancer-causing PAHs.

Dairy Products

Brier Run Farm
Route 1, Box 73
Birch River, WV 26610
(304) 649-2975
Brier Run Farm goat cheese (chèvre) is certified organic and sold by mail nationwide. It can be found in Boston at Bread & Circus supermarkets; in

New York City at Zabar's, Balducci's, Dean and Deluca, and other shops; in Washington, D.C., at Sutton Place Gourmet and other shops. Other stores in Pennsylvania, Virginia, Ohio, North Carolina, and Connecticut carry Brier Run products as well. Call the number above for stores in your area.

Nest Eggs

Nest Eggs, at stores nationwide, come from humanely raised chickens. For more information about where to find Nest Eggs brand in your area, write or telephone:

Food Animal Concerns Trust
(FACT)
P.O. Box 14599
Chicago, IL 60614-9966
(312) 525-4952

Baby Foods

Earth's Best
P.O. Box 887
Middlebury, VT 05753
(800) 442-4221

Canadian National Directory of Organic Food Sources

The Directory is a source book for finding suppliers of organic foods from produce to meat and poultry to convenience foods. It lists farms and stores. It can be bought by writing or calling:

Canadian Organic Growers
(COG)
P.O. Box 6408, Sta. "J"
Ottawa, Ontario, Canada
K2A 3Y6
(416) 253-5885

Beverages

Water Testing

These firms can test your water for lead, bacteria, metal, minerals, nitrates, industrial solvents, and pesticides.

National Testing Laboratories
6555 Wilson Mills Road
Cleveland, OH 44143
(800) 458-3330
(216) 449-2525
Complete line of water testing kits, reasonably priced.

Suburban Water Testing
Laboratories
4600 Kutztown Road
Temple, PA 19560
(800) 433-6595
(215) 929-3666
Offers a complete line of water testing services. Kits shipped to customers with sampling instructions.

Organic Wine

Chartrand Imports
Paul Chartrand
P.O. Box 1319
Rockland, ME 04841
(800) 473-7307
(207) 594-7300
Mail-order distributor for French and California organic wines.

Fitzpatrick Winery and Lodge
Brian Fitzpatrick
7740 Fairplay Road
Somerset, CA 95684
(209) 245-3248
A variety of organic wines by mail throughout the United States. They limit their use of sulfites.

Four Chimneys Farm Winery
211 Hall Road
Himrod-on-Seneca, NY
14842
(607) 243-7502
Excellent vintages with no added sulfites, available by mail throughout the country.

Frey Vineyards
14000 Tomki Road
Redwood Valley, CA 95470
(707) 485-5177
Organic wines available nationwide. Call for information on local availability.

The Organic Wine Company
54 Genoa Place
San Francisco, CA 94133
(415) 433-0167
Mail-order distributor for French and California organic wines.

Wine Link
440 Talbet Street
Daly City, CA 94014
(800) 231-1171
A wide selection of domestic and imported organic wines. Ships throughout the United States.

Organic Certification Groups

One of these groups will be able to tell you about organic produce growers and retailers in your area.

California Certified Organic
Farmers (CCOF)
303 Potrero Street, Suite 51
Santa Cruz, CA 95060
(408) 423-2263

Mercantile Foods Company
Farm Verified Organic
Program
Carpenter Road
Philmont, NY 12565
(518) 672-0190

Maine Organic Farmers'
& Gardeners' Association
(MOFGA)
P.O. Box 2176
Augusta, ME 04338
(207) 622-3118

Natural Organic Farmers'
Association (NOFA)—
Connecticut
153 Bowers Hill
Oxford, CT 06483
(203) 888-9280

NOFA—Massachusetts
153 N. Mail Street
(Rte. 16, S. Natick Ctr. retail)
Natick, MA 01760
(508) 655-2204

NOFA—New Hampshire
Route 1, Box 516
Andover, NH 03216
(603) 648-2521

NOFA—New York
Mulligan Farms
5403 Barber Road
Avon, NY 14414
(716) 226-6412

New England Farmers
Association
15 Barre Street
Montpelier, VT 05602
(802) 229-4940

Ohio Ecological Food and
Farm Association
7300 Bagley Road
Mount Perry, OH 43769

Organic Crop Improvement
Association (OCIA)
Agrisystems
125 West Seventh Street
Wind Gap, PA 18091
(215) 863-6700

Organic Food Production
Association of North America
(OFPANA)
P.O. Box 31
Belchertown, MA 01007
(413) 774-7511

Organic Growers and Buyers
Association
1405 Silver Lake
New Brighton, MN 55112
(612) 636-7933

Organic Growers of Michigan
7300 Leg Road
Kingston, MI 48741
(517) 683-3161

Ozark Organic Growers
Association
P.O. Box 1528
Fayetteville, AR 72702

Texas Department
of Agriculture
Organic Certification Program
Shashank Nilakhe
P.O. Box 12847
Austin, TX 78711
(512) 463-1145

Tilth Producers'
Cooperative—Oregon
P.O. Box 218
Tualatin, OR 97062
(503) 692-4877

Tilth Producers'
Cooperative—Washington
1219 East Sauk Road
Concrete, WA 98237
(206) 863-8449

Virginia Association of
Biological Farmers
Box 252
Flint Hill, VA 22727

Reporting Injuries and Adverse Reactions

If you suffer an acute injury, adverse reaction, or illness because of a household product, cosmetic, personal care product, food, or beverage, it is important to report the problem. However, reporting problems to the manufacturer or producer is only partially helpful. Sometimes the manufacturer or producer refuses to disclose complaints to proper government agencies. So you should also send complaints or reports to the proper government agency. (Unfortunately, there is no requirement for reporting long-term illnesses such as cancer.) Include detailed information such as the following:

PRODUCT DESCRIPTION

- Type of product
- Exact product name
- Any numbers of letters stamped on the label, cap, or container
- Product price
- Date bought

CONDITIONS OF APPLICATION AND USE

- Duration of use or exposure to the specific product
- Duration that you have used the brand or similar brand
- Part of the body the cosmetic was applied to or part of the body that was inadvertently exposed to the household product
- Whether the product was applied personally or professionally (e.g., in a beauty shop, by a professional pest exterminator, lawn care company, or painter)
- Frequency of use

ACTUAL PROBLEM

- Location of problem (eye, leg, left arm, etc.)
- Symptoms (itching, swelling, redness, burning, light-headedness, diarrhea, stomach upset, etc.)
- Length of time symptoms lasted
- Time from application, consumption, or exposure until the symptoms appeared
- Whether similar symptoms have been triggered by other products or foods
- Whether medical treatment was required

To report a household product-related injury write to the U.S. Consumer Product Safety Commission, Washington, DC 20207. You may call the commission's toll-free hotline in the continental United States at (800) 638-CPSC (2772). Operators are on duty from 10:30 A.M. to 4:00 P.M. Eastern time, Monday through Friday.

Call the FDA MedWatch line at 1-(800)-FDA-1088 to report adverse reactions to cosmetics and personal care products. MedWatch will provide a form for the physician to fill out and send to the manufacturers and the FDA, and will offer additional information, if needed.

To report cases of food-related poisoning, call the FDA office of Emergency and Epidemiological Operations at (301) 443-1240 to initiate an investigation into the suspect food or beverage.

Making the Marketplace Democratic

THE RIGHT TO KNOW—PART OF THE CONSUMER'S BILL OF RIGHTS

This book arises out of the need for labeling and the consumer's right to full disclosure until toxic chemicals can be phased out of consumer products. *The Safe Shopper's Bible* is a book that should never have been needed, but Congress reflects trends rather than creates them, and neither the White House nor Congress, especially in light of massive deregulatory legislation of the mid-1990s, is likely to actively inform shoppers of the presence of hazardous chemicals in consumer products and initiate a phaseout without massive grassroots efforts. Industry certainly will not phase out or label products for hazardous chemicals without pressure from government and the public. Indeed, both goals are synergistic: Full label disclosure will provide the impetus for a phaseout of all carcinogenic, neurotoxic, teratogenic, and immunotoxic chemicals from consumer products and the workplace. Full label disclosure is the all-important first step.

The national health care system would benefit because there would be fewer carcinogenic and other disease-causing chemicals endangering the health of consumers and workers. Furthermore, since a democracy is based in large part on the unencumbered flow of information and the right to know, the marketplace would be "democratized," with the results being informed consumers better able to direct their dollars.

Enacting the policy recommendations described in this section will make consumer products, as well as foods and beverages, safer for consumers. Moreover, it will begin shifting the nation toward safer production, manufacturing, and agricultural practices, while ensuring economically priced and effective consumer goods and a wholesome, plentiful food supply. Finally, such label information will help create a groundswell of public support for phaseout of carcinogenic and other highly toxic chemicals in consumer products.

CALIFORNIA'S PROPOSITION 65

There is a new climate in America with new possibility for change. Consider what is happening in California. Thanks to California's passage of Proposition 65 in 1986, which required disclosure of chemicals in the workplace and consumer products known to cause cancer or reproductive effects, products nationwide have become safer for all consumers. Old El Paso canned tamale chili gravy and Progresso canned tomatoes, manufactured by Whitman, eliminated their lead-soldered cans; Sears, Roebuck & Co. had dozens of products, including car wax and carburetor cleaner, reformulated to replace toxic chemicals with safer alternatives. Wine bottles sold in California soon will no longer have lead foil wrappers, protecting consumers from wine with unacceptably high levels of lead. Meanwhile, major manufacturers have asserted that Proposition 65, with its labeling demands, has "provided an opportunity to improve product performance."

POLICY RECOMMENDATIONS

The equation for change is simple and powerful. Informed shoppers at the grassroots level pressuring Congress for labeling legislation will, in turn, put pressure on industry to phase out hazardous substances from consumer products. Concerned people should pressure public officials to enact the following legislation:

Full Label Disclosure

Clearly, if the present cancer epidemic is to be reversed, health care costs cut, and the health of the nation's citizens improved, right-to-know consumer labeling legislation and regulation are imperative. Such legislation guarantees consumers the right to be warned when they are being exposed to carcinogens, neurotoxins, and teratogens being intentionally added to, or present as contaminants in, household products, cosmetics, foods, and other consumer products. Such legislation would fulfill the dual purpose of optimizing public health standards and creating the climate for reduced environmental pollution.

A March 1993 poll commissioned by Public Voice for Food and Health Policy found that 86 percent of the public "strongly agreed" that Americans have a right to know about the chemicals used on the foods they buy in their supermarket; 79 percent said they "strongly favor tough laws requiring clear labeling of the chemicals and pesticides used to grow a food product."

A successful legislative effort in this area, however, would do more than simply warn people when they are being exposed to hazardous chemicals. Labeling products as an interim measure would be the first step toward a phaseout of toxic chemicals in consumer products and foods. Such legislation would give industry a strong incentive to make the workplace, products, and foods safer.

Such warnings should be placed on product labels or containers. If direct labeling is impossible because of limited space on the product's label, the warning should be displayed on counters, shelves, or signs near the products. The warnings should clearly and prominently include a statement such as WARNING: THIS PRODUCT CONTAINS ONE OR MORE TOXIC CHEMICAL SUBSTANCES KNOWN TO CAUSE CANCER [OR BIRTH DEFECTS OR BRAIN DAMAGE]. The label might also include a symbol for non–English speakers.

Such warnings should *not* be based on the rubber numbers of quantitative risk assessments, which fail to represent the real cumulative damage resulting from exposure to low levels of chemical toxins. Instead, warnings should state the identity of such chemicals if they are simply present.

Warning regulations and requirements for labeling should also extend to businesses that use such substances in the workplace. There should be no "coding" of hazardous ingredients. They should be listed by their common or proper chemical name, as well as their toxic effects.

Furthermore, provisions should be made for requiring substitution of safer alternative ingredients when available.

Consumer right-to-know labeling will not significantly affect the cost of doing business. If businesses are not exposing people to chemicals that can cause cancer, neurotoxicity, or birth defects, complying with the right-to-know legislation will not cost anything because they will not need to provide warnings. The cost of adding a health warning to a product label is small. After all, companies change their product labels every time they create new advertising slogans. The passage of Proposition 65 in California has imposed minimal costs on business. Former EPA Administrator William Reilly wrote in a letter to Louis Sullivan, former Secretary of the Department of Health and Human Services, "In December 1988 a White House (Council of Economic Advisors) Working Group looked at the economic costs of Proposition 65 and concluded that these costs were 'relatively minimal.'"

The penalty for failure to warn people of such substances should be a fine of up to $25,000 and a penalty of up to four years in jail.

The Phaseout of the Manufacturing, Use, and Disposal of Hazardous Ingredients in Consumer Products

The use of hazardous ingredients in consumer products should be phased out. Only a sharp phaseout and ultimately a ban on the manufacture, use, and disposal of carcinogenic chemicals, replacing them with noncarcinogenic alternatives and technologies, is likely to reverse the burgeoning toll of childhood cancers. Such action could also reverse the cancer epidemic now striking more than one in three and killing more than one in four Americans. The highly politicized federal agencies and a lethargic, confused, and divided Congress, however, are unlikely to act without effective grassroots citizen action.

Legislation should be complemented by marketplace pressures based on tax penalties for the manufacture and use of carcinogens, especially when noncarcinogenic substitutes are available, and the use of tax incentives for the development of benign substitute products and processes.

If you agree that hazardous substances should be phased out and labeled in consumer products, call your senators and congressional representatives, and state legislators. Your senators' address is: U.S. Senate, Washington, DC 20510. Your representative's address is: House of Representatives, Washington, DC 20515. The Congressional switchboard phone number is (202) 224-3121.

Better yet, get together with a like-minded group of your neighbors and call on your senators and representatives when they are in town. If you have five to ten people, they cannot turn down your request for a meeting. Put the pressure on. In the meeting say, "I'd like you to support legislation that will phase out carcinogenic chemicals from consumer products and foods, and right-to-know legislation. Will you do it? Will you cosponsor it? Will you help pass this bill?" Let them know that you will support them, too, if they support such a bill—whether they are Democrats or Republicans! And follow up with letters and telegrams.

Also write or call people in the media including:

- Paul Harvey, 333 N. Michigan Avenue, 6th Floor, Chicago, IL 60601; Fax: (312) 899-4088.
- Larry King, 820 First Street NE, Washington, DC 20002; Phone: (202) 898-7690.
- Rush Limbaugh, EFM Media Management, Inc., 342 Madison Avenue, Suite 920, New York, NY 10173; Fax: (212) 661-7945.
- Jim Hightower, Hightower Radio; Phone: (512) 477-5588.
- Gary Null and Associates, P.O. Box 918, Planetarium Station, New York, NY 10024; Phone: (212) 799-1246.

TAKING ACTION

Support proconsumer reforms. Proconsumer reform legislation and policies require massive grassroots support. Support for reform should come through letters to key public officials, including the president. A model letter follows.

The President
The White House
1600 Pennsylvania Avenue, N.W.
Washington, DC 20500

Dear Mr. President:

Consumers have a right to be informed of carcinogenic, neurotoxic, and reproductive toxins added to their household products, cosmetics, and foods. This information is crucial in view of the escalating incidence of cancer. Cancer will strike eighty-three million Americans living today. Some thirty years ago, one in four Americans was stricken with cancer and one in five died. Today, one in three Americans is stricken and one in four will die from this disease. Cancer incidence is predicted to increase to one in two Americans. Clearly, prevention of cancer is the best policy.
    I urge you to support legislation that will:

- Phase out manufacturing, use, and disposal of all carcinogens, neurotoxins, and reproductive toxins and replace them with safer, nontoxic alternatives.
- Provide full and complete label information that informs consumers of all physical and chemical carcinogens, neurotoxins, and reproductive toxins present in consumer products, cosmetics, and foods—until these substances are phased out. Such information should be provided for all such substances intentionally added to consumer products and foods irrespective of their concentration in the product or on the food.
- Provide America's farmers and ranchers economic incentives for switching to sustainable, organic methods of agriculture.
- Protect and expand the Delaney amendment of the Food, Drug, and Cosmetic Act to ensure that it not only retains its original powers, but also expands them to include consumer products and the workplace.
Sincerely,

In addition to writing letters to legislators, consider getting involved with any group listed below.

Cancer Prevention Coalition
520 N. Michigan Avenue
Chicago, IL 60611
(312) 467-0600

A coalition of over fifty-five experts on cancer prevention, public health, and preventive medicine together with representatives of a wide range of labor, public interest, citizen, women's, and consumer groups. One of its key programs is the development of local and national initiatives for labeling and full disclosure of avoidable carcinogens in food and other consumer products.

Citizen Action
1730 Rhode Island Avenue, NW
Washington, DC 20009
(202) 775-1580
(202) 466-3980

A three-million-member consumer activist group working in all areas discussed in this book. An important organization to join and support.

Community Nutrition Institute
2001 South Street, NW, Suite 530
Washington, DC 20009
(202) 462-4700

Food Animals Concerns Trust (FACT)
P.O. Box 14599
Chicago, IL 60614-9966
(312) 525-4952

FACT is actively involved in taking farm animals out of crates and cages and putting them in more humane settings. Write or call for sources of humanely raised veal.

Feingold Association of the U.S.
P.O. Box 6550
Alexandria, VA 22306
(703) 768-3287

An international organization providing information on food additives, chemical sensitivity, and related health problems. Write or call for the location of the nearest Feingold support group in your area. Publishes an excellent newsletter, Pure Facts, *ten times annually.*

Greenpeace
1436 U Street, NW
Washington, DC 20009
(202) 319-2472

The Humane Farming Association
1550 California Street, Suite 6
San Francisco, CA 94109
(415) 485-1495
The Humane Farming Association has been in the forefront of the movement to treat farm animals humanely.

Mothers and Others for a Livable Planet
40 West 20th Street
New York, NY 10011
(212) 727-4474

National Coalition Against Misuse of Pesticides (NCAMP)
701 East Street, SE, Suite 200
Washington, DC 20003
(202) 543-5450
Dedicated to standing up for victims of pesticide poisoning, disseminating information, and acting as the national umbrella group for the many local grassroots groups working to change pesticide laws in their states and counties.Publishes a newsletter.

Natural Resources Defense Council (NRDC)
71 Stevenson Street, Suite 1825
San Francisco, CA 94105
(415) 777-0220

Northwest Coalition for Alternatives to Pesticides (NCAP)
P.O. Box 1393
Eugene, OR 97440
(503) 344-5044
Five-state coalition of the Northwest that has fought the U.S. Forest Service on herbicide spraying. Publishes the Journal of Pesticide Reform, *a quarterly.*

Pesticide Action Network (PAN)
North America Regional Center
116 New Montgomery, Suite 810
San Francisco, CA 94105
(415) 541-9140
Worldwide umbrella organization of people and groups from across the globe who are opposed to the proliferation of pesticide use.

The Pure Food Campaign
1130 17th Street, NW, Suite 300
Washington, DC 20036
(202) 775-1132

Union of Concerned Scientists
1616 P Street, NW, Suite 310
Washington, DC 20036
(202) 332-0900

Notes

INTRODUCTION

The Case for Concern

page 2:   Two of the greatest health risks: L. B. Stammer, "Clean air quest—an inside job: when it comes to human health, pollution in homes and offices may be the greatest threat," *Los Angeles Times,* 26 December 1989, p. A1.

page 2:   Increased sensitivity to synthetic chemicals in consumer products and furnishings: M. Weisskopf, "Hypersensitivity to chemicals called rising health problem: some cannot adapt to low doses of toxics, study says," *Washington Post,* 10 February 1990.

page 2:   Cancer and nervous system damage: U.S. EPA, *Chemicals Identified in Human Biological Media. A Data Base,* EPA 560/13-80-036B, PB81-161-176 (Washington, D.C., 1980).

page 2:   Leukemia and non-Hodgkin's lymphoma cases linked to hair-color products: K. P. Cantor et al., "Hair dye use and risk of leukemia and lymphoma," *American Journal of Public Health* 78, no. 5 (1988): 570–71; S. H. Zahm et al., "Use of hair coloring products and risk of lymphoma, multiple myeloma, and chronic lymphocytic leukemia," *American Journal for Public Health* 82, no. 7 (1992): 990–97.

page 2:   Leukemia and home and garden pesticides: R. A. Lowengart et al., "Childhood leukemia and parents' occupational and home exposures," *Journal of the National Cancer Institute* 79, no. 1 (1987): 39–46.

page 2:   Childhood brain cancer and pesticides: J. R. Davis et al., "Family pesticide use and childhood brain cancer," *Archives of Environmental Contamination and Toxicology* 24 (1993): 87–92.

page 2:   Hospital admissions because of household cleaner-related poisonings: Consumer Product Safety Commission (CPSC), "1990 Product Summary Report: National Electronic Injury Surveillance System" (Washington, D.C.: National Injury Information Clearinghouse), p. 7.

page 2:   Hospital admissions because of pesticide-related poisonings: ibid., p. 15.

Are Government and Industry Not Telling Us What We Need to Know to Make Informed Purchases?

page 4:   FDA enforcement record criticized: General Accounting Office (GAO), *Pesticides: Need to Enhance FDA's Ability to Protect the Public from Illegal Residues* (Washington, D.C.: GPO, 1986); General Accounting Office (GAO), *Pesticides: Better Sampling and Enforcement Needed on Imported Food* (Washington, D.C.: GPO, 1988; General Accounting Office (GAO), *Food Safety and Quality: FDA Surveys Not Adequate to Demonstrate Safety of Milk Supply,* Report to the Chairman, Human Resources and Intergovernmental Relations Subcommittee, *Committee on Government Operations, House of Representatives,* GAO/RCED-91-26 (Washington, D.C.: GPO, 1990).

page 4:   USDA enforcement record criticized: National Research Council (NRC), *Meat and Poultry Inspection: The Scientific Basis of the Nation's Program* (Washington, D.C.: National Academy Press, 1985); U.S. Department of Agriculture (USDA), *Residue Monitoring Program Yearly Data Summary (Domestic/Imports for the Years 1983–1988),* (Washington, D.C.: Food Safety and Inspection Service); G. Anthan, "Contamination rate reaches 80 percent at some U.S. poultry plants," *Des Moines Register,* 12 April 1987.

page 4:   Contaminated meat: USDA, *Residue Monitoring Program, 1983–1988.*

page 5:   EPA's own estimates would result in sixty-four thousand excess cancers a year: S. S. Epstein, & J. Feldman, "Opening the door for carcinogens: assaults on nation's food-safety laws multiply," *Los Angeles Times,* 27 February 1989.

page 5:   Unpredictable synergistic interactions: S. S Epstein, "Book review: Cancer Risk Assessment: A Quantitative Approach," *Cancer Cell* 3, no. 5 (May 1991): 195–96.

page 5:   Overall rising cancer incidence: S. S. Epstein, "Losing the war against cancer: who's to blame and what to do about it," *International Journal of Health Services* 20, no. 1 (1990): 53–71; S. S. Epstein, "Evaluation of the national cancer program and proposed reforms," *American Journal of Industrial Medicine* 24 (1993): 109–33.

page 5: Higher cancer rates in industrialized countries and for workers: Epstein, "War against cancer."

page 5: Cancer overtakes heart disease as leading killer: United Press International (UPI), "Cancer now the leading killer of middle-aged studies show," *Los Angeles Times,* 26 December 1990.

page 6: Baby boom generation at higher cancer risk than its grandparents: D. Davis et al., "Decreasing cardiovascular disease and increasing cancer among whites in the U.S. from 1973 through 1987," *Journal of the National Cancer Institute* 271 (February 1994): 431–37.

page 6: Swedish study and baby boomers' higher risk of cancer: C. Laino, "With cancer rates up, environment is blamed," *Medical Tribune* 34, no. 8 (29 April 1993).

page 7: The war against cancer stalled: *Cancer at the Crossroads:* NCI, National Cancer Advisory Board, *Cancer at a Crossroads: A Report to Congress for the Nation* (September 1994).

page 7: Disclosure will remain minimal: Federal Register 57, no. 197 (9 October 1992): 46627; P. Dickey, "Long-term health hazards to be identified on many consumer product labels," *Alternatives* 11, no. 4 (Winter 1992).

page 7: Largest organic farmer in the United States is now Gallo: D. Zwerdling, "Organic Farming" (Washington, D.C.: National Public Radio, 1–4 November 1993).

page 8: Hot dogs and leukemia: J. M. Peters et al., "Processed meats and risk of childhood leukemia (California, USA)," *Cancer Causes and Control* 5 (1994): 195–202.

PART I. HOUSEHOLD PRODUCTS

Homemaking Can Be a Dangerous Job!

page 17: Production rates for synthetic chemicals have burgeoned: Epstein, "War against cancer."

page 18: Methylene chloride is carcinogenic: International Agency for Research on Cancer (IARC, 1987), *IARC Monographs on the Evaluation of Carcinogenic Risks to Humans. Overall Evaluations of Carcinogenicity: An Updating of IARC Monographs,* vols. 1–42, suppl. no. 7 (Lyon, France: World Health Organization, 1987), pp. 194–95.

How We Evaluated Household Products

page 19: People who have been "sensitized" are especially vulnerable: N. Ashford & C. Miller, *Chemical Exposures: Low Levels and High Stakes* (New York: Van Nostrand Reinhold, 1990).

page 20:   CPSC alleges consumer exposure is minimal: personal communication with the authors from Ken Giles of the Consumer Product Safety Commission, 3 May 1993.

page 20:   No safe threshold for carcinogens. Epstein, S. S., "Evaluation of the national cancer program and proposed reforms." *American Journal of Industrial Medicine,* no. 24 (1993): 109–33.

CHAPTER 1. CLEANING PRODUCTS

Cleansers (Scouring Powders and Soft Scrubs)

page 54:   Crystalline silica causes cancer: *IARC Monographs,* 1987, supplement 7, pp. 341–42.

Furniture Polishes

page 67:   Cleaning and polishing recipes: Total Environment Center and Australian Consumers' Association. *A-Z of Chemicals in the Home.* (Sydney, Australia: 1990), pp. 97–98.

Laundry Detergents and Soaps

page 73:   Brands that are petroleum-free: A. Berthold-Bond, "The laundry quandary, part 2," *Green-keeping* 1, no. 2 (May/June 1991): 4–7.

CHAPTER 2. PAINT AND RELATED PRODUCTS

Paints

page 93:   Paints cause mucous membrane and skin irritation: A. Van Faassen & P. J. A. Borm, "Composition and health hazards of water-based construction paints: results from a survey in the Netherlands," *Environmental Health Perspectives* 92 (1991): 147–54.

page 93:   Painters suffer from nonallergic contact dermatitis, chronic bronchitis, and asthma: International Agency for Research on Cancer (IARC). *IARC Monographs on the Evaluation of Carcinogenic Risks to Humans. Some Organic Solvents, Resin Monomers and Related Compounds, Pigments and Occupational Exposures in Paint Manufacture and Painting,* vol. 47 (Lyon, France: World Health Organization, 1989), p. 424.

page 93:   Paints cause allergic sensitization: ibid.

page 93:   Painters suffer from allergic contact dermatitis: ibid.

page 93:   Cancer risk associated with occupational exposures in painting: ibid., pp. 423–24.

page 94: Crystalline silica is carcinogenic: *IARC Monographs,* 1987, pp. 341–42.

page 94: Greatest risk for exposure to lead in paint: N. Irving Sax & Richard J. Lewis, Sr., *Hazardous Chemicals Desk Reference.* (New York: Van Nostrand Reinhold, 1987), p. 582.

page 94: Kelly-Moore products contain mercury-based fungicides: "Material Safety Data Sheets," Kelly-Moore Paint Co. See Acrylic Primer Sealer.

page 94: Ethylene glycol and ethylene glycol ethylether are absorbed by the lungs and skin and are teratogenic: "Material Safety Data Sheets," Dutch Boy Products, July 1988, p. 13.

page 94: Acetoxyphenylmercury is found in paints and is teratogenic: "Material Safety Data Sheets," Kelly-Moore Paint Co. See Acrylic Primer Sealer; Sax & Lewis, p. 115.

Paint Removers and Strippers

page 99: Methanol can cause blindness: Sax & Lewis, p. 611.

page 100: Methylene chloride can cause irregular heartbeat: "Paint removers: new products eliminate old hazards," *Consumer Reports* (1991): p. 340.

page 100: 1,1,1-trichloroethane can cause irregular heartbeat: Sax & Lewis, p. 828.

CHAPTER 3. PESTICIDES

Home and Garden Pesticides

page 107: Pesticides that cause severe eye, skin, and respiratory irritation: National Coalition Against the Misuse of Pesticides (NCAMP), statement of Jay Feldman, national coordinator, before the Subcommittee on Toxic Substances, Environmental Oversight, Research and Development Committee on Environment and Public Works, U.S. Senate, 9 May 1991. NCAMP, Washington, D.C.

page 108: Pesticides that cause allergic reactions and sensitization: ibid.

page 109: A highly increased risk for leukemia found for children whose parents used pesticides: Lowengart et al., "Childhood leukemia."

page 109: Childhood brain cancer associated with pesticides: Davis et al., "Family pesticide use."

page 109: Another study found relationship between insecticides and weed killers and leukemia: S. Richardson et al., "Occupational risk factors for acute leukemia: a case-control study," *International Journal of Epidemiology* 21, no. 6 (1992): 1063–73.

page 109: DDVP is carcinogenic: "No-pest strip insecticide poses an unacceptably high risk of cancer in people and pets," *Journal of Pesticide
Reform* (Spring 1988): 29.

page 109: EPA estimates members of a household using the pest strips face a
cancer risk ten times greater than pest control workers who apply
DDVP: ibid.

page 109: Flea collars put pets at increased cancer risk: ibid.

page 109: Pesticides that are carcinogenic: R. Engler, "List of chemicals evaluated for carcinogenic potential," Office of Prevention, Pesticides and
Toxic Substances, U.S. Environmental Protection Agency (Washington, D.C.: GPO, 14 October 1992).

page 110: Pesticides that are neurotoxic: NCAMP, 1991.

page 110: Pesticides capable of causing reproductive effects: ibid

page 112: EPA does not "approve" pesticides: ibid.

CHAPTER 4. PET SUPPLIES

Cat Litter

page 121: Crystalline silica is irritating to the lungs: Sax & Lewis, pp.772–73.

page 121: Crystalline silica is carcinogenic: *IARC,* 1987, pp. 341–42.

Flea and Tick Products

page 124: D-limonene is hazardous when used on cats: S. A. Briggs & Rachel
Carson Council, *Basic Guide to Pesticides: Their Characteristics and
Hazards* (Washington, D. C.: Taylor & Francis, 1992), p. 211.

page 124: Foggers and bombs contain flammable propellants or solvents: "Guide
to a pest-free pet," *Consumer Reports* (August 1991): p. 563.

page 124: Each time a pet is treated, human exposure occurs: National Research
Council (NRC), *Animals as Sentinels of Environmental Health Haz-
ards,* Committee on Animals as Monitors of Environmental Hazards,
Board of Environmental Studies and Toxicology, Commission on Life
Sciences, Natural Research Council (Washington, D.C.: National
Academy Press, 1991), pp. 72–73.

page 125: Dipping pets causes muscle weakness: R.G. Ames et al., "Health symp-
toms and occupational exposure to flea control products among
California pet handlers," *Journal of the American Industrial Hygiene
Association* 50, no. 9 (1989): 466–72.

page 125: Sponging associated with convulsions and mental confusion: Ames,
"Health symptoms and occupational exposure."

page 125: Workers who use protective clothing not at increased risk: ibid.

page 126: Supplements with primrose oil cure canine dermatitis: D. H. Scarff
& D. H. Lloyd, "Double blind, placebo-controlled, crossover study

of evening primrose oil in the treatment of canine atopy," *The Veterinary Record* (1 August 1992): 97–99.

page 127: Don't handle ticks: *Consumer Reports* (1991): 565.

page 127: Best tick medicine is prevention: *Consumer Reports* (1991): p. 565.

page 127: Lyme disease concentrated in eight states: ibid.

page 127: Repeat mineral oil treatment to eliminate new generations of ear mites: ibid.

CHAPTER 5. AUTO PRODUCTS

Antifreeze and Coolants

page 135: Thousands of animals die from ethylene glycol poisoning: Sta-Clean Antifreeze, "Did you know the right antifreeze can protect you from more than just extreme temperatures?" Sta-Clean Antifreeze, undated.

page 135: Half of all poisoning deaths of dogs and cats associated with ethylene glycol: ARCO Chemical Company, "Propylene glycol antifreeze: The safer alternative," ARCO Chemical Company, undated.

CHAPTER 6. ART AND CRAFT SUPPLIES

Art and Craft Supplies

page 145: A study found only 36 percent of art products included a hazardous ingredient statement: L. Sikes, Public Interest Research Group, Art & the Craft of Avoidance: *Toxic Art Supplies Lack Warnings Despite Federal Labeling Law* (Washington, D.C.: Public Interest Research Group [PIRG], September 1991).

page 146: Significantly elevated risks for cancers among male and female artists: B. A. Miller et al., "Mortality patterns among professional artists: a preliminary report," National Cancer Institute, 1985.

page 146: Results from a case-control study support association between cancer and employment as artistic painter: B. A. Miller et al., "Cancer risk among artistic painters," *American Journal of Industrial Medicine* 9 (1986): 281–87.

page 146: Arsenic, cadmium, and lead are carcinogenic: *IARC*, 1987, pp. 100–106, 139–42, 230–32.

page 146: Crystalline silica is carcinogenic: ibid., p. 341–42.

page 146: Lead and cadmium are carcinogenic: ibid., pp. 139–42, 230–32.

page 146: Methylene chloride is carcinogenic: ibid., pp. 194–95.

page 147: Vinyl chloride is carcinogenic: ibid., pp. 373–76.

page 147: Di(2-ethylhexyl)phthalate is carcinogenic: ibid., p. 62.

page 147: Chromium and lead are carcinogenic: ibid., pp. 165–68, 230–32.

page 147: Carbon monoxide is neurotoxic: Sax & Lewis, p. 298.

page 147: Acetylene phosgene is neurotoxic: ibid., pp. 119, 298.

page 147: Mercury antifungal agents cause nervous system damage: ibid., pp. 604–05.

page 147: Methyl ethyl ketone and toluene are neurotoxic: ibid., pp. 263, 821-22.

page 147: Lead is teratogenic: ibid., p. 580.

page 147: Pigments in paints including lead are teratogenic: ibid.

page 148: "Art Materials Recommended Especially for Children": Adapted from U.S. Public Interest Research Group, *Art & the Craft of Avoidance* (Washington, D.C.: PIRG, 1991).

page 150: Pickling bath should be vented to outside: M. McCann, A. Babin, & C. I. H. Olmstead, "Health and safety in metal jewelry," *Art Hazards News* 15, no. 1 (1992): 3–6.

CHAPTER 7. MISCELLANY

Air Filters

page 154: Some plants remove toxic chemicals: B. C. Wolverton et al., "Interior landscape plants for indoor air pollution abatement. Final report— September 1989," National Aeronautics and Space Administration, John C. Stennis Space Center, Mississippi.

page 154: Natural gas for cooking and heating releases benzene: Southern California Gas Company, "Proposition 65 Warning," March 1993.

Carpets and Carpet Backing

page 154: Levels of VOCs and 4-phenylcyclohexane: The Carpet and Rug Institute, *Carpet and Indoor Air Quality in Commercial Installations,* (Dalton, GA: The Carpet and Rug Institute, 1994).

page 155: For chemically sensitive people, carpets have "terrifying" health effects: C. Duehring, "Unraveling the carpet toxicity problem. Part 1," *Environment and Health* (Winter 1993).

Cotton Clothing

page 157: Organic cotton farmers achieve virtually same yields as chemically dependent neighbors: D. Zwerdling, "Organic Farming" (Washington, D.C.: National Public Radio, 1–4 November 1993).

page 158: Thirty-five million tons of pesticides applied to cotton crop: *Organically Grown Cotton. Basic Collection,* vol. 2 (South Hackensack, NJ: Ecosport, n.d.).

page 158: Textile industry is sixth most polluting industry in world: *1993 Catalog Supplement* (South Hackensack, NJ: Ecosport).

page 158: Clothing made with naturally colored cotton: O. Strong, "Dressing green. Big firms spot profit in 'organic' clothes," *Los Angeles Times,* 20 October 1992; J. Makower, "Behind the seams: the budding crop of earth-minded clothing," *Co-op America Quarterly* (Summer 1993): 5.

page 158: Electroplating creates millions of tons of hazardous waste: Zwerdling, "Organic Farming."

Electromagnetic Fields

page 159: Much exposure to EMFs results from everyday appliances: J. Raloff, "EMFs run aground. Mapping magnetic fields from water pipes and other homely sources," *Science News* 144 (21 August 1993): 124.

page 159: EMFs change biological tissue: L. Alvin et al., "Electric and magnetic fields: measurements and possible effects on human health from appliances, powerlines, and other common sources: what we know, what we don't know in 1990," Special Epidemiological Studies Program, California Department of Health Services, 1991.

page 159: Swedish standards for VDTs: Environmental Protection Agency (EPA), Office of Radiation and Indoor Air, *EMFs in Your Environment: Magnetic Field Measurements of Everyday Electrical Devices* (Washington, D.C.: GPO, December 1992), p. 21.

page 159: Carcinogenicity of EMFs: R. Stone, "Polarized debate: EMFs and cancer," *Science* 258 (1992): 1724–25; "Danish studies offer new support for EMF-cancer link," *Microwave News* 12, no. 6 (1992): p. 5; Raloff, "EMFs run aground," p. 124; G. M. Matanoski et al., "Electromagnetic field exposure and male breast cancer," *The Lancet* 337 (1991): 737; T. Tynes & A. Anderson, "Electromagnetic fields and male breast cancer," *The Lancet* 336 (1990): 1596.

page 159: Prenatal exposure to electric blankets associated with leukemia and brain cancer: D. A. Savitz et al., "Magnetic field exposure from electric appliances and childhood cancer," *American Journal of Epidemiology* 131, no. 5 (1990): 763–73.

page 160: A modest statistically insignificant increase in breast cancer risk from electric blankets: J. E. Vena et al., "Use of electric blankets and risk of postmenopausal breast cancer," *American Journal of Epidemiology* 134, no. 2 (1991): 180–85.

page 160: EMFs alter sodium balance of brain: R. O. Becker "Electromagnetic fields: what you can do. How to protect yourself from the possible health effects," *East West* (May 1990): p. 55.

page 160: Exposure to radiation from television causes reproductive effects: ibid.

page 160: Exposure to radiation from VDTs may cause miscarriages: ibid.

page 160: Women using computers had higher miscarriage rates: ibid.
page 160: Finnish researchers found a higher miscarriage rate among women exposed to VDT magnetic fields: "Finnish pregnancy study," *Microwave News* 12, no. 6 (1992): 14.
page 160: Miscarriage incidence higher among women exposed in home with electric heat cables installed in ceilings: Becker, "Electromagnetic fields," p. 110.

Pool, Spa, and Hot Tub Chemicals

page 164: Chlorinated pool water causes respiratory distress: M. Shaffer, "Chlorine may spur swimmers' asthma," *Medical Tribune* (24 July 1992): p. 34.
page 164: Prolonged exposure to chlorine causes sensitization: ibid.
page 165: Pregnant women should avoid saunas and hot tubs: A. Milunsky et al., "Maternal heat exposure and neural tube defects," *Journal of the American Medical Association* 268, no. 7 (1992): 882–85.

Toys

page 167: One out of six toys should not have been offered for sale: H. C. Kelley et al., *The 1993 Toy Safety Report* (Upper Marlboro, MD: The Institute for Injury Reduction, 18 November 1993).
page 168: An estimated 123,000 children treated in hospitals for toy-related injuries: Consumer Product Safety Commission (CPSC), "Toy-related deaths and injuries," Memorandum (Washington, D.C.: 23 October 1990).

Water Filters

page 170: Some 940,000 people are made ill annually from contaminated water: Natural Resources Defense Council (NRDC), *Think Before You Drink. The Failure of the Nation's Drinking Water System to Protect Public Health* (New York: September 1993), p. i; J. Rose, "Waterborne pathogens: assessing health risks," *Health & Environment Digest* 7, no. 3 (1993): 1–6.
page 170: Radiation not effectively regulated: NRDC, *Think Before You Drink,* p. v.
page 171: Nearly one million people become sick each year from contaminated drinking water: ibid.
page 174: Screen filters are important where there is known or suspected contamination with microorganisms: R. Gabler, *Is Your Water Safe to Drink?* (Mount Vernon, NY: Consumers Union, 1988), p. 190.

page 175: Activated carbon filters do not remove radioactive contaminants other than radon: E. J. Sternglass, personal communication to the authors, 17 November 1993.

page 175: Under-the-sink models remove up to 99 percent of contaminants: J. C. Stewart, *Drinking Water Hazards: How to Know if There Are Toxic Chemicals in Your Water and What to Do if There Are* (Hiram, OH: Envirographics, 1990), p. 211.

page 175: Phenol removal rating is best if under thirty parts per million: Gabler, *Is Your Water Safe to Drink?* pp. 196–97.

page 175: Filters made from bituminous coal are most effective: Stewart, *Drinking Water Hazards,* p. 210.

page 176: For every gallon of water produced, up to nine gallons go down the drain: ibid., p. 216.

PART II. COSMETICS AND PERSONAL CARE PRODUCTS

Healthy Beauty

page 181: Men and women used cosmetics to attract lovers, disguise effects of aging: L. C. Parish & J. T. Crissey, "Cosmetics: a historical review," *Clinics in Dermatology* 6, no. 3 (1988): 1–3.

page 181: Egyptian women used lead sulfate: ibid., pp. 1–3.

page 181: Hebrews used oils for emollients and sun protection: ibid., p. 2.

page 181: Quote from Juvenal: ibid., p. 2.

page 181: Cosmetics least regulated products under FFDCA: D. T. Duffy, "Classification and regulation of cosmetics and drugs: a legal overview and alternatives for legislative change," a memorandum to Congressman Ron Wyden from the American Law Division of the Congressional Research Service (Washington, D.C.: The Library of Congress, 4 May 1990).

page 181: FFDCA does not require premarket safety testing: ibid.

page 181: FDA enforcement action occurs only after cosmetics enter into commerce: ibid.

page 182: FDA would not ban AETT-containing products: A. Hampton, *Natural Organic Hair and Skin Care* (Tampa, FL: Organica Press, 1987), p. 262.

page 182: Hair-coloring products used by up to 40 percent of women: S. Zahm et al., "Use of hair-coloring products and the risk of lymphoma, multiple myeloma, and chronic lymphocytic leukemia," *American Journal of Public Health* 82, no. 7 (1992): 990–97.

page 182: Use of hair-coloring products place women at increased cancer risk: J. A. Markowitz et al., "Hair dyes and acute nonlymphocytic leukemia

(ANLL)," *American Journal of Epidemiology* 122 (1985): 523, Abstract; K. P. Cantor et al., "Hair dye use and risk of leukemia and lymphoma," *American Journal of Public Health* 78, no. 5 (1988): 570–71; Zahm et al., "Use of hair-coloring products," pp. 990–97; L. M. Brown et al., "Hair dye use and multiple myeloma in white men," *American Journal of Public Health* 82 (1992): 1673–74; International Agency for Research on Cancer, *IARC Monographs on the Evaluation of Carcinogenic Risks to Humans. Occupational Exposures of Hairdressers and Barbers and Personal Use of Hair Colourants; Some Hair Dyes, Cosmetic Colourants, Industrial Dyestuffs and Aromatic Amines,* vol. 57 (Lyon, France: World Health Organization, 1993); M. J. Thun et al., "Hair dye use and risk of fatal cancers in U.S. women," *Journal of the National Cancer Institute* 86, no. 3 (1994): 210–15.

page 182: Hair-coloring products account for up to 20 percent of all non-Hodgkin's lymphoma cases in U.S. women: Zahm et al., "Use of hair-coloring products," pp 990–97.

page 182: Suggestive evidence of an association between hair dye use and breast cancer: National Cancer Institute (NCI), "Bioassay of 2, 4-diaminotoluene for possible carcinogenicity," Carcinogenesis Technical Report Series, No. 162, 1979; National Cancer Institute (NCI), "Bioassay of 2,4-diaminoanisole sulfate for possible carcinogenicity," Carcinogenesis Technical Report Series, No. 84, Series, 1978; W. Rojanapo et al., "Carcinogenicity of an oxidation product of *p*-phenylenediamine," *Carcinogenesis* 17, no. 12 (1986): 1997–2002; N. Shafer & R. W. Shafer, "Potential of carcinogenic effects of hair dyes," *New York State Journal of Medicine* 76 (1976): 394–96; L. J. Kinlen et al., "Use of hair dyes by patients with breast cancer: a case-control study," *British Medical Journal* ii (1977): 366–68; R. E. Shore et al., "A case-control study of hair dye use and breast cancer," *Journal of the National Cancer Institute* 62 (1979): 277–83; C. H. Hennekens et al., "Use of permanent hair dyes and cancer among registered nurses," *The Lancet* (1979): 1390–93; P. C. Nasca et al., "Relationship of hair dye use, benign breast disease, and breast cancer," *Journal of the National Cancer Institute* 64 (1980): 23–28.

page 182: Cosmetic manufacturers lack adequate data on safety and refuse to disclose test results: *Cosmetics Regulation: Information on Voluntary Actions Agreed to by FDA and the Industry.* U.S. General Accounting Office, March 1990 (GAO/HRD-90-58).

page 182: Only a tiny percentage of cosmetic distributors file reports with the government of injuries to consumers: ibid.

page 182: Less than 40 percent of manufacturers are registered: ibid.

page 182:   Industry participation has actually declined: ibid.

page 183:   FDA has committed no resources to assessing safety of chemicals in cosmetics: ibid.

page 183:   It is difficult for FDA to remove unsafe ingredients: J. Bailey, 9 October 1992, personal communication from Dr. John E. Bailey, acting director, Office of Cosmetics and Colors, FDA.

page 183:   Some thirty-eight thousand cosmetic-related injuries required medical treatment in the U.S.: Consumer Product Safety Commission (CPSC), "Product summary report: National Electronic Surveillance System" (Washington, D.C.: National Injury Information Clearinghouse, 1990).

page 183:   Some chemicals penetrate the skin in significant amounts: R. L. Bronaugh et al., "Extent of cutaneous metabolism during percutaneous absorption of xenobiotics," *Toxicology and Applied Pharmacology* 99 (1989): 534–43.

Contact Dermatitis Hazards: Allergens, Sensitizers, and Irritants

page 184:   As many as two million people in U.S. suffer from contact dermatitis: R. Nader, "The regulation of the safety of cosmetics," in *Consumer Health and Product Hazards: Cosmetics and Drugs, Pesticides, Food Additives,* ed. S. S. Epstein & R. D. Grundy (Cambridge: Massachusetts Institute of Technology, 1974), vol. 2, pp. 87–141.

page 185:   Two leading causes of allergy: R. M. Adams & H. I. Mailbach, "A five-year study of cosmetic reactions," *Journal of the American Academy of Dermatology* 13, no. 6 (1985): 1062–69.

page 185:   Commonly reported symptoms: K. I. N. Stevens, "How safe are perfumes?" *The Human Ecologist* (Fall 1990): p. 15; "Perfume survey," Candida Research and Information Foundation (CRIF) (Winter 1989–90); CRIF is conducting a national survey of the effects of perfume exposure. Write to P.O. Box 2719, Castro Valley, CA 94546.

page 185:   Chemicals in fragrances designated as hazardous: I. Wilkenfeld "Perfume or pollutant?" *Green Alternatives* (November/December, 1992): 34.

page 185:   Fragrance ingredients that cause contact dermatitis: Research Institute for Fragrance Materials, A. A. Fisher, *Contact Dermatitis,* 2d ed. (Philadelphia: Lea & Febiger, 1973), p. 237.

page 186:   95 percent of mix in fragrances is synthetic: D. Zemp, "Scents of trouble: for the sensitive, fragrances can trigger problems," *Los Angeles Times,* 18 September 1991, pp. E1–E2.

page 186:   Fragrances derived from mixtures of six hundred or more raw materials and synthetic chemicals: D. L. Opdyke, "The RIFM story," in *The Cosmetic Industry: Scientific and Regulatory Foundations,* ed. Norman F. Estrin (New York: Marcel Dekker, 1984), p. 234.

page 186:   84 percent of ingredients in fragrances never tested or tested minimally: Ashford & Miller, p. 61.

page 186:   FDA quoted: Stevens, "How safe are perfumes?" p. 17.

page 186:   Scents troubling for asthmatics: Zemp, "Scents of trouble," p. E1.

page 186:   Three-fourths of asthma patients suffer adverse reactions to perfume: C. Shim & M. H. Williams, *American Journal of Medicine* 80 (1986) p. 18–22.

page 186:   Perfume in cat litter causes asthma: Ugeskr Laeger 153, no. 13 (1991): 939–40.

page 187:   Less likely to suffer allergies from one oil or a blend of two or three than synthetic fragrances: M. E. Ardita, personal communication with the authors by Marie E. Ardita, cosmetic chemist with Earth Science, Inc., of Corona, CA, 1992.

page 187:   Synthetic fragrance used in best-selling fragrance: P. Calistro & L. Van Gelder, "Is natural better?" *Allure* (April 1992): 48.

page 188:   Following ingredients that release formaldehyde or break down into formaldehyde: T. Conry, *Consumer's Guide to Cosmetics* (Garden City, NY: Anchor Press/Doubleday, 1980), p. 73; G. R. Kantor, et al., "Acute allergic contact dermatitis from diazolidinyl urea (Germall II) in a hair gel," *Journal of the American Academy of Dermatology* 13,(1985): 116–19; T. J. Stephens et al., "Experimental delayed contact sensitization to diazolidinyl urea (Germall II) in guinea pigs," *Contact Dermatitis* 16 (1987): 164–68; R. Winter, *A Consumer's Dictionary of Cosmetic Ingredients* (New York: Crown, 1989), p. 120; M. Johansen & H. Bundgaard, "Kinetics of formaldehyde release from the cosmetic preservative Germall 115, *Arch. Pharm. Chem. Sci.* 9 (1981): 117–22; Winter, *Consumer's Dictionary,* 1989, p. 256.

page 188:   Other preservatives can also cause allergic reactions or irritation: Winter, *Consumer's Dictionary,* 1981, p. 201; M. Hannuksela, "Rapid increase in contact allergy to Kathon™ CG in Finland," *Contact Dermatitis* 15 (1986): 211–14; Winter, *Consumer's Dictionary,* 1986, p. 222.

page 188:   Preservatives that cause fewest allergic reactions: *Natural Body Care Reports* 2 no. 1 (June 1991): 3. Published by Earth Science, Inc., Corona, CA. This report discusses each of the ingredients listed; also Hampton, *Natural Organic Hair and Skin Care,* 1987; Winter, *Consumer's Dictionary,* 1989, pp. 43, 232, 307, 318.

Cancer Risks

page 189: Most nitrosamines are carcinogenic: "Nitrosamine-contaminated cosmetics; call for industry action; request for data," *Federal Register* 44, no. 70 (10 April 1979): 21365.

page 189: FDA urges removal of DEA and TEA: ibid.

page 189: 37 percent of products contain nitrosamines: Food and Drug Administration, Division of Colors and Cosmetics, "Progress report on the analysis of cosmetic products and raw materials for nitrosamines," 1 March 1988 (Washington D.C.: GPO, 1988).

page 190: Germany discourages use of DEA and TEA: International Agency for Research on Cancer (IARC), *Occupational Exposures of Hairdressers and Barbers,* p. 62.

page 190: Bronopol causes formation of carcinogens: Conry, *Consumer's Guide to Cosmetics,* p. 73.

page 190: Chanel uses Bronopol: See, for example, Chanel's Teint Natural Liquid Makeup SPF 8 and Chanel Teint Pur Mat Matte Makeup SPF 8.

page 190: Not known if padimate-O's nitrosamines are carcinogenic: M. A. Pathak & P. Robins, "A response to concerns about sunscreens: a report from The Skin Cancer Foundation," *J. Dermatol. Surg. Oncol.* 15, no. 5 (1988): 486–87.

page 190: Cosmetics contaminated with 1,4-dioxane: Food and Drug Administration (FDA), Cosmetic Handbook (Washington, D.C.: GPO, n.d.).

page 191: Polysorbate 60 and 80 contaminated with 1,4-dioxane: Winter, *Consumer's Dictionary,* 1989, p. 242.

page 191: Blue 1 and Green 3 are carcinogenic: *Federal Register* 47, no. 188 (28 September 1982): 42563–66; *Federal Register* 47 no. 224 (19 November 1982): 52140–44.

page 191: Impurities in Red 33, Yellow 5, and Yellow 6 cause cancer: *Federal Register* 53, no. 168 (30 August 1988): 33110–21; *Federal Register* 50 (4 September 1985): 35774; *Federal Register* 51 (19 November 1986): 41765.

page 191: Some coal tar colors contain carcinogenic impurities: *Federal Register* (28 September 1982).

page 191: FDA alleges color additives do not pose hazards: *Federal Register* (30 August 1988).

page 191: Use of hair-color products associated with human cancer: Markowitz et al., "Hair dyes"; Cantor et al., "Hair dye use"; Zahm et al., "Use of hair-coloring products"; Brown, "Hair dye use in white men"; *IARC,* 1993; Thun et al., "Hair dye use and fatal cancers"; Shafer & Shafer, "Potential of carcinogenic effects"; Kinlen et al., "Use of hair dyes and breast cancer"; Shore et al., "A case control study"; Hennekens et al.,

"Use of permanent hair dyes"; Nasca et al., "Relationship of hair dye use."

page 191: Lanolin contaminated with carcinogenic pesticides: S. Milstein, personal communication in 1992 to the authors from Dr. Stan Milstein, special asistant to the director, Office of Cosmetics and Colors.

page 191: Sixteen pesticides identified in lanolin in 1988: National Research Council. *Pesticides in the Diets of Infants and Children* (Washington, D.C.: National Academy Press, 1993), p. 313.

page 192: Chemicals likely to migrate through skin: Milstein communication.

page 192: NAS's concern over lanolin contamination: NRC, 1993, p. 313.

page 192: Talc is carcinogenic: National Toxicology Program, *Toxicology and Carcinogenesis Studies of Talc (CAS No. 14807–96-6) in F344/N Rats and B6C3F₁ Mice (Inhalation Studies),* Technical Report Series, no. 421, September 1993.

page 193: Crystalline silica is carcinogenic: IARC, 1987, p. 341–42.

page 193: Inadequate data on amorphous silica: ibid.

page 193: Hazard of silica is primarily via inhalation: U. Saffiotti, personal communcation to the authors, 22 July 1993. Saffiotti is chief of the National Cancer Institute Laboratory for Experimental Pathology.

How We Evaluated Cosmetics and Personal Care Products

page 194: Data on cosmetic reactions: R. M. Adams & H. I. Mailbach, "A five-year study of cosmetic reactions," *Journal of the American Academy of Dermatology* 13, no. 6 (1985): 1062–69.

page 198: Bronopol is a carcinogen precursor: Conry, *Consumer's Guide to Cosmetics,* p. 73.

page 198: BHA is carcinogenic: IARC, 1987, p. 59.

page 198: Formaldehyde is carcinogenic: ibid., pp. 211–16.

page 198: Padimate-O is inadequately tested: Pathak & Robins, "Concerns about sunscreens," pp. 486–87.

page 199: TEA is a carcinogen precursor: *Federal Register* 44, no. 70 (10 April): 21365.

page 199: BHT is inadequately tested: IARC, 1987, p. 59.

page 199: Coal tar is carcinogenic: ibid., 76.

page 199: D&C Green 5 evidence of carcinogenicity: *Federal Register* 47, no. 108 (4 June 1982): 24278–86.

page 199: D&C Orange 17 evidence of carcinogenicity: *FDA's Regulation of Carcinogenic Additives: Hearing Before a Subcommittee of the Committee on Government Operations. House of Representatives. One Hundredth Congress.* First Session (Washington, D.C.: GPO, 24 June 1987), p. 2.

page 199: D&C Red 19 evidence of carcinogenicity: N. I. Sax, *Cancer Causing Chemicals* (New York: Van Nostrand Reinhold, 1981), p. 394.

page 199: D&C Red 33 evidence of carcinogenicity: *Federal Register* (30 August 1988).

page 199: DEA evidence of carcinogenicity: *Federal Register* 44, no. 70 (10 April 1979): 21365.

page 199: FD&C Blue 1 evidence of carcinogenicity: *Federal Register* (28 September 1982).

page 199: FD&C Green 3 evidence of carcinogenicity: *Federal Register* (19 November 1982).

page 199: FD&C Red 4 evidence of carcinogenicity: N. I. Sax, *Cancer Causing Chemicals,* p. 394.

page 199: FD&C Red 40 evidence of carcinogenicity: Winter, Consumer's Dictionary, 1989, p. 139. Hampton, *Natural Organic Hair,* p. 416.

page 199: FD&C Yellow 5 evidence of carcinogenicity: *Federal Register* (4 September 1985).

page 199: FD&C Yellow 6 evidence of carcinogenicity: *Federal Register* (19 November 1986).

page 199: Fluoride evidence of carcinogenicity: National Toxicology Program, *Toxicology and Carcinogenesis Studies of Sodium Fluoride (CAS No. 7681-49-4) in F344/N Rats and B6C3F$_1$ Mice (Drinking Water Studies)* (Research Triangle Park, NC: NIH Publication no. 91-2848, December 1990).

page 199: Lead acetate evidence of carcinogenicity: IARC, 1987, pp. 230–32.

page 199: Methyl methacrylate inadequate evidence of carcinogenicity: IARC, 60 (1994): pp. 445–74.

page 199: Saccharin evidence of carcinogenicity: *IARC,* 1987, pp. 334–39.

page 199: Silica evidence of carcinogenicity: ibid., pp. 341–42.

page 199: Talc evidence of carcinogenicity: National Toxicology Program: *Toxicology and Carcinogenesis Studies of Talc.*

CHAPTER 8. EYE AND FACE MAKEUP

Foundations

page 205: Foundation and makeup products are third leading cause of contact dermatitis: Adams & Mailbach, "Study of cosmetic reactions."

page 205: Cosmetic acne affects about one-third of all women: Conry, *Consumer's Guide to Cosmetics,* p. 221.

page 205: Ingredients with potential to cause cosmetic acne: ibid., pp. 221–22.

Mascara

page 212: 1,964 hospital admissions as a result of mascara-related injuries: CPSC, "1990 Product Summary Report," p. 16.

page 212: Eye maladies caused by eye makeup: S. J. Taub, "What goes on under your makeup if you are allergic to cosmetics," *Eye, Ear, Nose and Throat Monthly* 54, no. 5 (1975): 211.

page 213: Quaternium 15 is an eye irritant: Conry, *Consumer's Guide to Cosmetics,* p. 333.

page 213: Phenylmercuric acetate is an allergen and skin irritant: Conry, *Consumer's Guide to Cosmetics,* pp. 308, 332.

Lipsticks, Glosses, and Lip Pencils

page 217: Contact dermatitis cases caused by cosmetic pigments: M. B. Sulzberger, J. Goodman, L. A. Byrne, & E. D. Mallozzi, "Acquired specific hypersensitivity to simple chemicals. II. Cheilitis, with special reference to sensitivity to lipstick," *Archives of Dermatology* 37 (1938): 597–615. C. D. Calnan & I. Sarkany, "Studies in contact dermatitis; II. Lipstick cheilitis," *Transactions of the St. John's Hospital Dermatological Society* 39 (1957): 28–36. C. D. Calnan, "Reactions to artificial colouring materials," *Journal of the Society of Cosmetic Chemists* 18 (1967): 215–23.

page 217: Use of coal tar colors causes nausea and other allergic symptoms: "Petroleum-based FD+C colors: are you at risk?" *Paul Penders Personal Care Bulletin* (Fall 1991): 1.

page 217: Additional allergens found in lipsticks: R. Hayakawa, M. Kayoko, M. Suzuki, Y. Arima, & Y. Ohkio, "Lipstick dermatitis due to C18 aliphatic compounds," *Contact Dermatitis* 16 (1987): 215–19.

page 217: Causes of drying or cracking lips: Conry, *Consumer's Guide to Cosmetics,* pp. 222–23.

page 217: Eosin dyes used today: ibid., p. 223.

page 218: Avoid products containing various colors, preservatives, and artificial sweeteners: U.S. General Accounting Office, *Report to Congress: Lack of Authority Hampers Attempts to Increase Cosmetic Safety,* No. HRD-78-139 (Washington, D.C.: GPO., 8 August 1978), pp. 107–111.

CHAPTER 9. HAIR CARE

Shampoos

page 228: Shampoos reported to FDA for various minor irritations: Winter, *Consumer's Dictionary,* 1989, p. 269.

page 228: Polyethylene glycol and DMDM hydantoin form formaldehyde: S. Fregert, "Contact allergens and prevention of contact dermatitis," *Journal of Allergy and Clinical Immunology* 78 (1986): 1071–72; D. H. Liem, "Analysis of antimicrobial compounds in cosmetics," *Cosmetics and Toiletries* 92 (1977): 59–72.

page 229: EDTA an irritant: Winter, *Consumer's Dictionary*, 1989, pp. 131–32.

page 229: D&C Green 5 an irritant: Winter, *Consumer's Dictionary*, 1989, p. 95.

page 229: Selenium sulfide an irritant: ibid., p. 267.

page 229: Ingredients that provide aggressive cleaning: Conry, *Consumer's Guide to Cosmetics,* pp. 67–69.

page 229: Milder cleansers: ibid.

page 229: Gentle cleansers: ibid.

page 230: Ingredients that break down into formaldehyde: Fregert, "Contact allergens"; Liem, "Analysis of compounds."

Hair-Coloring Products for Women

page 241: Hair coloring products cause irritation: J. F. Corbett, "Hair Coloring," *Clinics in Dermatology* 6, no. 3 (1988): 96–101.

page 241: Hair-coloring products cause cancer: Markowitz et al., "Hair dyes"; Cantor et al., "Hair dye use"; Zahm et al., "Use of hair-coloring products"; Brown, "Hair dye use in white men"; *IARC,* 1993; Thun et al., "Hair dye use and fatal cancers"; Shafer & Shafer, "Potential of carcinogenic effects"; Kinlen et al., "Use of hair dyes and breast cancer"; Shore et al., "A case control study"; Hennekens et al., "Use of permanent hair dyes"; Nasca et al., "Relationship of hair dye use."

CHAPTER 10. DENTAL AND ORAL HYGIENE

Mouthwashes

page 251: Salicylate is allergenic: Winter, *Consumer's Dictionary*, 1989, p. 265.

page 251: High-alcohol mouthwash contributes to cancer: W. J. Blot, et al., "Mouthwash use and oral conditions in the risk of oral and pharyngeal cancer," *Cancer Research* (June 1991); Wynder et al., "Oral cancer and mouthwash use," *Journal of the National Cancer Institute,* 70 (1983); W. J. Blot, et al. "Oral cancer and mouthwash," *Journal of the National Cancer Institute* 70 (1983); Weaver, et al., "Mouthwash and oral cancer: carcinogen or coincidence? *Journal of Oral Surgery* 37 (1979).

CHAPTER 11. FEMININE HYGIENE

Douches, Feminine Deodorants, and Hygiene Products

page 257: Douches with the highest potential for irritation: Conry, *Consumer's Guide to Cosmetics,* 1989, p. 269.

page 257: Other problem ingredients include phenol and sodium lauryl sulfate: Winter, *Consumer's Dictionary,* 1989, p. 232; Conry, *Consumer's Guide to Cosmetics,* p. 267.

page 258: Vaginal douches and cervical cancer: J. W. Gardner et al., "Is vaginal douching related to cervical carcinoma?" *American Journal of Epidemiology* 133, no. 4 (1991): 368–75.

Feminine Care and Body Powders (Talc and Cornstarch)

page 259: Use of talcum powder associated with ovarian cancer: D. W. Cramer, et al., "Ovarian cancer and talc: a case-control study," *Cancer* 50, no. 2 (15 July 1982): 372–76; B. L. Harlow, et al., "Perineal exposure to talc and ovarian cancer risk," *Obstetrics & Gynecology* 80, no. 1 (July 1992): 19–26; D. L. Longo & R. C. Young, "Cosmetic talc and ovarian cancer," *The Lancet* (18 August 1979): 349–51.

page 259: Cosmetic talc is carcinogenic. Cancer Prevention Coalition. Citizen Petition to the FDA for Banning Talc-Containing Cosmetic Products. November 17, 1994. Chicago, IL: Cancer Prevention Coalition.

CHAPTER 12. NAIL PRODUCTS

Nail Polishes, Hardeners, and Protectors

page 263: Use of sculptured nails causes paresthesia: A. A. Fisher, "Adverse nail reactions and paresthesia from 'photobonded acrylate sculptured nails,'" *Cutis* 45 (1990): 293–94.

page 263: Women contaminate their facial skin with irritants in nail products: J. S. Jellinek, *Formulation and Function of Cosmetics* (New York: Wiley Interscience, 1970), p. 438.

page 263: Solvents in nail products are neurotoxic: "9225. Toluene," "1519. n-Butyl Acetate," "3685. Ethyl Acetate," *Merck Index,* 9th ed., ed. Martha Windholz (Rahway, NJ: Merck & Co., 1976), pp. 125, 196, 494–95. As cited in Conry, *Consumer's Guide to Cosmetics,* 1980.

page 264: Twenty-nine hundred children admitted to hospital because of nail preparation–related poisonings: CPSC, "1990 Product Summary Report," p. 16.

CHAPTER 13. SKIN PRODUCTS

Antiperspirants and Deodorants

page 265: Antiperspirants and Alzheimer's disease: A. B. Graves et al., "The association between aluminum-containing products and Alzheimer's disease," *Journal of Clinical Epidemiology* 43, no. 1 (1990): 35–44.

page 266: FDA warns of triclosan's long-term health hazards: "OTC Topical Antimicrobial Products," *Federal Register* (6 January 1978): 1231–32.

page 266: Irritants found in antiperspirants: Conry, *Consumer's Guide to Cosmetics,* p. 246.

page 266: Quaternium 18 acts as sensitizer: ibid., p. 242.

Soaps

page 285: Glycerin soaps are mildest: American Medical Association (AMA). *AMA Book on Skin and Hair Care,* ed. L. A. Schoen, (Philadelphia: J. B. Lippincott, 1971), p. 162.

page 285: Tallow soaps less irritating than coconut soaps: M. I. Oestreicher, "Detergents, bath preparations, and other skin cleansers," *Clinics in Dermatology* 6, no. 3 (1988): 32.

page 285: Gentlest to least gentle soaps: P. J Frosch & A. M. Kligman, "The soap chamber test. A new method for assessing the irritancy of soaps," *Journal of the American Academy of Dermatology* 1 (1979): 35–41.

PART III. FOODS AND BEVERAGES

Danger of Carcinogens in the Food Supply

page 295: Two important studies: National Research Council, *Pesticides in the Diets of Infants and Children* (Washington, D.C.: National Academy Press, 1993); R. Wiles & C. Campbell, *Pesticides in Children's Food* (Washington, D.C.: Environmental Working Group, 1993).

page 295: A long line of reports detailing pesticide hazards since the 1960s: S. S. Epstein, *The Politics of Cancer* (San Francisco: Sierra Club Books, 1978).

page 295: Pesticide use has increased 125 percent: Public Voice for Food & Health Policy, "Pesticide reform necessary to address consumer concerns" (Washington, D.C.), 21 June 1993.

page 296: Kessler quoted: M. Burros, "U.S. is taking aim at farm chemicals in the food supply. Emphasis is on children. Policies of three agencies and a new study signal a shift in government's stance," *New York Times,* 26 June 1993.

page 296: 1993 study found women with highest levels of DDT had four times the breast cancer risk: M. S. Wolff et al., "Blood levels of organochlorine residues and risk of breast cancer," *Journal of the National Cancer Institute* 85, no. 8 (1993): 648–52.

page 296: One of many studies to associate pesticides with breast cancer: S. S. Epstein, "Environmental pollutants as unrecognized causes of breast cancer," *International Journal of Health Services* 24, no.1 (1994): pp. 145–50.

page 296: Growing evidence that breast cancer is caused by pesticides: J. Raloff, "EcoCancers: do environmental factors underlie a breast cancer epidemic?" *Science News* 144 (3 July 1993): 10–13; Epstein, "Environmental Pollutants"; Epstein, *Politics of Cancer.*

page 296: The only study to exculpate pesticides as a cause of breast cancer was flawed: N. Krieger, et al., "Breast cancer and serum organochlorines: a prospective study among white, black, and Asian women," *Journal of the National Cancer Institute* 86, no. 8 (20 April 1994): 589–99; Epstein, S. S. "Pesticides not cleared of breast cancer link." *New York Times.* Letter to the Editor. 5 May 1994, sec. A, p. 18.

page 297: QCRA has been seriously challenged: S. S. Epstein, "Book review: *Cancer Risk Assessment: A Quantitative Approach,*" *Cancer Cell* 3, no. 5 (May 1991): 195–96.

page 297: There is no such thing as "safe" exposure to carcinogens: S. S. Epstein & J. Feldman, "Opening the door for carcinogens," *Los Angeles Times,* 27 February 1989; S. S. Epstein & J. Feldman, "'Negligible Risk' is still much too great," *Los Angeles Times,* 16 November 1989; S. S. Epstein & L. Yeomans, "What about 'putting people first'?" *Los Angeles Times,* 8 September 1993.

The Advantages of Organic Foods

page 298: Organic foods are purer than conventional crops: B. Baker & P. McGee, "CDFA pesticide residue analysis of organics. A special CCOF report," *California Certified Organic Farmers State Newsletter* 8, no. 4 (Fall 1991): 6.

page 298: Washington state reports no detectable pesticides on organic crop samples: D. Steinman, *Diet for a Poisoned Planet* (New York: Ballantine Books, 1992), p. 326.

page 298: Organically grown foods are more nutritious: B. Smith, "Organic foods vs. supermarket foods: element level," *Journal of Applied Nutrition* 45, no. 1 (1993).

page 300: Organically grown foods have higher amounts of vitamin C: W. Schuphan, "Nutritional value of crops as influenced by organic and inorganic fertilizer treatments—results of 12 years of experiments with vegetables," *Qual. Plant., Plant Foods Hum. Nutr.* 23 (1974): 333. Cited in Knorr, "Quality of ecologically grown food," *Cereal Foods World* 27 no. 4 (1982): 165–67

page 300: Organically grown foods have higher protein content: B. S. D. Pattersson, "A comparison between conventional and bio-dynamic farming systems as indicated by yields and quality," *Proc. Int. Res. Conf., International Federation of Organic Agricultural Movements* (Topsfield, MA, 1978), cited in Knorr, "Quality of ecologically grown food."

page 300: Three-year study with rabbits shows more live births among animals with the organic diet: D. Knorr, "Quality of ecologically grown food," 165–67.

page 300: Organic foods and benefits in the area of sexual reproduction: Abell, A., Ernst, E. & Bonde, J. P. "High sperm density among members of organic farmers' association." *The Lancet* 343 (1994): p. 1498.

page 301: Organic foods' increasing popularity: *Wall Street Journal.* "Shoppers seeking out organic produce." 23 September 1994, sec. B1.

How We Evaluated Foods and Beverages

page 301: Formula to determine which foods pose greatest cancer risk: NRC, 1993, pp. 267–322.

page 302: Many pesticides have cancer potency numbers: ibid., p. 335; Engler, "List of chemicals."

page 302: Q^* values for dieldrin, 2,4-D, and folpet: Engler, "List of chemicals."

page 302: Calculating risks at concentrations in the human diet: J. B. Swartz & S. S. Epstein, "Problems in assessing risks from occupational and environmental exposure to carcinogens," Banbury Report 9, *Quantification of Occupational Cancer* (Cold Spring Harbor Laboratory, 1981), pp. 559–75.

page 303: Sources for residues of contaminants in apples: Food and Drug Administration (FDA), "Listing of total diet data by food code and market basket for original and duplicate analyses," 14 August 1991; Wiles & Campbell, *Pesticides in Children's Food,* p. 67; NRC, 1993, p. 256.

page 304: Sources for residues of contaminants in oranges: FDA, "Listing of total diet data"; Food and Drug Administration (FDA), "Listing of pesticides, industrial chemicals, and metals data by fiscal year, origin, sample flag, and industry/product code. 1990." 10 September 1991.

How to Use the Shopping Charts

page 305: Carcinogenic contaminants commonly found in foods and beverages: Engler, "List of chemicals," pp. 1–8; Briggs & Rachel Carson Council, *Basic Guide to Pesticides.*

CHAPTER 14. FOODS

Fruits

page 309: Florida oranges are dyed but California oranges are not: "Very Orange Oranges," *Pure Facts: Newsletter of the Feingold Association of the United States* 16, no. 9 (November 1992): 5.

page 309: Citrus Red No. 2 is carcinogenic: *IARC,* 1987, p. 60.

page 310: Waxes contain carcinogenic fungicides: (ortho-phenylphenol) *IARC,* 1987, p. 70; (benomyl) Engler, "List of chemicals," p. 5.

page 310: Fruits most likely to be waxed: Center for Science in the Public Interest (CSPI), *The Wax Cover-Up: What Consumers Aren't Told About Pesticides on Fresh Produce* (Washington, D.C.: CSPI, 1989).

page 310: Apples retain pesticide residues: "When washing isn't enough," *National Gardening* (October 1988).

page 310: Washing and peeling can reduce pesticide residues: NRC, p. 257.

Nuts and Seeds

page 316: Aflatoxin is carcinogenic: *IARC,* 1987: 83–87.

page 316: Peanuts heavily contaminated with carcinogenic pesticide residues: Food and Drug Administration (FDA), *Total Diet Study, April 1982–April 1986: Dietary Intakes of Pesticides, Selected Elements, and Other Chemicals,* Association of Official Analytical Chemists (Arlington, VA); Food and Drug Administration (FDA), *Listing of Total Diet Data by Food Code and Market Basket for Original and Duplicate Analyses,* 14 August 1991.

Vegetables

page 317: Pickled vegetables linked with cancer: *IARC* 56 (1993), pp. 83–113.

page 318: Vegetables most likely to be waxed: CSPI, *The Wax Cover-Up.*

Grains

page 322: Increased cancer risk for people exposed to herbicides: L. Hardell, et al., "Malignant lymphoma and exposure to chemicals, especially organic solvents, chlorophenols, and phenoxy acids: a case-control study," *British Journal of Cancer* 43 (1981): 169; L. Hardell & N. O. Bengtsson, "Epidemiological study of socioeconomic factors and clinical findings in Hodgkin's disease, and reanalysis of previous data regarding chemical exposure," *British Journal of Cancer* 48 (1983): 217; S. K. Hoar et al., "Agricultural herbicide use and risk of lymphoma and soft-tissue sarcoma," *Journal of the American Medical Association* 256 (1986): 1141; S. K. Zahm & A. Blair, "Geographical variation in lymphoma incidence," letter to the editor, *British Journal of Cancer* 57 (1988): 443.

pages 323: Colors in cereals and evidence of carcinogenicity (in order of how they are listed): *Federal Register* 47, no. 188 (28 September 1982): 42563–66; *Federal Register* 47, no. 224 (19 November 1982: 52140–44; N. I. Sax, *Cancer Causing Chemicals*, p. 394; Winter, *Consumer's Dictionary*, p. 139; Hampton, *Natural Organic Hair and Skin Care*, p. 416; *Federal Register* 50 (4 September 1985): 35774; *Federal Register* 51 (19 November 1986): 41765.

Meat, Poultry, and Meat Substitutes

page 326: DDT and breast cancer: Wolff, "Blood levels of organochlorine residues."

page 326: Pesticide contaminants cause breast cancer: Epstein, "Environmental pollutants as unrecognized causes of breast cancer."

page 326: 143 drugs and pesticides known to leave residues in meat and poultry: Committee on Interstate and Foreign Commerce, Subcommittee on Oversight and Investigations, *Cancer Causing Chemicals in Food. Report together with Additional and Dissenting Views. Ninety-Fifth Congress. Second Session* (Washington, D.C.: GPO, 1978), p. 24.

page 326: Only 46 of 143 drugs and pesticides are monitored by USDA: ibid.

page 326: Four thousand new animal drugs could have adverse health effects: *Human Food Safety and the Regulation of Animal Drugs Report*, 99th Congress, 1st session (HR): 99-461, 1985.

page 326: Quote from industry executive: Mack Graves, former chief executive officer and president of the Coleman Meat Company, of Denver, Colorado, August 1993. Graves is a former executive with the Armour Food Company and Perdue, 1985–1988.

page 327: Sulfamethazine is carcinogenic: *Food Safety and Quality: FDA Surveys Not Adequate to Demonstrate Safety of Milk Supply*, Report to the Chairman, House of Representatives,GAO/RCED-91-26 (Washington, D.C.: General Accounting Office, November 1990), pp. 21–22.

page 327: Structural similarities increase probability of both substances causing cancer: ibid, p. 11.

page 327: Hormones leave residues in meat: National Research Council, *Meat and Poultry Inspection: The Scientific Basis of the Nation's Program* (Washington, D.C.: National Academy Press, 1985).

page 327: Hormones cause cancer: *IARC*, 1987, pp. 272–309.

page 327: Most meat and poultry containing illegal residues sold to public: Committee on Interstate and Foreign Commerce, Subcommittee on Oversight and Investigations, *Cancer Causing Chemicals in Food*, p. 24.

page 327:   Continued illegal use of DES: O. Schell, *Modern Meat* (New York: Random House, 1985), p. 255.

page 328:   Progesterone and testosterone are carcinogenic: *IARC*, 1987, pp. 57, 272–309.

page 328:   FDA admits residues could produce "adverse effects": S. S. Epstein, "The chemical jungle: today's beef industry," *International Journal of Health Services* 20, no.2 (1990): 277–80.

page 328:   Delicacy of body's hormonal balance: R. Hertz, "The estrogen-cancer hypothesis with special emphasis on DES," in *Origins of Human Cancer,* ed. H. H. Hiatt, J. D. Watson, and J. A. Winston, pp. 1665–82, vol. 4 of *Cold Spring Harbor Conference on Cell Proliferation* (Cold Spring Harbor Laboratory, 1977).

page 328:   Even a dime-sized piece of meat contains trillions of molecular carcinogens: S. S. Epstein, "The chemical jungle."

page 329:   Epidemic associated with increased rates of uterine and ovarian cancer: ibid.

page 329:   Hot dogs with nitrites cause increased risk of childhood leukemia: Peters et al., "Processed meats."

page 329:   Children born to mothers who consume hot dogs more likely to have brain tumors: S. Sarasia & D. A. Savitz, "Cured and broiled meat consumption in relation to childhood cancer: Denver, Colorado (United States)." *Cancer Causes and Control* 5 (1994): 141–48.

page 329:   As many as twelve of eighteen PAHs cause cancer: L. Lefferts, "Great grilling," *Nutrition Action Health Letter* (July–August 1989).

page 329:   NCI estimates HAs increase human cancers in U.S.: Michael Jacobson, *Safe Food* (Los Angeles: Living Planet Press, 1991) p. 111.

page 330:   Countries whose meat is least affected by Chernobyl: Department of Food and Agriculture, *Imported meat and poultry samples analyzed for radiocesium by the Food Safety and Inspection Service following the Chernobyl accident, May 1986 through December 1988* (Washington, D.C.: USDA).

page 331:   Microwave-cooking bacon lowers levels of nitrosamines: B.G. Österdahl & E. Alriksson, "Volatile nitrosamines in microwave-cooked bacon," *Food Additives and Contaminants* 7, no. 1 (1990): 51–54.

page 332:   Cooking with mesquite produces higher concentrations of PAHs: Lefferts, "Great grilling."

Seafood

page 336:   Seafood can be contaminated when uninformed shopping choices are made: S. S. Epstein & D. Steinman, "All we're doing is rearranging the deck chairs on a seafood Titanic," *Los Angeles Times*, 18 February 1994.

page 336: Cancer risk for average consumer is seventy-five times greater than normally acceptable guidelines: National Academy of Sciences, *Seafood Safety* (Washington, D.C.: National Academy Press, 1991).

Dairy

page 341: Testing methods inadequate: General Accounting Office (GAO), *Food Safety and Quality* (GAO/RCED-91-26), p 1.

page 341: Sulfamethazine residues found in milk: ibid., pp. 4, 11.

page 341: 46 percent of milk samples contained more than one sulfa drug: ibid., p. 5.

page 341: Metabolites of sulfamethazine cannot be detected: ibid., p. 11.

page 342: Chloramphenicol found in milk supply: ibid., p. 31.

page 342: Dioxin's carcinogenicity more potent than DDT: R. E. Keenan et al., "Pathology reevaluation of the Kociba et al. (1978) bioassay of 2,3,7,8-TCDD: implications for risk assessment," *Journal of Toxicology and Environmental Health* 34 (1991): 279–96.

pages 342–44: BGH sources of information: S. S. Epstein, "Growth hormones would endanger milk," *Los Angeles Times,* 27 July 1989; S. S. Epstein, "Potential public health hazards of biosynthetic milk hormones," *International Journal of Health Services* 20, no. 1 (1990): 73–84; S. S. Epstein, "Needless new risk of breast cancer," *Los Angeles Times,* 20 March 1994; S. S. Epstein, "Insulin-like growth factor I in biosynthetic milk is a potential risk factor for breast and gastrointestinal cancer," *International Journal of Health Services* (1995).

page 344: Milk prime route of exposure to radiation: E. J. Sternglass & J. M. Gould, "Breast cancer: evidence for a relation to fission products in the diet," *International Journal of Health Services* 23, no. 4 (1993): 783–804.

Eggs

page 348: Number of salmonella-poisoning cases has increased: M. Burros, "Eating well: salmonella study suggests that eggs should be treated with great caution," *New York Times,* 13 April 1988; A. Hanson & W. Bennett, "Trojan eggs," *New York Times Magazine,* 30 July 1989; W. Leary, "Research links eggs to recent outbreak of food poisoning," *New York Times,* 7 April 1988; W. Leary, "U.S. begins testing to fight rise in egg contamination," *New York Times,* 16 September 1988.

Condiments, Herbs, and Spices

page 355: Aluminum's neurotoxicity and role in hyperactivity in children: J. M. H. Howard, "Clinical import of small increases in serum aluminum," *Clinical Chemistry,* 30, no. 10 (1984): 1722–23.

page 355   Growing evidence aluminum plays a role in Alzheimer's disease. C. N. Martyn, et al. "Geographical relation between Alzheimer's disease and aluminum in drinking water." *The Lancet,* 14 January 1989: 59–62. H. D. Foster, "Aluminum and health." *Journal of Orthomolecular Medicine* 7 (4)(1992), 206–8.

Sweeteners, Syrups, and Additives

page 359:   PBOI's conclusions: General Accounting Office (GAO), *Food Additive Approval Process Followed for Aspartame. Report to the Honorable Howard M. Metzenbaum, U.S. Senate,* GAO/HRD-87-46 (Washington, D.C.: GPO, June 1987), pp. 38, 44.

page 359:   Cyclamates' evidence of carcinogenicity: *IARC,* 1987, p. 61.

page 359:   Saccharin's evidence of carcinogenicity: ibid., p. 71.

Baby Foods

page 360:   EPA tolerances calculated for adults: *Pesticides in Children's Food;* NRC, 1993.

page 360:   Recent report quoted: ibid.

CHAPTER 15. BEVERAGES

Tap Water

page 363:   Recent report quoted: Natural Resources Defense Council (NRDC), *Think Before You Drink,* p. v.

page 364:   Groundwater supplying drinking water to fifty million Americans potentially contaminated with agricultural chemicals: U.S. Department of Agriculture, *The Magnitude and Costs of Groundwater Contamination from Agricultural Chemicals: A National Perspective,* Agricultural Economic Report no. 576 (Washington, D.C.: USDA, October 1987), p. iii.

page 364:   Sources of exposure to VOCs in drinking water: Environmental Protection Agency, "Identification and evaluation of waterborne routes of exposures from other than food and drinking," Office of Water Planning and Standards, contract no. 68-01-3857, January 1979; A. T. Shehata et al., Bureau of Health, Maine Department of Human Services, "A multi-route exposure assessment of chemically contaminated drinking water and health significance with emphasis on gasoline," Report to Maine Department of Environmental Protection, undated; J. B. Andelman, "Inhalation exposure in the home to volatile organic contaminants of drinking water," *Science Total Environ.* 47 (1985): 443–60.

page 365:   2.5 million people drink water containing more than twenty-five ppb arsenic: J. Brown et al., *University of California at Berkeley and California Environmental Protection Agency, Review of Arsenic in Drinking Water Studies*, referenced in *Science News* (April 1992), p. 253, as cited in NRDC, *Think Before You Drink*, p. 20.

page 365:   Public water supplies of some two hundred million Americans chlorinated: International Agency for Research on Cancer, *IARC Monographs on the Evaluation of Carcinogenic Risks to Humans. Chlorinated Drinking-water; Chlorination By-products; Some Other Halogenated Compounds; Cobalt and Cobalt Compounds*, vol. 52 (Lyon, France: World Health Organization, 1991).

page 365:   Chlorinated drinking water causes cancer: R. D. Morris et al., "Chlorination, chlorination by-products, and cancer: a meta-analysis," *American Journal of Public Health* 82, no. 7 (1992): 955–63.

page 365:   More people die from THMs than from fires and handguns: NRDC, *Think Before You Drink*, p. i.

page 366:   Fluoride's evidence of carcinogenicity: NTP, 1990.

page 366:   VOCs increase cancer risk: J. Fagliano, "Drinking water contamination and the incidence of leukemia: an ecologic study," *American Journal of Public Health* 80, no. 10 (1990): 1209–12; S. W. Lagakos et al., "An analysis of contaminated well water and health effects in Woburn, Massachusetts," *Journal of the American Statistical Association* 81, no. 395 (1986): 583–96.

page 366:   Brass fittings on well pumps leach high levels of lead into well water: F. Clifford, "State acts to cut use of brass in well pumps," *Los Angeles Times*, 19 April 1994, A3.

page 366:   Mississippi River Basin contained atrazine at levels exceeding EPA's maximum contaminant level. United States Geological Survey (USGS), *Distribution of Selected Herbicides and Nitrate in the Mississippi River and Its Major Tributaries, April Through June 1991*, USGS Water Resources Investigations Report 91-4163, 1991.

page 366:   Nearly ten thousand community drinking water wells contain pesticides: U.S. Environmental Protection Agency (EPA), *National Survey of Pesticides in Drinking Water Wells: Phase I Report*, (Washington, D.C.: GPO, 1990).

page 366:   Fission products damage immune cells of the bone marrow: U.S. Environmental Protection Agency, *Addendum To: The Occurrence and Exposure Assessment for Radon, Radium 226, Radium 228, Uranium, and Gross Alpha Particle Activity in Public Drinking Water Supplies*, 30 September 1992, as cited in NRDC, *Think Before You Drink*, pp. 19–20.

page 366: Evidence that radiation-contaminated drinking water supplies are responsible for escalating breast cancer mortality: Sternglass & Gould, "Breast cancer."

page 366: Long Island breast cancer incidence related to drinking water: Sternglass & Gould, "Breast cancer."

Bottled Water

page 368: Bottled water from deep spring source better shopping choice: E. J. Sternglass, personal communication.

page 368: Surveys have found wide range of contaminants in bottled water: S. Marquardt et al., *Bottled Water: Sparkling Hype at a Premium Price* (Washington, D.C.: The Environmental Policy Institute, 1989).

Coffee, Tea, Soft Drinks, and Other Beverages
Containing Caffeine

page 369: Coffee possible cause of urinary bladder cancer: International Agency for Research on Cancer, *IARC Monographs on the Evaluation of Carcinogenic Risks to Humans. Coffee, Tea, Mate, Methylxanthines and Methylglyoxal,* vol. 51 (Lyon, France: World Health Organization 1991), p. 461.

page 369: Methylene chloride is carcinogenic: *IARC,* 1987, pp. 194–95.

page 369: Evidence for carcinogenicity of cyclamates and saccharin: ibid., pp. 178–82, 334–39.

page 370: Chloroform and THMs are carcinogenic: *IARC,* vol. 52, 1991.

page 370: High consumption of caffeine by fathers and pregnancy complications: P. S. Weathersbee et al., "Caffeine and pregnancy: a retrospective study," *Postgraduate Medicine* 62 (1977): 64–69, as cited in J. Elkington, *The Poisoned Womb* (New York: Viking Penguin, 1986).

page 370: Women who consumed seven cups of coffee or more daily have increased incidence of babies born with defects: Elkington, *The Poisoned Womb,* Penguin, p. 54.

page 370: Aspartame may cause a few cases of mental retardation a year: Jacobson, *Safe Food,* 1991. General Accounting Office (GAO), *Food Additive Process Followed for Aspartame.*

Alcoholic Beverages

page 371: Alcohol consumption associated with breast cancer: International Agency for Research on Cancer (IARC), *Alcohol Drinking* 44 (Lyon, France: World Health Organization, 1988) pp. 226–29; M. P.

Longnecker et al., "A meta-analysis of alcohol consumption in relation to risk of breast cancer," *Journal of the American Medical Association* 260, no. 5 (1988): 652–56.

page 371: Alcoholic beverages contain asbestos: *IARC,* 44, p. 98.

page 371: Wine contains carcinogenic pesticide residues: ibid., pp. 98–99.

page 371: Urethane is present in alcoholic beverages: ibid., p. 97.

page 371: Urethane is carcinogenic: A. Tannenbaum et al., "Multipotential carcinogenicity of urethane in the Sprague-Dawley rat," *Cancer Research* 22 (1962): 1362–71; *IARC* 7, 111–40.

CHAPTER 16. FOOD SAFETY ISSUES

Packaging

page 373: Cling film contains carcinogens that migrate into foods: N. Harrison, "Migration of plasticizers from cling-film," *Food Additives and Contaminants* 5, no. 1 (1988): 493–99.

page 374: Dimethyl terephthalate has shown limited evidence of carcinogenicity: D. Kriebel & B. Allar, letter to Dr. Jere Goyan, commissioner, FDA, 25 November 1980.

page 374: Vinylidene chloride is carcinogenic: "Vinyl Halides' Carcinogenicity." *NIOSH/OSHA Current Intelligence Bulletin* 28, 21 September 1978.

page 374: Foods cooked in aluminum have aluminum leached into them: M. Walker, "Aluminum-contaminated drinking water, milk, tea & cookware," *Townsend Letter for Doctors,* April 1993, pp. 288–92.

Mold

page 375: Foods that do not need to be thrown out with appearance of a little mold: Jacobson, *Safe Food,* p. 182.

page 375: Foods that should be thrown out with appearance of mold: ibid.

Irradiation

page 376: Information on irradiation: S. S. Epstein and J. Gofman, "Irradiation of foods," *Science* 223 (1984): 1354. M. Colby & S. S. Epstein, "Risks of radiation: too many questions about food safety," *USA Today,* 22 January 1992, p. A11; M. F. Jacobson & S. Schmidt, "Food irradiation. Zapping our troubles away?" *Nutrition Action* (April 1992): 5–7.

Index

ABOUT THE AUTHORS

David Steinman is a prize-winning investigative journalist, author of *Diet for a Poisoned Planet,* and co-author of *Seafood Safety.* He conducted one of the first U.S. studies of the concentrations of two carcinogenic chemicals, DDT and PCBs, in the blood of seafood consumers. His work has appeared in *Woman's Day, Self,* the *Los Angeles Times, Natural Health,* and other magazines. He has won awards from Sierra Club, California Newspaper Publishers Association, and Best of the West; his investigative reports have been nominated for a Pulitzer Prize. He is a member of the board of directors of the Cancer Prevention Coalition, editorial board member of the *Journal of Optimal Nutrition,* and a former member of the editorial advisory boards of *Greenkeeping* and *Environment and Health* magazines.

Samuel S. Epstein, M.D., professor of occupational and environmental medicine at the School of Public Health, University of Illinois Medical Center (Chicago), is past president of the Rachel Carson Council, author of the prize-winning *The Politics of Cancer* and *Hazardous Waste in America,* and a leading expert on the environmental causes of cancer and other chronic diseases, with some 300 scientific publications to his credit. He is former Chief of the Laboratories of Environmental Toxicology and Carcinogenesis at the Children's Cancer Research Foundation in Boston and Senior Research Associate in Pathology at Harvard Medical School.

SAFE AND HEALTHY NEWSLETTER

The authors of *The Safe Shopper's Bible* have developed *Safe and Healthy,* a monthly newsletter offering important up-to-date consumer information on a wide range of topics. For information or to subscribe, write to *Safe and Healthy,* PO Box 2267, Rockville, MD 20847.